ERCP

The Fundamentals

ERCP

The Fundamentals

EDITED BY

Peter B. Cotton MD FRCS FRCP

Digestive Disease Center
Medical University of South Carolina
Charleston, USA

Joseph Leung MD FRCP FACP MACG FASGE

Department of Gastroenterology and Hepatology
University of California, Davis School of Medicine
Sacramento, USA
and
Section of Gastroenterology
VA Northern California Health Care System
GI Unit, Sacramento VAMC
Mather, USA

SECOND EDITION

WILEY Blackwell

This edition first published 2015 © 2015 by John Wiley & Sons, Ltd.

Registered Office
John Wiley & Sons, Ltd, The Atrium, Southern Gate, Chichester, West Sussex, PO19 8SQ, UK

Editorial Offices
9600 Garsington Road, Oxford, OX4 2DQ, UK
The Atrium, Southern Gate, Chichester, West Sussex, PO19 8SQ, UK
111 River Street, Hoboken, NJ 07030-5774, USA

For details of our global editorial offices, for customer services and for information about how to apply for permission to reuse the copyright material in this book please see our website at www.wiley.com/wiley-blackwell

Library of Congress Cataloging-in-Publication Data

Advanced digestive endoscopy (2006)
   ERCP : the fundamentals / edited by Peter B. Cotton, Joseph Leung. – Second edition.
     p. ; cm.
   Preceded by: Advanced digestive endoscopy / edited by Peter B. Cotton and Joseph Leung. 2006.
   Includes bibliographical references and index.
   ISBN 978-1-118-76941-6 (cloth)
   I. Cotton, Peter B., editor. II. Leung, J. W. C., editor. III. Title.
   [DNLM: 1. Cholangiopancreatography, Endoscopic Retrograde–methods. 2. Biliary Tract Diseases–diagnosis. 3. Biliary Tract Diseases–surgery. 4. Pancreatic Diseases–diagnosis. 5. Pancreatic Diseases–surgery. WI 750]
   RC847.5.E53
   616.3'6–dc23

2014029622

A catalogue record for this book is available from the British Library.

Wiley also publishes its books in a variety of electronic formats. Some content that appears in print may not be available in electronic books.

Cover image: ©iStock.com/selvanegra

Set in 9.5/13pt Meridien by SPi Publisher Services, Pondicherry, India
Printed and bound in Singapore by Markono Print Media Pte Ltd

1 2015

Contents

Contributors

Lars Aabakken MD, PhD, BC
Professor of Medicine, Chief of GI Endoscopy
Oslo University Hospital—Rikshospitalet
Oslo, Norway

Alan Barkun MD, CM, FRCP(C), FACP, FACG, AGAF, MSc (Clinical Epidemiology)
Chairholder, the Douglas G. Kinnear Chair in Gastroenterology,
and Professor of Medicine, McGill University
Director of Digestive Endoscopy (adult section), Division of Gastroenterology,
Montreal General Hospital, McGill University and the McGill University Health Centre
Chief Quality Officer, Division of Gastroenterology,
McGill University and the McGill University Health Centre
Montreal, Canada

Todd H. Baron MD, FASGE
Director of Advanced Therapeutic Endoscopy
Professor of Medicine
Division of Gastroenterology & Hepatology
University of North Carolina at Chapel Hill
Chapel Hill, USA

Michael Bourke MBBS, FRACP
Clinical Professor of Medicine
University of Sydney
Sydney, Australia
and
Director of Gastrointestinal Endoscopy
Westmead Hospital
Westmead, Australia

Gregory A. Coté MD, MS
Assistant Professor of Medicine
Indiana University School of Medicine
Indianapolis, USA

Peter B. Cotton MD, FRCS, FRCP
Professor of Medicine
Digestive Disease Center
Medical University of South Carolina
Charleston, USA

John T. Cunningham MD
Samuel and Winifred Witt Professor of Medicine
Section of Gastroenterology and Hepatology
University of Arizona Health Sciences Center
Tucson, USA

Evan L. Fogel MD, MSc, FRCP(C)
Professor of Clinical Medicine
Director, ERCP Fellowship Program
Digestive and Liver Disorders
Indiana University Health, University Hospital
Indianapolis, USA

Moises Guelrud MD
Clinical Professor of Medicine
Tufts University School of Medicine;
Director of Advanced Endoscopic Therapy
Division of Gastroenterology
Tufts Medical Center
Tufts University School of Medicine
Boston, USA

Andres Gelrud MD, MMSc
Associate Professor of Medicine
Director, Center for Pancreatic Disorders
Director, Interventional Endoscopy of the Center for Endoscopic
Research and Therapeutics (CERT)
University of Chicago
Chicago, USA

Bronte A. Holt MBBS, BMedSc, FRACP
Interventional Endoscopist
Center for Interventional Endoscopy
Florida Hospital
Orlando, USA

Sundeep Lakhtakia
Asian Institute of Gastroenterology
Hyderabad, India

John G. Lee MD
Professor of Clinical Medicine
UC Irvine Health, H. H. Chao Comprehensive
Digestive Disease Center
Orange, USA

Joseph Leung MD, FRCP, FACP, MACG, FASGE
Mr. & Mrs. C. W. Law Professor of Medicine
Department of Gastroenterology and Hepatology
Davis School of Medicine, University of California,
Sacramento, USA
Chief, Section of Gastroenterology
VA Northern California Health Care System
GI Unit, Sacramento VAMC
Mather, USA

Wei-Chih Liao MD, PhD
Clinical Assistant Professor
Department of Internal Medicine
National Taiwan University Hospital
National Taiwan University College of Medicine
Taipei, Taiwan

Phyllis M. Malpas MA, RN, CGRN
Nurse Manager
Endoscopy Digestive Disease Service Line
Medical University of South Carolina
Charleston, USA

Derrick F. Martin FRCR, FRCP
Professor of Gastrointestinal Radiology
Wythenshawe Hospital
and
Department of Radiology
University Hospital of South Manchester
Manchester, UK

Julia McNabb-Baltar MD, FRCPC
Instructor of Medicine
Division of Gastroenterology, Hepatology and Endoscopy
Brigham and Women's Hospital
Harvard Medical School
Boston, USA

D. Nageshwar Reddy MD, DM, FRCP
Secretary General – World Endoscopy Organisation
Chairman and Chief of Gastroenterology
Department of Gastroenterology
Asian Institute of Gastroenterology
Hyderabad, India

Mohan Ramchandani MD, DM
Senior Consultant
Department of Gastroenterology
Asian Institute of Gastroenterology
Hyderabad, India

Wiriyaporn Ridtitid MD
Advanced Endoscopy Fellow
Indiana University School of Medicine
Indianapolis, USA
and
Chulalongkorn University
King Chulalongkorn Memorial Hospital
Thai Red Cross Society
Bangkok, Thailand

Joseph Romagnuolo MD, MSc, FRCPC
Professor
Medical University of South Carolina
and
Departments of Medicine, Public Health Sciences
Charleston, USA

Stuart Sherman MD
Professor of Medicine
Glen Lehman Professor in Gastroenterology
Digestive and Liver Disorders
Indiana University Health, University Hospital
Indianapolis, USA

Paul R. Tarnasky MD
Digestive Health Associates of Texas
Program Director, Gastroenterology
Methodist Dallas Medical Center
Dallas, USA

Shyam Varadarajulu MD
Medical Director
Florida Hospital Center for Interventional Endoscopy
Florida Hospital
Professor of Internal Medicine, University of Central Florida
Orlando, USA

John J. Vargo, II MD, MPH, FASGE
Vice Chair, Digestive Disease Institute
Chair, Department of Gastroenterology and Hepatology
Cleveland Clinic
Cleveland, USA

Hsiu-Po Wang MD
Professor
Department of Internal Medicine
National Taiwan University Hospital
National Taiwan University College of Medicine
Taipei, Taiwan

Mohammad Yaghoobi MD, MSc, AFS, FRCPC
Clinical Instructor
Advanced Endoscopy Program
Division of Gastroenterology and Hepatology
Medical University of South Carolina
Charleston, USA

Introduction: Developments in ERCP over 40 years

Peter B. Cotton

Digestive Disease Center, Medical University of SC, Charleston, USA

The history

Endoscopic cannulation of the papilla of Vater was first reported in 1968. However, it was really put on the map shortly afterward by Japanese gastroenterologists, working with instrument manufacturers to develop appropriate long side-viewing instruments. The term "ERCP" (endoscopic retrograde cholangiopancreatography) was agreed at a symposium at the World Congress in Mexico City in 1974. The technique gradually became established worldwide as a valuable diagnostic technique, although some were skeptical about its feasibility and role, and the potential for serious complications soon became clear. It was given a tremendous boost by the development of the therapeutic applications, notably biliary sphincterotomy in 1974 and biliary stenting 5 years later.

It is difficult for most gastroenterologists today to imagine the diagnostic and therapeutic challenges of pancreatic and biliary medicine 40 years ago. There were no scans. The pancreas was a black box, and its diseases diagnosed only at a late stage. Biliary obstruction was diagnosed and treated surgically, with substantial operative mortality.

The period of 20 or so years from the mid 1970s was a "golden age" for ERCP. Despite significant risks, it was quite obvious to everyone that management of duct stones and tumors was easier, cheaper, and safer by ERCP than by available surgical alternatives. Percutaneous transhepatic cholangiography (PTC) and its drainage applications were also developed during this time, but were used (with the exception of a few units) only when ERCP failed or was not available.

The situation has changed in many ways during the last two decades. Some new ERCP techniques have been developed, but the role of ERCP in general has been impacted markedly by improvements in radiology and surgery.

Radiology

Imaging modalities for the biliary tree and pancreas have proliferated. High-quality ultrasound, computed tomography, endoscopic ultrasonography, and magnetic resonance scanning (with magnetic resonance cholangiopancreatography (MRCP)) have greatly facilitated the noninvasive evaluation of patients with known and suspected biliary and pancreatic disease. As a result, ERCP is now almost exclusively used for the treatment of conditions already documented by less invasive techniques. There have also been some improvements in interventional radiology techniques in the biliary tree, which are useful adjuncts when ERCP is unsuccessful, or impractical.

Surgery

There has been substantial and progressive reduction in the risks associated with surgery, due to minimally invasive techniques, and better perioperative and anesthetic care. It is no longer correct to assume that ERCP is always safer than surgery. Surgery should be considered a legitimate alternative to ERCP, not only when ERCP is unsuccessful.

Patient empowerment

Another relevant development in this field is the increased participation of patients in decisions about their care. Patients are rightly demanding information about their potential interventionists, and the likely benefits, risks, and limitations of all the possible approaches to their problems.

The quality imperative

All of these developments are forcing the ERCP community to concentrate on the quality of their services, to make sure that the right things are done in the right way. These issues are important in all clinical contexts, but come into clearest focus where ERCP is still considered somewhat speculative, for example, in the management of chronic pancreatitis and of possible sphincter of Oddi dysfunction. There is increasing attention on who should be trained, and to what level of expertise. How many ERCPists are really needed? In earlier days, most gastroenterology trainees did some ERCP, and continued to dabble in practice. Now the focus is on ensuring that there is a smaller cadre of properly trained ERCPists with sufficient cases to maintain and enhance their skills.

This book

This is our second book devoted to ERCP. The first, entitled *Advanced Digestive Endoscopy: ERCP*, was published on gastrohep.com in 2002, and printed by Blackwell in 2006. This edition owes much to its predecessor, but the new title

ERCP: The Fundamentals emphasizes our attempt to provide core information for trainees and practitioners, rather than a scholarly review of the (now) massive literature. Note that we have largely separated the technical aspects (how it can be done, along with some videos) from the clinical aspects, to allow the authors of the latter chapters to review the complex questions of when it might be done (and when best not).

We greatly appreciate the efforts of all the contributors, and look forward to constructive feedback.

Peter B. Cotton and Joseph W. Leung

November 2013

About the companion website

This series is accompanied by a companion website:
www.wiley.com/go/cotton/ercp

The website includes:
- Video clips

SECTION 1
Preparation

CHAPTER 1

Training and assessment of competence (Preparing the endoscopist)

Joseph Leung[1,2] & Peter B. Cotton[3]

[1]Department of Gastroenterology and Hepatology, Davis School of Medicine, University of California, Sacramento, USA
[2]Section of Gastroenterology, VA Northern California Health Care System, GI Unit, Sacramento VAMC, Mather, USA
[3]Digestive Disease Center, Medical University of South Carolina, Charleston, USA

KEY POINTS

- ERCP includes a range of mainly therapeutic procedures of different levels of complexity.
- Training involves both clinical and technical aspects.
- Hands-on apprenticeship dominates, but various simulators can help.
- Competence should be assessed objectively, and the data made available to patients.

Background

ERCP is the most complex common endoscopic (digestive) procedure. It has great potential for benefits, but it also carries significant risk of failure, adverse events [1], and medico-legal jeopardy [2]. Clearly, it must be done as well as possible, and there has been more focus on quality recently. The key questions are:

- Who should be trained?
- What should be taught, and how?
- Who should teach?
- How are training and competence assessed?
- What level of performance is acceptable?

Who should be trained?

ERCP training is usually a part of the postgraduate training of selected gastro-enterologists, and a few surgeons. The number needed has fallen with the widespread use of magnetic resonance cholangiopancreatography (and also endoscopic ultrasound). In the structured British National Health System, the number of training positions is now tailored to the projected population needs. In many countries, and especially in the United States, there is no such limitation, with the result that some trainees are short-changed, and some have marginal volumes in ongoing practice. It is incumbent upon training programs to ensure that those they train are able to reach an acceptable level of competence for safe independent practice.

What should be taught, and how?

While we focus here mainly on the difficulties involved in teaching the necessary technical skills, it is essential to realize that optimal ERCP requires that practitioners are knowledgeable about pancreatic and biliary medicine and the many alternative diagnostic and therapeutic approaches, as well as being skilled in the basic tenets of patient care. These important aspects should be well covered in basic gastrointestinal (GI) training programs, such as the 3-year fellowships in the United States.

Levels of complexity

ERCP is not a single procedure. The term encompasses a large spectrum of interventions performed (mainly) through the papilla. The concept of levels of complexity or difficulty, introduced by Schutz and Abbot, has recently been updated by a working party of American Society for Gastrointestinal Endoscopy (ASGE) [3]. There are four levels (Table 1.1). Levels 1 and 2 together include the fundamental (mostly) biliary procedures, which are needed at relatively short notice at the community level. The more complex level 3 ("Advanced") and 4 ("Tertiary") procedures are mainly performed by relatively few highly trained endoscopists in higher-volume centers.

These distinctions are clearly relevant to training. No one should be trained to less than competence at level 2. Whilst some practitioners will gradually advance those skills in practice (with mentoring, self-study, and courses), there are increasing numbers of advanced positions (e.g., 4th year in the United States) providing training in the more complex procedures.

Table 1.1 Complexity levels in ERCP. Adapted from Cotton et al, 2011 [3]. Reproduced with permission of Elsevier.

Basic, levels 1 and 2
Deep cannulation of duct of interest, sampling
Biliary stent removal/exchange
Biliary stone extraction <10 mm
Treat biliary leaks
Treat extrahepatic benign and malignant strictures
Place prophylactic pancreatic stents

Advanced, level 3
Biliary stone extraction >10 mm
Minor papilla cannulation and therapy
Remove internally migrated biliary stents
Intraductal imaging, biopsy, needle aspiration
Manage acute or recurrent pancreatitis
Treat pancreatic strictures
Remove pancreatic stones mobile and <5 mm
Treat strictures, hilar and above
Manage suspected sphincter dysfunction (±manometry)

Tertiary, level 4
Remove internal migrated pancreatic stents
Intraductal guided therapy (photodynamic therapy, electrohydraulic lithotripsy)
Pancreatic stones impacted and/or >5 mm
Intrahepatic stones
Pseudocyst drainage, necrosectomy
Ampullectomy
Whipple, Roux-en-Y, bariatric surgery

Progressive training

Like other endoscopy procedures, basic ERCP training involves lectures, study courses, didactic teaching, and the use of books, atlases, and videos, in addition to hands-on supervised clinical practice [4–6]. Clinical teaching includes the elements of a proper history and physical examination with pertinent laboratory tests. Overall management will include work with in- and outpatients with pancreaticobiliary problems, with discussion on the various diagnostic and treatment options, and the assessment and mitigation of risk. This is best achieved in a multidisciplinary environment, with close cooperation particularly with surgeons and radiologists.

After a period of observation, technical training begins with learning the proper technique of scope insertion and positioning. Despite the fact that trainees may have performed many upper endoscopy and colonoscopy procedures, handling and manipulating a side-viewing duodenoscope requires a different skill set. It takes 20–30 cases before the novice endoscopist can master the basic skills of handling the side-viewing scope.

Selective cannulation of the desired duct (usually initially the bile duct) is the key challenge in ERCP, since it is essential for therapeutic interventions. Incompetence in this aspect causes failure and increases the risk of postprocedure pancreatitis. Deep cannulation allows passage of guide wires to support sphincterotomy, stenting, and balloon dilation. Training in these basic steps should be delivered in stages. The trainer demonstrates the technique and then gives verbal instructions to guide the hands-on trainee. In difficult cases, the trainer may take over part of the procedure to complete the more difficult steps and then allow the trainee to continue. The trainees will acquire basic ERCP experience by learning the different steps although not necessarily in a systematic manner. However, the trainee will be able to assimilate the experience and eventually be able to complete the entire procedure independently.

The extent to which a trainee can learn more complex skills will depend on many factors, not least the length of time available and the case mix in the training center.

It is also important for trainees to learn about all of the equipment that can be used during ERCP, including important aspects of radiology safety and image interpretation. ERCP is a team event, and it is necessary to appreciate the importance of well-trained and motivated staff.

Simulation training

The relative shortage of cases in many institutions and the risks involved in training have naturally encouraged the development of adjunctive alternatives to hands-on experience. Simulation practice provides trainees an opportunity to handle the scope and accessories and get familiar with the procedure before performing on patients. Preliminary data indicates that simulation practice can improve the clinical performance of novice trainee ERCPists [5].

In recent years, credentialing and governing bodies have recommended or mandated the use of simulation in training as part of residency education, and simulators have been used extensively in surgery. The essence of simulation in ERCP training is to provide trainees with the opportunities to understand the basic anatomy; become familiar with the equipment (accessories) and learn the basic techniques of scope handling, manipulation of accessories, and coordination with the assistant without involving a patient. Unless the alternative practice method offers the opportunity to use real scope and accessories with hands-on experience, trainees may not be able to reap the benefits of additional or supplemental training.

Different simulators are available for learning and practicing ERCP technique. Therefore, the IDEAL simulator/simulation training should incorporate the following: provide trainees with the learning opportunity to *I*mprove their basic skills, *D*emonstrate realism to help trainees understand anatomy and motility, *E*ase of incorporating into a training program (i.e., inexpensive and portable system that allows repeated practices without special setup), *A*pplication in training including teaching therapeutic procedures, and *L*earning with real scope and accessories including use of simulation fluoroscopy [7].

While ERCP practice on a live anesthetized pig offers the closest resemblance to the human setting, it is rarely used, since it is expensive, labor-intensive, and difficult to organize without special facilities, and carries potential ethical concerns. In general, three types of simulators are available—computer simulators, ex vivo porcine stomach models, and mechanical simulators (Table 1.2). Computer simulators, (e.g., GI Mentor II) are useful for learning the anatomy, including duodenal motility and basic orientation for cannulation [8]. However, the computer simulator uses special probes instead of real accessories and this lacks realism and does not offer the tactile sensation when it comes to the manipulation of the "accessories" for therapeutic ERCP.

A more commonly used training model is the ex-vivo porcine stomach model with attached biliary system that allows trainees to practice with real scope and accessories [9]. However, the anatomical variation, that is, close proximity of the papilla to the pylorus in the porcine model makes scope positioning and cannulation more difficult. Besides, there are separate biliary and pancreatic ductal openings, making it suboptimal to practice selective cannulation. To facilitate practice of biliary papillotomy, the porcine model is further improved by attaching a chicken heart (Neopapilla model) to a separate opening created in the second portion of the duodenum, which corrects for the anatomical difference and allows multiple (up to three) papillotomy practices to be performed on each chicken heart (artificial papilla) [10].

Another form of supplemental simulation training involves the use of mechanical simulators, namely, the ERCP mechanical simulator (EMS) or the X-vision ERCP simulator [11, 12]. Both utilize a rigid model with special papillae adapted to a mechanical duodenum. Selective cannulation can be achieved using injection of a color solution (X-vision) or using a guide wire with the help of a catheter or papillotome (EMS). The X-vision model allows practice papillotomy to be performed on artificial papillae made of a special molded material [13]. The EMS allows practice papillotomy using a foamy papilla soaked with a special conducting gel [14]. In addition, dilation of stricture, brush cytology and stenting, as well as basket stone extraction and mechanical lithotripsy can be performed using the EMS.

Table 1.2 A comparison of different simulator models for advanced ERCP training.

	EMS and X-vision	Computer	Live animal	Ex vivo porcine
References	7, 11, 13, 14, 15, 16, 17	8	5	9,10
Preprogrammed	No	Yes	No	No
Demonstrates anatomy	Simulated	Simulated	Yes*	Yes*
Demonstrates motility	No	Simulated	Yes	No
Basic equipment	Scope and diathermy	Probes and software	Scope and diathermy	Scope and diathermy
Real scope/accessories	Yes	No Modified probes	Yes	Yes
Papillotomy	Yes (artificial)	Simulated	Yes	Yes (Neopapilla[†])
Learning experience				
Tactile sensation	Very good	Good	Very good	Very good
Coordination/ teamwork	Yes	Maybe	Yes	Yes
Supervised training	Yes	Maybe	Yes	Yes
Scoring of experience	Yes (manual)	Yes (computerized)	Yes (manual)	Yes (manual)
Clinical benefits	Yes (EMS[‡])	Maybe	Maybe	Maybe
Technical support				
Anesthesia/technician	No/no	No/no	Yes/yes	No/yes
Assistant	Yes	No	Yes	Yes
Fluoroscopy	Simulated	No	Yes	Transillumination
Estimated cost of model	$3–5 K	$90 K	$1 K/animal	$250/set
Repeated practice	Yes	Yes	Yes (same day)[§]	Yes (same day)[§]
Special/animal lab	No	No	Yes	Yes
Varying levels of difficulties	Yes	Yes (programmed)	No	No
Objective assessment	Yes	Computer report	Yes	Yes
Documentation	Manual	Computerized	Manual	Manual
Reproducibility	Yes	Yes	Maybe	Maybe
Part of routine training	Easy	Easy	Difficult	Maybe

*Anatomical variation with pig stomach model; the papilla is close to the pylorus.
[†]Neopapilla modification allows for multiple papillotomy practices (up to three per "papilla").
[‡]EMS is the only model with two randomized controlled trials; results showing improvement of trainees' clinical performance with coached simulation practice.
[§]Live animal model allows for only one papillotomy per animal. Ex vivo model allows for only one papillotomy unless modified using the Neopapilla.

Despite different simulators being available to supplement clinical ERCP training, and two prospective trials showing their value [15, 16], their use has been largely restricted so far to special teaching workshops.

Who should teach?

A skilled endoscopist may not necessarily be a good teacher. The trainer needs to be able to recognize and correct the errors (mistakes) made by the trainee in terms of technical operation as well as clinical judgment, and to do it in a supportive and nonpunitive manner. The "Train the trainer" courses have been beneficial in highlighting the key elements. In the British system, attendance at such courses is now mandated, and trainees are required to assess their teachers in the e-portfolio system.

How are training and competence assessed?

Whatever training methods are employed, the key issue clearly is how well the trainee can perform. Trainees should keep logs of their procedures (on simulators as well as patients), and some metrics are suggested in Tables 1.3–1.5.

Objective assessment of performance is easier to document with practice on simulators (Table 1.2). Specific end points may include successful execution of the procedure and total procedure time taken including the use of simulated fluoroscopy time during the practice [11]. Documentation during computer simulation training is more complete with tracking of the time taken and number of attempts made to perform a particular procedure. Adjustment or modification in training can be done by using different computer software programs with varying levels of complexity, whereas the mechanical simulator can incorporate a different setup including changing position of the papilla or level of the bile duct stricture. Such changes can cater for procedures with varying levels of difficulties from basic cannulation to papillotomy and to the more advanced procedures such as multiple stents placement for a simulated bile duct stricture [17].

In general, trainer assessment is more subjective based on a summation of the overall clinical performance of the trainees (Tables 1.3 and 1.4), both technical and clinical. The Accreditation Council for Graduate Medical Education (ACGME) has devised objective end points for measuring the quality of ERCP training and success with the procedure, but strictly speaking, these end points cannot account for all of the different aspects of this technical procedure.

Table 1.3 Some suggested simulator practice scores to evaluate trainees' practice performance.

Cannulation			
Position—achieve proper orientation and axis	1	Failed cannulation	−2
Successful/deep cannulation of selected system	1	Number of attempts	
Wire manipulation			
Manipulate wire for cannulation and stricture	1	Loss wire/access	−1
Coordinated exchange of accessories	1	End of wire on floor	−1
Balloon dilation			
Proper preparation of insufflator	1	Excess air left in balloon	−1
Maintain position of balloon during dilation	1		
Cytology			
Control position of brush during cytology	1		
Document bare brush across stricture	1		
Stenting			
Able to measure stent length properly	1	Stent too short or too long	−2
Proper deployment of stent	1		
Deploy multiple stents in the common duct	1		
Demonstrates how to deploy self-expandable metallic stent	1		
Basket			
Proper stone engagement and removal	1	Stone pushed into IHBD	−1
Demonstrate how to free impacted basket and stone	1		
Demonstrate skill with use of mechanical lithotripter	1		
Retrieval balloons			
Able to control balloon size	1		
Papillotomy			
Maintain good position during cut	1	Deviated cut	−2
Control tension on cutting wire	1		
Shaping wire position if indicated	1		
Perform stepwise cut	1		
Sizing the papillotomy	1		
Assistance from trainer			
Verbal instructions only	1	Hands-on assistance 25%	−1
		50%	−2
		75%	−3

Table 1.4 Clinical assessment (to be filled in by trainer at completion of ERCP).

ERCP performance score

Trainee performed procedures *without* trainer's hands-on assistance

Selective cannulation	Yes	No	NA
Biliary sphincterotomy	Yes	No	NA
Pancreatic sphincterotomy	Yes	No	NA
Biliary stone extraction	Yes	No	NA
Balloon dilation	Yes	No	NA
Brush cytology	Yes	No	NA
Biliary plastic stent	Yes	No	NA
Pancreatic plastic stent	Yes	No	NA
Metal stent placement	Yes	No	NA
Mechanical lithotripsy	Yes	No	NA

(yes = 1, no = 0; actual ERCP performance score = sum/number of applicable categories, the score is used as a covariable for analysis.)

ERCP "error" score

Did the following occur during this trainee performed ERCP?

Failed cannulation	Yes	No	NA
Introduce air into ducts	Yes	No	NA
Overfilled (obstructed) ductal system	Yes	No	NA
End of guide wire on floor	Yes	No	NA
Loss wire/access	Yes	No	NA
Inappropriate length (too short) stent used	Yes	No	NA
Failed to document bare brush across stricture	Yes	No	NA
Uncontrolled papillotomy cut	Yes	No	NA
Stone being pushed into IHBD	Yes	No	NA
Stone and basket impaction	Yes	No	NA

(yes = 0, no = 1; actual ERCP "error" score = sum/number of applicable categories; this score is used as a covariable for analysis.)

Clinical performance assessment (excellent, good, poor, not assessed)

Preparation of the patient before the procedure
Care after the procedure
Assessment of prior imaging
Interpretation of ERCP radiographs
Communication with the patient
Communication with the family
Communication with referrers

Overall assessment of current competence in standard ERCP skills (%):

Table 1.5 Trainer assessment score of trainees' performance (five-point score).

5. (Excellent) Demonstrates good knowledge in operating the accessories, able to successfully complete procedure in >80% of cases, no iatrogenic induced failure or complication, or performance as good as an attending
4. (Good) Demonstrates good knowledge, good skills, needs only occasional assistance from trainer
3. (Average) Understands the operation of accessories, demonstrates only reasonable knowledge in actual operation of accessory, average skills, requires assistance from trainer
2. (Fair) Can handle the side-viewing duodenoscope, understands the operation of accessories, unsure about actual operation or performance of accessories, requires >50% help from trainer
1. (Poor) Good control of upper GI scope, struggles with side-viewing scope, some knowledge of accessories but does not understand the operation or control of accessories or wires, needs a lot of attention and assistance from trainer

Numbers

The question "How many hands-on cases does a trainee need to become competent?" has dominated and confused the field for decades. The original guess by ASGE that 100 might be sufficient was shown to be seriously inadequate by the seminal study by Jowell and colleagues that showed that their trainees were only approaching 80% competency after 180–200 procedures [18]. The ASGE recommends that trainees should have performed 200 ERCP procedures with 80% success of cannulation with more than half of the procedures being therapeutic before they are considered competent or rather ready for assessment of competency [19]. The Australians have an even tougher criterion which requires trainees to have performed 200 successful solo procedures without trainer involvement [20].

These assessments are usually made by a sympathetic trainer at "home base," and are a complex amalgam of subjective information. We usually think that the trainee is "reasonably OK," but we do not know how they actually perform once in practice with less experienced staff (and maybe unfamiliar equipment), and with some peer pressure to succeed.

The only important numbers (in practice and in training) are the actual outcomes, using agreed quality metrics, such as deep biliary cannulation success and pancreatitis rates. Thus, we have long recommended that practitioners collect these data (report cards) [21], and have the opportunity to compare them with peers (benchmarking) [22]. These systems also include complexity levels, so that the spectrum of practice can be documented.

Because of the need for X-ray, ERCP is the one endoscopic procedure that is done only in hospitals. Hospitals have the responsibility for ensuring that their credentialing and privileging systems allow only competent endoscopists into their units. These systems need to be improved.

How else can we move forward? The assessment at the end of training could be made by people other than their trainers, by a combination of logbooks, videos, references, and observation of procedures (live and simulated) in their home environment or elsewhere. Ideally, there should be some form of certification at the national level, incorporating the complexity levels.

What level of performance is acceptable?

There are significant variations in the quality of ERCP performance. Taking deep biliary cannulation as a key metric, we know that experts achieve greater than 95% success, but not all cases can or should be done by experts. So what is acceptable, and who decides? Professional societies have usually suggested 85 or 90% in general, but much depends on the clinical circumstances and setting. A less expert endoscopist will be acceptable, and may be life-saving, in an emergency (e.g., acute cholangitis), but patients with more complex and elective problems may prefer (if given the option) referral to a tertiary center. Patients should not be afraid to quiz their potential interventionists about their experience, and ask to see the report card [21]. These aspects are discussed further in Chapter 25.

Conclusion

ERCP now constitutes a variety of procedures, which require excellent clinical and technical skills with an experienced team in a supportive environment. The structures of training and practice are gradually being improved so as to raise the quality of ERCP practice worldwide, and patients are increasingly knowledgeable about the issues. We hope to see fewer, poorly trained, low-volume ERCPists in the future [23].

Appendix

Some examples of how to gauge trainees' performance during clinical practice

Cannulation

Understanding the use of contrast (different concentrations), priming the catheter and eliminating air bubbles, preparing a wire-guided papillotome (and if necessary, shaping the catheter or papillotome)

Able to achieve proper positioning with correct orientation and alignment with the axis for respective ducts for selective and deep cannulation of respective system, appropriate use of contrast injection, avoid overfilling of pancreas or obstructed biliary systems, and able to capture good radiograph for documentation

Guide wire manipulation

Understanding the use of different guide wires and their application, able to manipulate a guide wire with coordinated exchange of accessories, good control during exchange and avoid losing wire position, if necessary, able to shape tip of guide wire to negotiate difficult bile duct stricture, selective placement of guide wire in intrahepatic system and/or pancreatic duct

Dilation (rigid or balloon)

Understanding the use of rigid catheter dilator versus pneumatic balloons, understand how to fill insufflator with contrast and get rid of air in syringe and operate insufflator, choice of balloon size, good coordination with exchange and maintaining position of balloon during dilation

Understand the use of Soehendra stent retriever for dilation under special circumstances

Cytology

Understanding the use of double-lumen cytology and/or single-lumen cytology brush, choice of brush in different situations (biliary versus pancreatic), able to control (and document) the position of the brush during cytology specimen taking, understand how to prepare specimen slides and samples

Stenting

Understand the difference between straight versus double-pigtail stents, choice of stents, know and demonstrate how to measure stent length based on different methods, choice of guide wire for difficult stenting (intrahepatic bile duct (IHBD) stricture), special stent (for left hepatic duct) and proper deployment of stent (position and length), and able to deploy multiple stents in the common duct and right and left hepatic ducts

Basket

Understand the operation of different types of basket, wire-guided basket, lithotripsy basket, understand and demonstrate proper stone engagement and removal, demonstrate how to free an impacted basket and stone, understand and demonstrate skill with use of mechanical lithotripter, understand and know how to steer the basket into intrahepatic system

Retrieval balloons

Understand how to operate a stone retrieval or occlusion balloon, know how to control the volume of air inflated into the balloon, avoid overinflating the balloon and know how to adjust balloon size during course of action

Papillotomy

Understand the axis of the bile duct and pancreatic duct, know how to perform a controlled cut along the respective axis, know how to correct a deviated cut and know when to stop cutting, demonstrate understanding and perform different hemostasis methods to control postpapillotomy bleeding and able to insert biliary stent to ensure drainage

References

1 Cotton PB. Complications of ERCP. In Cotton PB and Leung J. Eds. Advanced Digestive Endoscopy: ERCP, Blackwell Science, Massachusetts, MA, USA, 2005.
2 Cotton PB. Analysis of 59 ERCP Lawsuits; Mainly about Indications. Gastrointest Endosc 2006;63:378–382.
3 Cotton P, Eisen G, Romagnuolo J, et al. Grading the Complexity of Endoscopic Procedures: Results of an ASGE Working Party. Gastrointest Endosc 2011;73:868–874.
4 Cohen J. Training and Credentialing in Gastrointestinal Endoscopy in Endoscopy Practice and Safety. In Cotton Ed. Advanced Endoscopy (e-book), Gastrohep.com, 2005: 1–50.
5 Leung J, Lim B. Training in ERCP. In Cohen J. Ed. Successful Training in GI Endoscopy, Wiley-Blackwell, Sommerset, NJ, USA, 2010;85–96.
6 Chutkan RK, Ahmad AS, Cohen J, et al. ERCP Core Curriculum. Gastrointest Endosc 2006;63(3):361–376.
7 Leung JW, Yen D. ERCP Training – The Potential Role of Simulation Practice, J Interv Gastroenterol 2011;1:14–18.
8 Bar-Meir S. Simbionix Simulator. Gastrointest Endosc Clin N Am. 2006 Jul;16(3):471–478, vii.
9 Neumann M, Mayer G, Ell C, et al. The Erlangen Endo-Trainer: Lifelike Simulation for Diagnostic and Interventional Endoscopic Retrograde Cholangiography. Endoscopy 2000;32:906–910.
10 Matthes K, Cohen J. The Neo-Papilla: A New Modification of Porcine Ex-vivo Simulators for ERCP Training (with videos). Gastrointest Endosc. 2006;64(4):570–576.
11 Leung JW, Lee JG, Rojany M, et al. Development of a Novel ERCP Mechanical Simulator. Gastrointest Endosc 2007 Jun; 65(7):1056–1062.
12 Frimberger E, von Dellus S, Rosch T, et al. A Novel and Practicable ERCP Training System with Simulated Fluoroscopy. Endoscopy, 2008;40:517–520.
13 von Delius S, Thies P, Meining A, et al. Validation of the X-Vision ERCP Training System and Technical Challenges during Early Training of Sphincterotomy. Clin Gastroenterol Hepatol 2009;7(4):389–396.
14 Leung J, Yen D, Lim B, Leung F. Didactic Teaching and Simulator Practice Improve Trainees' Understanding and Performance of Biliary Papillotomy. J Interv Gastroenterol 2013;3: 51–55.

15 Lim B, Leung J, Lee J, *et al*. Effect of ERCP Mechanical Simulator (EMS) Practice on Trainees' ERCP Performance in the Early Learning Period: U.S. Multi-Center Randomized Controlled Trial. Am J Gastroenterol 2011;106:300–306.

16 Liao W, Leung J, Wang H, *et al*. Coached Practice using ERCP Mechanical Simulator Improves Trainees' ERCP Performance: A Randomized Controlled Trial. Endoscopy 2013;45:799–805.

17 Leung JW, Lee W, Wilson R, *et al*. Comparison of Accessory Performance using a Novel ERCP Mechanical Simulator. Endoscopy 2008;40:983–988.

18 Jowell PS, Baillie J, Branch MS, *et al*. Quantitative Assessment of Procedural Competence. A Prospective Study of Training in Endoscopic Retrograde Cholangio-pancreatography. Ann Int Med 1996;125(12):983–989.

19 Baron T, Petersen BT, Mergener K, *et al*. Quality Indicators for Endoscopic Retrograde Cholangiopancreatography. Gastrointest Endosc 2006;63(4):S29–S34.

20 Conjoint Committee for Recognition of Training in Gastrointestinal Endoscopy. www.conjoint.org.au (accessed on July 31, 2014).

21 Cotton PB. How Many Times have you Done this Procedure, Doctor? Am J Gastroenterol 2002;97:522–523.

22 Cotton PB, Romagnuolo J, Faigel DO, *et al*. The ERCP Quality Network: A Pilot Study of Benchmarking Practice and Performance. Am J Medical Quality 2013;28(3):256–260.

23 Cotton PB. Are Low-Volume ERCPists a Problem in the United States? A Plea to Examine and Improve ERCP Practice-NOW. Gastrointest Endosc 2011 Jul;74(1):161–166.

CHAPTER 2

Preparing the facilities and equipment

Joseph Leung

Department of Gastroenterology and Hepatology, Davis School of Medicine, University of California, Sacramento, USA
Section of Gastroenterology, VA Northern California Health Care System, GI Unit, Sacramento VAMC, Mather, USA

KEY POINTS

- An organized purpose-designed room provides a functional floor plan, with places for fixed equipment, work space for various staff, and ready access to accessories.

- The endoscopy and fluoroscopy display monitors should be placed side by side at eye level directly opposite to the endoscopist and assistant to facilitate ERCP procedures.

- A large 4.2-mm channel duodenoscope that accepts 10 Fr accessories is preferred for most procedures in adults.

- Understanding the setup and functions of diathermy units is crucial for a successful sphincterotomy.

- Close coordination between the endoscopist and assistant is necessary for exchange with the long wire system.

- Endoscopists should be familiar with the advantages of using short guide wire systems.

ERCP is a team event with many contributing elements. The key issues for endoscopists, trainees, nurses, anesthesia, radiology, and reporting are covered in separate chapters. Here we address the physical facilities and equipment.

Room setup and floor plan

Having a room dedicated to ERCP is ideal, but ERCPists and centers with relatively low volumes often have to share space in radiology. Apart from issues of scheduling, there are several reasons why that arrangement may be problematic. The room may be too small to accommodate comfortably all of the equipment and personnel

---

ERCP: The Fundamentals, Second Edition. Edited by Peter B. Cotton and Joseph Leung.
© 2015 John Wiley & Sons, Ltd. Published 2015 by John Wiley & Sons, Ltd.
Companion Website: www.wiley.com\go\cotton\ercp

(including anesthesia when needed). The layout may be such as to expose team members to more radiation than ideal. Another important issue is the position of the monitors. ERCPists need to have the fluoroscopy and endoscopy monitors side by side, which may be difficult to arrange. In addition, it is tedious and inefficient to have to transport all of the potentially needed equipment for each case. The same issues arise when ERCP has to be done in other places, such as operating rooms and intensive care units.

The principal design features of a dedicated ERCP room and the main items of equipment are described.

The ERCP room should be large enough (at least 450 sq ft) to house all of the endoscopy equipment, monitors, anesthetic equipment, in addition to the fluoroscopy unit, and the staff. The space should be allocated into convenient functional areas for the many people who may be involved, that is, the endoscopist(s) nurse/assistant(s), radiology tech, sedation/anesthesia staff, plus any trainees and observers (Figure 2.1).

Accessories should be organized and stored to facilitate easy retrieval during procedures (Figure 2.2).

The endoscopy and fluoroscopy monitors should be placed side by side (Figure 2.3) (or combined in one screen) and ceiling-mounted at eye level across the X-ray table (to the right behind the patient's head) for the convenience of both the endoscopist and the key assistant. Some units have the endoscopy monitor mounted on the

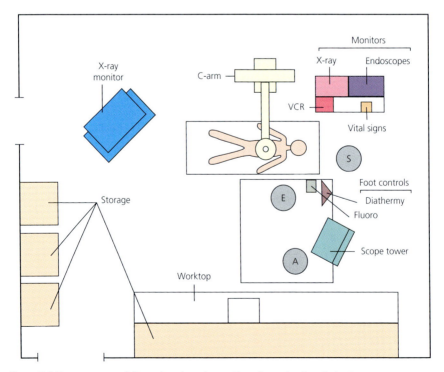

Figure 2.1 Room setup and floor plan. A, assistant; E, endoscopist; S, sedationist.

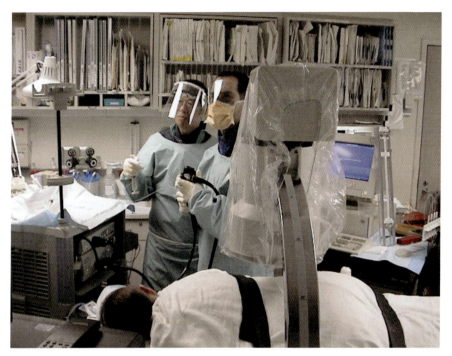

Figure 2.2 Space for endoscopists and trainee or assistant. Accessories organized and within easy reach of endoscopist.

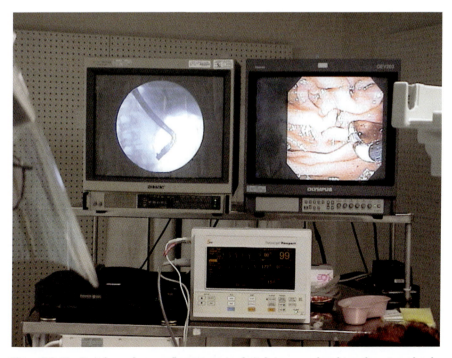

Figure 2.3 Monitors for endoscopy, fluoroscopy, and vital signs are placed together at eye level.

endoscopy cart placed by the head of the patient. This setup requires the endoscopist to turn more to the right and away from the patient, which can predispose to scope displacement or straining of the back and neck If the fluoroscopy monitor cannot be moved (as in some older machines), it may be necessary to tap the signal and display it on another monitor placed together with the endoscopy monitor.

Endoscopy tower/support system

The endoscopy support system includes the light source, video processor, and recording equipment. This is all best mounted on a beam suspended from the ceiling (which avoids having wires trailing across the floor). Alternatively, a purpose-designed cart can be used. The position of this equipment can be adjusted to the preference of the endoscopist, but is usually placed to the right of the endoscopist, with sufficient room left in between for the assistant to manipulate accessories.

Duodenoscopes

Video endoscopes are available from several manufacturers, mainly Olympus, Pentax, and Fujinon. We prefer to use the larger "therapeutic" endoscope with a 4.2-mm channel for most procedures in adults because it can accept the larger 10 Fr accessories. The smaller endoscope with a 3.2-mm channel can be used when luminal narrowing is expected, and in children above the age of two. Smaller pediatric duodenoscopes (with a 2.0-mm channel) are available for examination in neonates.

In patients with a distorted anatomy or postsurgical changes, it may be necessary to use a forward-viewing scope such as the pediatric colonoscope for Billroth II gastrectomy or an enteroscope for patients with Roux-en-Y hepatico-jejunostomy. An upper endoscope can sometimes be used to traverse a prior choledochoduodenostomy to access the intrahepatic ducts. The Spyglass system is a free-standing unit that goes through the large channel scope and allows cholangioscopy to be performed by a single operator. Extralarge channel endoscopes are available for passage of "baby" choledochoscopes and pancreatoscopes.

The designs of the common duodenoscopes are broadly similar. One Olympus model incorporates a notch at the elevator (V-notch) that allows the elevator to grip the guide wire during exchange of accessories.

Accessories

The commonly used ERCP accessories are listed in Table 2.1 and are discussed here. Other more complex or advanced accessories and their applications will be described individually in the chapter on techniques.

Table 2.1 ERCP accessories.

Item	Examples	Function
Cannulation		
Catheter (S, LW)	Bullet tip(C), Taper tip (C), 5-4-3 (B)	Single channel for diagnostic injection of contrast; and assist in passage of guide wire for selective cannulation (use with special adaptor)
Needle tip catheter (S)	Cramer (C)	For minor papilla cannulation (pancreas divisum)
Catheter (D,SW)	Fusion glow tip (C), RX (B)	Separate channel for contrast injection and passage of short guide wire (special design)
Sphincterotomy		
Sphincterotome (D,T), (LW,SW)	Cannulatome (C), DASH papillotome (C), Clever cut (O) Truetome (B), Autotome (B)	Facilitate insertion of guide wire for selective cannulation; biliary and pancreatic sphincterotomy
Precut sphincterotome (D, LW), (SW)	Needle knife, Huibregtse (C), Microknife (B)	Precut sphincterotomy for impacted stone or stent guided sphincterotomy and minor papilla sphincterotomy
Stone extraction		
Stone extraction basket (D,C)	22Q (O), WEB (C), Trapezoid (B)	Removal of biliary and pancreatic stones (lithotripsy compatible)
Special basket	Flower (O)	Removal of small stones or stone fragments
Stone extraction balloon (D,T,A)	Escort (C), Fusion (C), Extractor RX(B), Extractor XL (B)	For occlusion cholangiogram; sizing of strictures and sphincterotomy; stone extraction; deflection of guide wire for selective cannulation of intrahepatic system
Special devices for stone extraction		
Lithotripsy basket	Fusion basket (C), Trapezoid (B)	Stone extraction with the option of lithotripsy if required
Lithotripter sheath	Soehendra lithotripter (C)	For stone fragmentation in the event of unexpected stone and basket impaction
Mechanical lithotripter	BML (O)	Special basket with built-in metal sheath and handle for fragmentation of large stones
Electrohydraulic	Walz	Intraductal lithotripsy using choledochoscopy
Laser	Holmium laser	Intraductal lithotripsy in combination with choledochoscopy
Cholangioscope	Mother and baby scope (O), Spyglass (B)	Choledochoscopy to facilitate biopsy and intraductal therapy including selective cannulation and intraductal lithotripsy

(Continued)

Table 2.1 (*Continued*)

Item	Examples	Function
Stricture dilation		
Dilation catheter (S)	Cotton/Cunningham (C)	Dilation of tight biliary or pancreatic strictures
Dilation balloons (D,Con)	Quantum (C), Fusion Titan (C), Hurricane RX (B), Maxforce (B)	Dilation of biliary or pancreatic strictures; balloon sphincteroplasty
Cytology brush (D)	DL brush (C), RX cytology (B)	Brush cytology of biliary or pancreatic strictures
Drainage		
Plastic biliary stents (S)	Cotton Leung (C), Advanix (B). Olympus stent	Drainage for biliary decompression in acute cholangitis; drainage for malignant biliary obstruction; drainage and dilation of benign biliary stricture; drainage for pancreatic stricture or stone obstruction
Plastic pancreatic stents (S)	Geenen (C), Zimmon (C)	Drainage of PD to prevent post-ERCP pancreatitis; dilation of PD stricture, assists with needle knife precut of biliary sphincterotomy or minor papillotomy
Stent introducer system	OASIS (C), Naviflex (B) Fusion OASIS (C)	Deployment of biliary or pancreatic stent for drainage
Open-mesh SEMS	Wallflex (B), Zilver (C), Evolution (C)	Drainage for malignant biliary obstruction
Fully covered SEMS	Wallflex (B)	Drainage for malignant biliary obstruction; selected cases with benign bile duct stricture
Nasobiliary catheter (S) Nasopancreatic drain	Pigtail, angled tip (C) Straight tip (C), Flexima NB catheter (B)	Temporary drainage of bile duct in acute cholangitis and stone obstruction; less commonly used for PD drainage
Miscellaneous		
Stent retriever (snare)	Mini micro snare (C)	Snare for removal of indwelling stent
Stent retriever	Soehendra stent retriever (C)	Adapted for dilation of tight biliary or pancreatic strictures
Injector	Sclerotherapy needle (C)	Injection therapy; control of postsphincterotomy bleeding

D, double lumen; LW, long wire; SW, short wire; T, triple lumen; S, single lumen.
Inflation with contrast: Con, air: A.
Manufacturer: (B), Boston Scientific; (C), Cook Endoscopy; (O): Olympus.

Cannulas/catheters

These are simple long plastic tubes, usually of 5-Fr gauge, with a tapered or rounded radio-opaque tip. They are used for injection of contrast and for insertion of guide wires. These functions can be done by exchange in a single channel, but catheters with two channels are easier to use. Similar catheters are used for aspiration of bile or fluids, irrigation, and insertion of cytology brushes.

Sphincterotomes

Standard "pull-type" sphincterotomes are plastic catheters with an exposed 2–3-cm wire for coagulation and cutting. They also have one or two channels for injection and guide wires. Traction on the cutting wire can facilitate selective cannulation by deflecting the tip. The "needle knife" sphincterotome is a simple catheter with a central short extendable cutting wire. It can be used to obtain access to the bile duct when standard approaches fail (with or without an indwelling stent), and to initiate drainage of a pseudocyst.

Stone extraction balloons and baskets

These are used for removing stones from the bile duct or pancreatic duct depending on the size and location of the stones and the exit passage. Balloons can be used to perform an occlusion cholangiogram and for testing the adequacy of a sphincterotomy or dilation of bile duct strictures. Baskets typically have four wires in a hexagonal configuration. Those designed for lithotripsy have stronger wires, an outer metal sheath, and a crank handle to apply traction to crushing the stone against a metal sheath.

Dilation catheters and balloons

These are used over guide wires to dilate strictures in the bile duct and pancreatic duct. The dilation catheters are stiff (often Teflon) with a tapered tip, and a radio-opaque maker at the maximum size. Dilating balloons are usually 4 cm in length, and 4, 6, 8 or 10 mm in diameter.

Plastic stents

These are used for either palliative drainage of malignant obstructive jaundice or temporary drainage of the biliary system in patients with obstructing stones and/or cholangitis. Multiple stents have been placed for the continuing dilation of benign bile duct stricture after balloon dilation. Smaller stents with a different design are used for drainage of the pancreatic duct. The commonest biliary stents are 7 and 10 Fr, either "straight" (actually slightly curved) with retaining flaps at both ends or with pigtails.

Self-expandable metal stents (SEMS)

SEMS are larger than plastic stents and are being used for biliary drainage. Open-mesh SEMS are used mainly for palliation of malignant obstructive jaundice. They are used especially for hilar obstruction to avoid blocking the opposite side. Fully covered (fc)SEMS are mostly used for drainage of distal CBD obstruction. Because they can be removed endoscopically, fcSEMS are now being used for refractory benign bile duct strictures.

Cytology brushes and biopsy forceps

These are used to obtain cytological/tissue samples for the confirmation of underlying malignancy. Cytology brushes are contained within a catheter, placed over a guide wire, and then exposed to obtain tissue. Small biopsy forceps can be inserted free hand into the bile duct to obtain tissue samples under fluoroscopic guidance.

Nasobiliary catheters

Nasobiliary catheters are designed to provide drainage of the bile duct for a few days, and can be used for flushing or repeat cholangiography. They are simply long plastic tubes that are placed at ERCP over a guide wire. The tip (pigtail or sharp bend) is anchored in an intrahepatic duct, and the proximal end is brought out of the mouth, and then rerouted to the nose. Nasopancreatic catheters are similar but rarely used.

Guide wires

Guide wires are important adjuncts for many if not all therapeutic procedures. There are many different sizes and materials. Fundamental differences exist in their length ("short" = 200–260 cm, or "long" = 400–460 cm), diameter (0.018–0.035 in.), coating (hydrophilic or not), and tip flexibility. Their merits and specific uses are described in Chapter 7.

Accesory storage and organization of the work top

Accessories should be stored in such a way as to allow easy retrieval as well as stock-keeping. A limited supply of commonly used items should be kept in the procedure room (and restocked after use), with clear labels, and displayed on shelves like books in a library (Figure 2.4). It may be preferable to group similar items together while keeping the special items separately. The accessories in use or likely to be used for a particular case are placed on work tops, which can be on a separate cart and/or on pull-out shelves from the suspending beam. To minimize cross-contamination it is necessary to separate the clean and soiled (used) items. It is important to ensure that the opened accessories are properly kept and maintained during the procedure and to avoid contamination so that they can be reused safely if needed. Long accessories such as guide wires tend to uncoil and they are best kept looped and restrained with a clip or a piece of wet gauze. Others have used clean plastic bags to hold the coiled-up accessories when they are not in use. Most of the accessories used today are disposable (one-time use only) but are meant for one patient use and not one attempt.

It is helpful to establish a preprocedure "game plan" with the assistant so that the necessary accessories can be pulled before the start of a procedure.

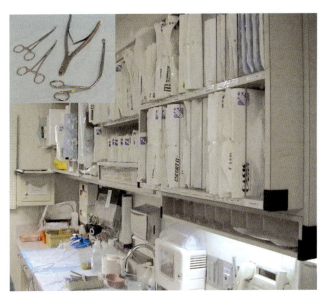

Figure 2.4 Organize accessories within easy reach for retrieval. Do not stack up, "file" like books in a library with large clear "correct" labels. Categorize in groups. Special accessories and tools.

Electrosurgical unit (diathermy)

The diathermy unit provides both cutting and coagulation currents, either separately or in combination (blended mode). Depending on the model, the power setting on the diathermy machine can be preset (e.g., ERBE unit) or adjusted according to the individual's preference (e.g., ValleyLab or Olympus unit).

The power setting on different diathermy units varies depending on the energy output of the units. For the Olympus diathermy (e.g., PSD-20 or equivalent), the power is set at 3–3.5 with a blended current; the setting on a ValleyLab diathermy machine (a 60-W unit) is a power setting of 30–40 W on cut with a blended I current. The power setting on the ERBE unit is already preset for ERCP sphincterotomy (Endocut mode). It has a unique design that initially coagulates followed by cutting of the papilla, thus allowing the sphincterotomy to be performed in a controlled manner. The cut can be controlled also by the endoscopist using the foot pedal or alternatively by the built-in microcomputer when the unit is activated by the foot pedal.

Additional items

Resuscitation equipment should be readily available nearby.

Contrast should be drawn up in clearly labeled syringes prior to the procedure and be ready for use. It is preferable to have at least two 20-ml syringes filled with contrast of normal and half normal concentration. A 20-ml syringe is handy for contrast injection because it is easy to handle, contains sufficient volume, and permits injection by the endoscopist.

Other items to facilitate ERCP include a small pot of 30% alcohol in sterile water (nonflammable), which is used for cleaning the gloves (finger tips) or to wipe down the guide wire during exchanges and to remove any bile or contrast, which can become sticky when dried. The dilute alcohol solution also reduces friction at the biopsy valve and facilitates insertion of larger accessories; 4 in. × 4 in. gauze pads are used for cleaning and wiping.

Sterile water with simethicone can be flushed down the channel to remove gas bubbles in the duodenum to improve visualization during the procedure.

Additional 20-ml syringes are used for aspiration of bile for culture and/or cytology. Sterile water is sometimes used to flush the catheters prior to insertion of hydrophilic wires and for exchanges, and also for irrigation and flushing of the bile ducts to remove sludge and stone fragments.

A pair of McGill forceps is useful in assisting with rerouting of nasobiliary catheter.

A mucus trap is useful for collecting duodenal aspirate, which represents the bile sample for culturing purposes.

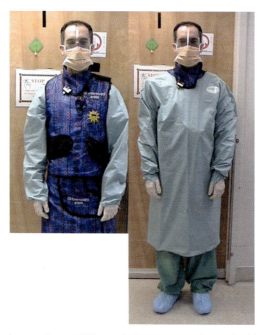

Figure 2.5 Personnel protection—OSHA regulations. Gowns, gloves (double), shoe cover, face shield or mask, lead apron (skirt and vest) and collar, X-ray badge, and lead lining for room and warning signs. It is preferable to have the impervious gown on the outside to protect the lead apron.

Personnel protection

Details of radiation protection equipment and practices are given in Chapter 12. External impervious gowns should be worn on the outside of the lead apron (to minimize contamination) in addition to (double) gloves, and shoe covers as appropriate. Staff should wear a face shield or mask to avoid splash injury (Figure 2.5).

Conclusion

Proper physical organization of the room and all equipment, and good coordination with the team, are essential for ERCP. The choice of accessories will depend on the type of procedures and the endoscopist's preference but familiarity with all of the equipment is crucial to success.

CHAPTER 3

ERCP team and teamwork

Phyllis M. Malpas

Endoscopy Digestive Disease Service Line, Medical University of South Carolina, Charleston, USA

KEY POINTS

- Endoscopic retrograde cholangiopancreatography (ERCP) is a team event, involving the talents of several disciplines, both inside and outside the procedure room.
- Good outcomes depend on staff education, mutual respect, and multiple levels of support.
- The patient's needs and privacy must be protected.
- The ERCP team is only one section of the whole unit.

Back in the mid to late 1980s ERCP was coming into its own as a therapeutic specialty of gastrointestinal (GI) medicine and nursing. As a team member in ERCP, I was working alongside devotees such as Jeffrey Ponsky and Roy Ferguson and in the proximity of great names, like Cotton, Cunningham, Leung, Geenen, Soehendra, and Huibregste. These names appeared in our conversation and on our devices. It was natural that ERCP became a critical focus of our work. Because we were all sailing in previously uncharted waters, we often did not recognize the "hows," "whos" and "whys" of what we needed to create or develop. This chapter, therefore, is to be taken for what it is—an honest chapter with some words of wisdom gained from long experience, as an endoscopy and ERCP team member, and as a nurse manager. It is critical for those seeking to build great ERCP teams to take the time and make the effort needed to grasp the current state as well as the future vision of the organization. Failure to bridge any cultural divide can hamper ERCP teams. These gaps may seem slight and appear to be only surface deep. In the long run, however, they can widen into chasms affecting procedure volume and timing, staffing levels, education and expectation of staff training, financing of capital equipment and procurement constraints, physician scheduling and anesthesia and radiology expectations, and, most importantly, patient care and safety.

ERCP is the most complex procedure performed on a regular basis in most endoscopy units, and is the quintessential team event. It might be compared to a musical concert. Whilst some members of the orchestra are more prominent,

ERCP: The Fundamentals, Second Edition. Edited by Peter B. Cotton and Joseph Leung.
© 2015 John Wiley & Sons, Ltd. Published 2015 by John Wiley & Sons, Ltd.
Companion Website: www.wiley.com\go\cotton\ercp

it is the combination of talents that produces the best music. Equally, it can be ruined if only one member performs badly. Recognizing and valuing the contributions of all members of the team is essential for continuing success.

Leaders of ERCP and endoscopy in medicine, nursing, and administration must define and at times redefine their combined vision and goals, "the culture," in the existing and specific organizational structure. Collaboration to translate vision into reality over time provides the solid foundation needed to develop these goals and to orchestrate them well. Building this core is as necessary as development of the individuals in the procedure room, the appropriateness of the devices we handle, and arguably the skill of the physicians and staff. It is the stage on which the entire orchestra is set, and from which the most harmonious music of the best teams is produced.

The ERCP front line consists of those in the room with the patient, that is, the endoscopist(s), primary "table" assistants, a nurse or technician, the radiology tech, the monitoring nurse, and the anesthesia provider. In close clinical support nearby in the unit are those involved in preparing and helping in the patient's recovery and caring for family members. Behind the scenes are those who make sure that all the necessary equipment and accessories are available and safe to use. Some of the details may vary according to the site and size of the ERCP practice, but the fundamentals are consistent.

The nurse manager and medical director of the unit have the responsibility to ensure that all the elements are in place, and that all involved have the necessary initial and ongoing training, while at the same time providing the same level of support to the remainder of the unit. There should be no room for "prima donnas."

Endoscopy staff

Registered nurse
Each procedure team should include at least one person licensed as a registered nurse as first or second assistant. Through education and experience the registered nurse continuously assesses the patient and hones critical thinking skills, providing the foundation for patient safety in any situation. In the United States and Canada, an Society of Gastroenterology Nurses and Associates (SGNA) sister organization, the GI Nursing Board (American Board of Certification for Gastroenterology Nurses), certifies the registered nurse in gastroenterology (Certified Gastroenterology RN) through examination. The level of education and training, as well as the nomenclature, will vary between countries.

GI technicians, technologists, assistants, associates
Nonnursing assistants play an important role in the ERCP team (Figure 3.1). Their training and education varies widely. In the United States, the SGNA recognizes the role of education and training, as well as the nomenclature through completion of

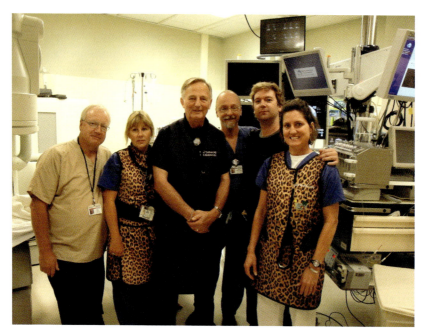

Figure 3.1 The team at Dr Cotton's last ERCP in May 2011.

an education series. Delineation of the role of assistive personnel is available as a guideline from SGNA and is updated regularly. Determination of the scope of practice for assistants must be vetted by the particular organization, as well as the rules and regulations of all the governing bodies.

First assistant

From the endoscopist's perspective, the most important immediate staff member is the person (often called the "table nurse" or "table tech") who sets up the equipment and accessories and manages them throughout the procedure. Educated smooth coordination between this assistant and the endoscopist is essential for success.

In the United States, depending on the setting, this person may be a registered nurse or a GI technician assistant or specialist. This is often their main role in the unit. Larger-volume units may need a cadre of two to four or more such experts, and especially if there is any significant chance of needing to perform procedures out of normal working hours.

Second assistant

A second assistant backing up the table nurse or technician is also critical for circulating in the room, keeping careful observation of the patient including positioning and comfort, arranging accessories and documenting the procedures. These individuals often become very competent at multitasking; indeed, they can provide useful continuity while other team members change. They may also become responsible for maintaining the inventory of accessories.

Anesthesia/sedation/monitoring

Many standard ERCP procedures can be and are done under moderate (conscious) sedation given by another registered nurse under the endoscopist's supervision. However, there is a trend toward the increasing use of anesthesia (modified or full), especially for complex procedures in sick patients (see Chapter 6).

Radiology

Fluoroscopy and filming are usually done by a radiology technologist (radiographer) in collaboration with the endoscopist. Busy units are able to appoint their own, who can become very knowledgeable and helpful. Trying to do complex procedures with a technologist who is rotating through the unit and unfamiliar with ERCP can be very frustrating. Radiation safety is an important consideration. More details are given in Chapter 12.

Team outside the procedure room

Lead ERCP endoscopist

High-volume units with several ERCP endoscopists should appoint a lead endoscopist who can work with the nurse manager to ensure that procedures and training go smoothly. This individual also has the task of effective liaison with equivalent leaders in other involved disciplines, especially Anesthesia and Radiology.

Clinical support in the unit

Preparation and recovery of ERCP patients is little different from those undergoing other procedures, and are handled by the same staff. Careful monitoring after ERCP is important because of the risk of serious adverse events, especially pancreatitis and perforation.

Technical support in the unit

Those responsible for reprocessing endoscopes are key members of the team. Reprocessing lapses are responsible for serious outbreaks of infection after ERCP. Equally important are those who manage and maintain all of the other equipment, including the increasing amount and complexity of IT.

Outside the unit

The staff who see the patients in the clinic before ERCP, and those who schedule the procedures, have important roles in ensuring that all relevant clinical data (e.g., imaging **discs** and reports) are available, and for helping educate the patients and family members. Finally we should acknowledge the contribution of our industry partners, who provide the equipment we need, and, in some instances, collaborate on developing new devices.

Education

Nurses and technologists chosen to work in ERCP are usually selected from the whole unit staff, and thus have a broad understanding and some extensive experience of the technical and clinical aspects of the practice of endoscopy in general. They may confirm their interest in becoming part of the ERCP team by watching some procedures and absorbing the often complex dynamics in the room. Specific training is required concerning some key facts of ERCP practice

- Pancreatic and biliary anatomy and diseases
- The range of ERCP therapeutic procedures
- The specialized accessories
- Radiation safety
- The specific risks and how to minimize them

Most of this can be learned by reference to the plethora of available text in books, journals, and websites (especially those of the major national and international professional societies), as listed in Section "Further Reading." In medical schools, staff may join didactic sessions in concert with other trainees, such as fellows. Clearly, staff needs time for these educational activities. At the end of the chapter the reader finds the foundation of an **ERCP Education and Training Plan**, which includes steps for all staff who may work in the ERCP arena, followed by steps of bench training for those advancing to key procedure roles, and training suggestions for mentored hands on ERCP intraprocedure training (Figure 3.2). This structure can be adapted to meet the particular needs in each setting.

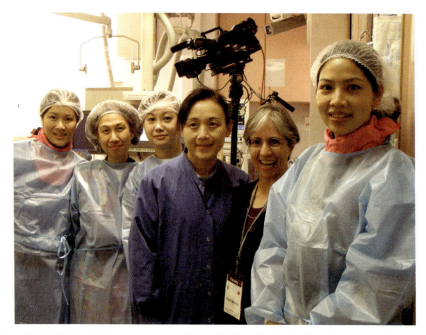

Figure 3.2 With the ERCP nursing team at Prince of Wales Hospital in Hong Kong, December 2010.

Education and training plan

Didactics, for any staff assigned to ERCP room
- Overview: utilization related to common diagnoses and treatments
- Patient details including anesthesia and positioning
- Detailed anatomy and some physiology
  - Drawings of pancreatobiliary system and surrounding anatomy
  - Photographic and fluoroscopic images, still and video
- Overview of general equipment/accessory types
- Procedure room observation with preceptor, not hands on
  - Endoscope, diagnosis, therapy
  - include endoscopic and fluoroscopic images
  - Observational focus on care of patient and room turnover
  - Focus on basic device setup and table management
  - Coordination between endoscopist and table assistant

On the Bench, Table Top, Dry Run—for staff who will take on a technical role
- Teach on the basics of endoscopy; build on solid foundation
- Build equipment platforms in a step-by-step fashion
  - Diagnostic basics: cannulas, guidewires, sphinctertomes
- Add variation(s) and specifics
- Include advancing platforms, e.g., dilation, stone extraction
- Talk through procedure use based on prior endoscopy experience
  - ERCP didactic and in room observation
- Dry run "hands on" encourage question and answer format
- Present industry information, manuals, and instructions for use
  - Obtain samples or training devices
- Component fit, sizing, progression, and transfer of devices
  - Utilize color guides, package indicators
- Demonstrate position of side-view scope and landmarks
  - Use models when appropriate and available

*Hands On in Procedure—*for table staff following solid mastery of bench training. *Must* be accompanied by key mentor/preceptor
- Set goals for precepted procedure numbers
- Enlist the assistance of the ERCP endoscopist in advance
- Seek therapeutic procedures related to patient diagnosis
- "Huddle" prior to case schedule to discuss upcoming procedures
- Mentor and trainee work closely together with dialogue
  - Handle specialty and infrequently used instruments
- Utilize industry partners for training when necessary
- Design tools to determine competency following training

Engaged physicians, nurses, and technologists who are regular members of the ERCP team are expected to support trainees and share their expertise by providing thoughtful information and instruction. All questions from learners and observers should be respectfully entertained within inevitable time constraints.

How to manage specialized accessories should be taught with an experienced mentor, initially "on the bench," and then with sequential responsibility during actual procedures. Training advances safely in a step-by-step fashion in an atmosphere of being "walked and talked" through techniques alongside a mentor as skill develops. The endoscopist(s) also need to be sympathetic and supportive during this phase. Experienced nurses and technicians should have the opportunity to attend regional and national meetings.

Industry partners

Endoscope and accessory manufacturers and suppliers are (not surprisingly) anxious to participate in the education of the staff, and can be very helpful by supplying teaching materials and organizing demonstrations. However, there are some potential pitfalls if the relationship is not managed effectively. There may be undue influence on purchasing decisions regardless of cost or actual clinical need, and there can be problems with patient confidentiality. These problems can be overcome by having strict rules concerning these interactions. In particular, product representatives should be admitted to the unit only by appointment with a specific agreed agenda.

Motivation; team building

General principles apply here as anywhere: respect for each team member's skills and contributions and sensitivity to their agendas. This applies particularly to members with different reporting streams, for example, Anesthesia and Radiology. Scheduling clashes are a potent cause of friction and unhappiness.

Endoscopists should realize that compliments on a job well done are always appreciated, but criticism is best given in private after the event. Those who (sadly) still posture and denigrate during procedures poison the atmosphere and lay the groundwork for further errors.

A list of procedures is likely to go better if the key people understand what is planned ahead of time. Thus, many successful teams have a "huddle" each morning to describe the cases and likely needs. In addition, there should always be a "time-out" before each procedure. Whilst this was introduced for safety reasons (wrong patient, radiation protection, etc.), it can be expanded to explain the specifics of the case, so that each member is on message.

Staff will appreciate some feedback about previous cases, whether good or bad. Whenever possible, key staff members should be included in other aspects of the ERCP service. Thus, they may be invited to attend case conferences and meetings about ERCP-related research.

Pitfalls

In addition to the risks already mentioned, to succeed day by day it is important to maintain focus on the primary reason for all of these activities—the individual patient. In the rush and excitement of high-tech procedures it is easy to lose track of their specific needs and privacy. Constant vigilance must be maintained to recognize and prevent the development of a casual atmosphere of "we have done this before." A team culture to quickly address such a tendency is significant, in particular for preceptor/mentor nurses and technicians and key physician ERCP partners. ERCP teams must continue to recognize that they constitute only one section of the whole unit orchestra—that their expertise as individual players in the orchestra does not then lead to the perils of excessive ownership or the "arrogance" of a niche specialty, drowning out the melodies the orchestra is geared to create. The closed door needed for radiology should not promote a closed door mentality for the staff.

Resources

Endoscopy units should have a library, including details of local policies and procedures and educational resources, both printed and online. Units lucky enough to have a formal nurse educator will be able to manage these and add key journal articles, support the development of further training opportunities, and monitor progress over time.

Wrap-up

Although teams involve any number of people, they appear only in relation to the commitment of each person. The greatest teams are both highly individualistic and solidly united. ERCP teams and teamwork involve ownership by all those involved, inside and outside the room. And the proof is in the pudding! The team advances safely, knowledgeably, efficiently, and compassionately, combining high technology and the human touch for all with whom we come in contact. It is my hope that this chapter contributes to current and future high-functioning teams, who are valued and recognized for their contribution every day in support of the patients we serve.

Further Reading

Books
Advanced Digestive Endoscopy: Practice and Safety. Ed, Cotton PB. Blackwell, Malden, MA, 2006.
Gastroenterology Nursing: A Core Curriculum, 5th Edition, Society of Gastroenterology Nurses and Associates, Chicago, IL, 2013.

Manual of Gastrointestinal Procedures, 6th Edition, Society of Gastroenterology Nurses and Associates, Chicago, IL, 2009.

Practical Gastrointestinal Endoscopy: The Fundamentals, 7th Edition. Haycock A, Cohen J, Saunders B, Cotton PB, Williams CB. Wiley Blackwell, Malden, MA, 2014.

The Johns Hopkins Manual for GI Endoscopic Nurses, 3rd Edition. Eds, Khashab M, Robinson T, Kalloo A. Slack Incorporated, Thorofare, NJ, 2013.

Journals (many of which include society guidelines and technology assessments)

Endoscopy

Gastrointestinal Endoscopy

Gastroenterology Nursing Journal

Professional Societies

American College of Gastroenterology (ACG). www.gi.org (accessed on August 6, 2014).

American Society for Gastrointestinal Endoscopy (ASGE), United States. www.asge.org (accessed on August 6, 2014).

Canadian Society of Gastroenterology Nurses and Associates (CSGNA). www.csgna.com (accessed on August 6, 2014).

European Society of Gastroenterology and Endoscopy Nurses and Associates. www.esgena.org (accessed on August 6, 2014).

Society for Gastrointestinal Nurses and Associates (SGNA), United States. www.sgna.org (accessed on August 6, 2014).

Society of Gastrointestinal Nurses and Endoscopic Associates, International. www.signea.org (accessed on August 6, 2014).

CHAPTER 4

Patient education and consent

Peter B. Cotton

Digestive Disease Center, Medical University of South Caroline, Charleston, USA

KEY POINTS

- Patient education is primarily the responsibility of the endoscopist offering ERCP.
- Staff can assist, and brochures and certain websites may be useful.
- The interaction should be in a relaxed clinical environment, with time for questions and reflection.
- Information must include expected benefits, potential risks, known limitations, and any alternatives.
- The consent process must be clearly documented.

ERCP can be very beneficial, but can also result in serious injury. No one can dispute the need to make sure that patients (and those upon whom they rely for support) understand precisely what is being proposed and why, so that they make an informed decision whether or not to proceed. Consent is an education process, not a piece of paper to be signed at the last minute. It can be achieved only in the context of an effective provider–patient relationship.

Except in urgent cases, this process should start well before the planned procedure, and not on the same day. In fact, the widespread use of anticoagulant and antiplatelet agents may make it necessary to make informed decisions a week or two ahead of time. These are not trivial issues. Balancing the risk of bleeding against the risk of stroke needs thoughtful consideration and often specialist consultation.

The education process should involve a face-to-face sit down fully clothed consultation with the endoscopist concerned, and include a family member if possible. The endoscopist should explain the reason why he or she is proposing the procedure, based upon full disclosure of all of the key elements, that is, the potential benefits (what it should achieve), the known limitations (why it may not work), the major risks, and any relevant alternatives. Note that one of the

---

ERCP: The Fundamentals, Second Edition. Edited by Peter B. Cotton and Joseph Leung.
© 2015 John Wiley & Sons, Ltd. Published 2015 by John Wiley & Sons, Ltd.
Companion Website: www.wiley.com\go\cotton\ercp

alternatives in complex patients is to offer referral to a tertiary center. The consent process must include adequate time for questions.

Additional useful information can be provided beforehand (and afterward) by nurses and other staff, and with explanatory brochures. Many are available from professional and other bodies, but I recommend developing one that is tailored to the local environment and practice. Figures 4.1 and 4.2 show the materials that we use. Feel free to copy and adapt it. The consent form to be signed eventually includes the statement "I have read the explanation material and have had the opportunity to ask questions."

ERCP stands for Endoscopic Retrograde CholangioPancreatography

ERCP is a way for a specialist doctor to get access to the bile duct and pancreatic duct, to confirm diagnoses and to provide treatments. It uses a flexible endoscope which is a long narrow tube with a camera at the end. The doctor passes the endoscope through your mouth (under sedation/anesthesia) to get to the papilla of Vater, a small nipple in your upper intestine (duodenum). This papilla is the drainage hole for your bile duct and the pancreatic duct, which bring digestive juices from your liver, gallbladder and pancreas. X-rays are taken to show whether there are any lesions such as stones or blockages. If so, the doctor may be able to treat them right away with instruments passed through the endoscope. The most common treatments are:

Sphincterotomy. This involves making a small cut in the papilla of Vater to enlarge the opening to the bile duct and/or pancreatic duct. This is done to improve the drainage or to remove stones from the ducts. Removed stones are usually dropped in the intestine, and pass through quickly.

Stenting. A stent is a small plastic tube, which is left in a blocked or narrowed duct to improve drainage. The narrowing may need to be stretched (dilated) before the stent is placed. Some stents are designed to pass out into the intestine after a few
weeks when they have done their work. Other stents have to be removed or changed after 3–4 months. There are also permanent stents made out of metal.

Other treatments are used occasionally. Your doctor will explain these if necessary.

Limitations and risks? There are some drawbacks to ERCP. Discuss these with your doctor.
• The test and treatments are not perfect. Occasionally, important lesions may not be seen, and treatment attempts may be unsuccessful.
• Working on the pancreas and bile duct can cause complications, even in the best hands. Your doctor will explain these and answer your questions.

The most common complication is
• Pancreatitis (swelling and inflammation of the pancreas). This occurs in about one patient in twenty, and results in the need to stay in hospital for pain medications and IV fluids. This usually lasts for a few days, but can be much more serious.

Other rare complications (less than 1 per 100) include, but are not limited to:
• Heart and lung problems.
• Bleeding (after sphincterotomy).
• Infection in the bile duct (cholangitis).
• Perforation (a tear in the intestine).
Severe complications (about 1 case in 500) may require prolonged stays in hospital and major surgery. Fatal complications are very rare.
In addition
• The sedation medicines may make you feel sick.
• A tender lump may form where the IV was placed. Call your doctor if redness, pain or swelling appears to be spreading.
• You will receive a low dose of radiation from the x-rays.

Alternatives? There may be some different approaches to your problem. Discuss them with your doctor. Note that most diagnoses can now be made with scans, such as CT and MRCP, or a test called Endoscopic Ultrasound (EUS). ERCP is usually done only when they have shown something that is best treated by ERCP. Possible alternative treatments include surgical operations, or, in some cases, interventional radiology.

Address any questions to the Pancreato-biliary office at........

Figure 4.1 The ERCP explanation sheet used at MUSC.

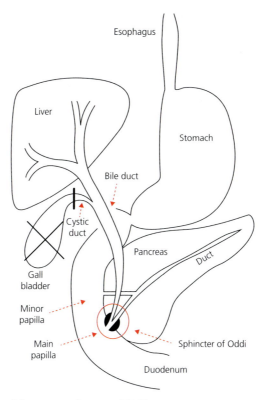

Figure 4.2 Diagram of the organs relevant to ERCP.

The Internet is rife with material, not all of it accurate or helpful, but there is at least one intriguing interactive site that provides a record of the patient's time and educational journey on the site (www.emmisolutions.com).

It is smarter to underplay the potential benefits, and overstate the risks, rather than the reverse. Those who say "Just sign here. We do this every day, don't worry about it" are asking for trouble.

Emergency situations do arise, when patients are more aware of their predicament, but they still need relevant information before making a decision.

Documenting the process is important

Modern electronic report writers make it possible to generate several sentences about obtaining consent at a single keystroke. Plaintiffs and their lawyers are often skeptical about the accuracy of that information when there is a dispute about what was said in a lawsuit. Thus, it is wise to hand-write or personally dictate what you do, and preferably have it witnessed by a staff member.

Doing the consent process properly is good medical practice, but it is also very helpful when (not if) there are bad outcomes. It is then possible and helpful to be able to say "the x-ray confirms a perforation; you remember that we talked about that rare possibility yesterday, don't you?" [1]

Conclusion

The task of preparing patients emotionally and intellectually for therapeutic interventions is a serious and enjoyable obligation. It is part of the privilege of being a doctor, not just a technician. Do it well.

Reference

1 Frakes JT, Cotton PB. Medico-legal aspects of ERCP. 2013. In T. Baron, R. Kozarek, D carr-Locke (Eds), *ERCP* (2nd edition). Philadelphia, Elsevier.

CHAPTER 5

Risk assessment and reduction

Joseph Romagnuolo

Medical University of South Carolina, Charleston, USA

Departments of Medicine, Public Health Sciences, Charleston, USA

> **KEY POINTS**
>
> - The most common adverse events (AEs) after endoscopic retrograde cholangiopancreatography (ERCP) are pancreatitis, cardiopulmonary events, bleeding, infection, and perforation, and rarely these events can cause disability or be fatal.
>
> - The actual risks in an individual case depend upon the context of the procedure, the characteristics of the patient, the skills of the procedure team, and the appropriate use of prophylactic interventions.
>
> - Understanding these interacting issues and managing them are key to making wise clinical decisions and improving patient education and informed consent.

One of the most important concerns about ERCP is its high risk in comparison to other endoscopic procedures. With post-ERCP pancreatitis rates, in good hands, ranging from 2 to 5% for low-risk procedures and 10 to 20% for high-risk procedures (even after risk-reducing maneuvers), and a mortality of about 1 in 1000 (mainly due to severe pancreatitis), this seems to be an appropriate concern; bleeding (about 1%), perforation (<0.5%), infection (1–2%), and cardiorespiratory AEs can also occur [1]. The risk involved in an individual ERCP case can vary widely. Thus, a biliary stent change in a healthy middle-aged man can be orders of magnitude different than manometry, dual sphincterotomy with pancreatic stenting in a young women with prior post-ERCP pancreatitis; not all ERCPs are the same and not all ERCPists have had the same case spectrum in their training and practice. This AE profile makes it important to ensure training is appropriate for both the endoscopist and the team/unit, to ensure indications are sound, non-invasive alternatives are appropriately considered, and patients are appropriately consented with respect to the risks, benefits, and alternatives.

A critical step toward reducing risks is to understand their predictors [2, 3]. Some factors may be modifiable and their identification allows time for that modification to occur. For the ones that are not modifiable, identifying the risks

---

ERCP: The Fundamentals, Second Edition. Edited by Peter B. Cotton and Joseph Leung.

© 2015 John Wiley & Sons, Ltd. Published 2015 by John Wiley & Sons, Ltd.

Companion Website: www.wiley.com\go\cotton\ercp

may lead to a change in plan (perhaps to an alternative to ERCP) or hypervigilance during and after the procedure.

This chapter will focus on the identification of patient and procedural and periprocedural factors that increase risk, and will not focus on definition of risks, documentation of risk or events, or the ideal ERCP technique that might lower risk, as those are discussed in more detail in other chapters. Some procedural factors are mentioned briefly however, to give perspective on their importance with respect to nonprocedure factors. Table 5.1 summarizes predictors of AEs after ERCP.

Table 5.1 Predictors of adverse events after ERCP(Adapted from Romagnuolo *et al*, 2011. [2 and 3]).

Adverse event	Modifying factor	Risk magnitude (OR)	Reference(s)	Comment(s)
Infection	Liver transplant	5.2	[4]	Very rare (0.25–0.5%) (risk decreasing with time: OR 0.9/year)
	Fistulas, nondrainable ducts (e.g., hilar, intrahepatic strictures) Ductoscopy		[5, 6]	
	Jaundice	1.4	[7]	
	Small center	1.4	[7]	
Bleeding (delayed)	Sphincterotomy	4.7	[8]	Very rare; can also occur with large-balloon sphincteroplasty No increased risk with antiplatelets, especially aspirin monotherapy [9, 10]
	Small center	1.1	[7]	
	Intraprocedural bleeding*	1.7	[11]	
	Coagulopathy*	3.3	[11]	Defined as >2 s prothrombin time, hemodialysis, or platelet count <80,000/mm³
	Anticoagulation within 3 days*	5.1	[11]	
	Cholangitis*	2.6	[11]	
	Small-volume endoscopist*	2.2 (1 or fewer per week)	[11]	

(Continued)

Adverse event	Modifying factor	Risk magnitude (OR)	Reference(s)	Comment(s)
Perforation	Postsurgical anatomy	2.5	[7, 8]	
	Precut sphincterotomy	2.0	[7]	
	Intramural contrast	1.9	[7]	
	Sphincterotomy			Rare
Pancreatitis[†]	Suspected SOD	1.9–9.7	[12, 13, 8, 14]	Biliary sphincterotomy is not a risk factor [7, 13, 15]
	Female	1.8–3.5	[12, 15, 16, 14]	
	Post-ERCP pancreatitis (prior)	5.4	[12]	
	Younger age	1.1 per 5-year decrease [8]; 1.1 (age < 70) [5]; 1.6 (age < 60) [7]	[7, 13, 15]	
	Normal bile duct	1.05	[7]	
	Normal bilirubin	1.9	[12]	
	No chronic pancreatitis	1.9	[12]	
	Nonuniversity center	2.4	[7]	
	Difficult cannulation	1.8–9.4	[12, 15, 16, 14]	Early precut sphincterotomy may reduce risk versus persistence [17, 18]
	Pancreatic sphincterotomy	1.5–3.8	Standard [12, 8, 19], minor papilla [13, 8]	
	Pancreatic injection	1.04–1.5	[7, 12, 13, 19–21]	Most studies define as any injection; in [13], defined as ≥2; extent of filling important [21]
	Lack of pancreatic stenting	1.4–3.2	[8, 22–24]	Significant in high-risk ERCP, especially SOD
	Trainee involvement	1.5	[13]	
	Balloon sphincteroplasty	2.0	[25]	For stone disease, heterogeneous studies
Cannulation failure (with/ without precut)	Grade 3 difficulty	1.4	[26]	
	ASA grade III–V	1.9		
	Trainee (1–50% involvement)	2.0		

(Continued)

Table 5.1 (*Continued*)

Adverse event	Modifying factor	Risk magnitude (OR)	Reference(s)	Comment(s)
	Indications:			
	Jaundice	2.2		
	Postsurgical disease	1.9		
	Pancreatitis	Acute (2.2), chronic (1.6)		
	Lower-volume endoscopist	2.79 for <90/year versus >239/year		
	Inefficient X-ray (>3 min/ low-difficulty case)	1.72		
	Moderate sedation	1.49 versus deeper		
Cardiopulmonary events[‡]	Age	1.02 (per year)	[27]	Events are very rare, 1.1–1.2% [27–29]
	ASA	1.8, 3.2, 7.5 (ASA III, IV, V)	[27, 28]	
	APACHE II	12 (for score >15), in EGD	[26, 30]	Potentially confounded by recent MI in high APACHE group
	Type of anesthesia	0.3 (MAC versus GAP in ASA I–II); no difference if ASA ≥ III	[28, 31–34]	A Cochrane review concluded there was no difference between propofol and nonpropofol sedation regarding adverse events, but not stratified by GAP versus MAC [32]
		0.5 (Propofol versus moderate sedation)		
	Inpatient	1.5	[27]	
	Setting (VA, nonuniversity)	1.2, 1.4	[27]	
	Supplemental oxygen	1.2	[27]	
	Trainee involvement	1.3	[27]	Risk factors within trainees also studied [35]
	Pulmonary disease	Sleep apnea, severe COPD or requiring home oxygen	[36, 37]	Undiagnosed sleep apnea does not appear to predict transient hypoxia during moderate sedation [37]

(*Continued*)

Adverse event	Modifying factor	Risk magnitude (OR)	Reference(s)	Comment(s)
	Cardiac disease	5.2 for recent MI (within 30 days)	[26, 30, 36, 38, 39]	Potential confounding by higher APACHE II in MI patients; [26, 30] others found EGD risk only increased within a few days of MI [38]
		Prior MI Prior or current/ recent CHF Rhythm other than sinus Severe valvular disease	[35, 40–42]	
	Obesity	~1.5 for hypoxemia	[43]	Body mass index may predict hypoxemia, but not necessarily AEs
	Other comorbidities	Diabetes, renal failure, uncontrolled hypertension, prior stroke or other neuro impairment, inability to do a 4–6 METS activity (walk up a flight of stairs)	[35, 42]	

APACHE, acute physiology score and chronic health evaluation; ASA, American Society of Anesthesiologists physiological classification; CHF, congestive heart failure; COPD, chronic obstructive pulmonary disease; EGD, esophagogastroduodenoscopy; GAP, gastroenterologist-administered propofol; MAC, monitored anesthesia care (generally with propofol); METS, metabolic equivalents; MI, myocardial infarction; SOD, sphincter of Oddi dysfunction; VA, veteran's affairs.
*These risk factors were determined only within the sphincterotomy subgroup, and do not necessarily predict bleeding in all ERCPs.
†As is evident in this section, some factors have more consensus than others on their role as a risk factor for post-ERCP pancreatitis; factors only found significant in one of many studies may or may not be true risk factors.
‡Mostly based on non-ERCP, or even nonendoscopy, patients.

Assessing and reducing the risks

As mentioned, there are five main risks attributed to an ERCP—pancreatitis, bleeding, infection, perforation, and cardiopulmonary events. The thresholds for calling these events an "incident" versus a true "adverse event" are detailed elsewhere [44]. In addition, two other nonclassical risks have recently been given more attention: the risk of technical failure and exposure to radiation. ERCP in pregnancy has its own set of risks.

Pancreatitis and postprocedural pain

There are many studies looking at predictors of post-ERCP pancreatitis, but still some controversies. Normal caliber bile duct [7], bilirubin level [12], prior post-ERCP pancreatitis [12], nonuniversity center [7], and trainee involvement [13] were found to be predictors in some studies, but not in others. Inconsistencies may be due to lack of control for confounding factors like suspected sphincter of Oddi dysfunction (SOD) and pancreatic therapy in some studies: suspected SOD and pancreatic therapy patients likely have independently higher risk, and tend to have a normal bilirubin and normal caliber bile ducts.

Several other factors are agreed upon. The list of independent predictors for post-ERCP pancreatitis includes female sex (OR 1.8–3.5) [12, 15, 16], suspected SOD (OR 1.9–9.7) [8, 12–14], younger age [7, 13, 15], pancreatic injection (OR 1.04–1.5) [7, 12, 13, 19–21] (especially filling to the tail) [21], and pancreatic sphincterotomy (OR 1.5–3.8).[12, 13, 8, 19]. In addition, simply having difficulty with cannulation (OR 1.8–9.4) increases the risk [12, 14–16] and implies that one's skill set in cannulation and the patient factors that might make cannulation difficult are important cofactors. Advanced chronic pancreatitis [12] probably reduces risk, given the lower gland reserve; minimal-change pancreatitis probably does not, so these patients should not be reassured that their risk is lower. Pancreatic stenting and rectal nonsteroidal anti-inflammatories (NSAID) in high-risk cases have been shown in randomized trials to be beneficial in reducing risk, and lack of pancreatic stenting in high-risk cases (OR 1.4–3.2), [8, 22–24] and lack of rectal NSAID prophylaxis [45] are associated with increased risk.

It is notable that biliary sphincterotomy does not appear to independently increase the risk of pancreatitis. It also appears that precut/needle-knife sphincterotomy likely does not add risk beyond that of the difficulty of cannulation itself; in fact, early precut may even reduce risk, as compared to conventional persistence, according to a meta-analyses of randomized trials [17, 18]. Balloon sphincteroplasty may increase risk (OR 2.0), [25] but is not a consistent finding; as such, it is generally reserved for patients on anticoagulation that cannot come off them, but need sphincter ablation, and for giant stone cases. When this was done, a longer balloon dilation time, which presumably more effectively destroys the sphincter muscle (rather than irritating it which may lead to spasm and pancreatitis), was recently shown in a meta-analysis to be helpful [46].

Many patients have some pain after ERCP, but without diagnostic criteria for pancreatitis. It may be caused a combination of bloating from air insufflation, activation of visceral hypersensitivity, subclinical pancreatitis, and other factors. Recently, the use of carbon dioxide (instead of room air) at ERCP has been shown to decrease postprocedural pain in a meta-analysis [47]. Brain stimulation may also decrease post-ERCP pain [48].

Since pancreatitis is the highest morbidity and mortality event for ERCP, the factors that predict its occurrence need to be accounted for in determining whether the strength of the indications and chance of benefit matches the risk; in our institution, it also helps choose who stays overnight for observation and IV fluids. A "simple" diagnostic ERCP in a high-risk patient (young women with normal ducts) is still a high-risk ERCP; avoiding the biliary sphincterotomy does not avoid the risk. Skilled cannulation, selective pancreatic stenting and rectal NSAID, and avoiding balloon dilation of the orifice if possible will together decrease the risk of pancreatitis (but not eliminate it). Using carbon dioxide might decrease post-ERCP pain.

Bleeding

Bleeding is generally only a concern for therapeutic ERCP procedures, mainly those involving sphincterotomy. Intraprocedural bleeding that is managed without altering the ability to complete the procedure is not considered an AE [44]. Not surprisingly, sphincterotomy (OR 4.7) [8] has been found to be an independent predictor of bleeding after ERCP. Performance of the procedure in a small center (OR 1.1) [7] has also been found to predict bleeding after ERCP. The reasons for this latter association are unclear; perhaps there is confounding by ERCP volume by the endoscopist at those centers, or lack of unit expertise in controlling intraprocedural bleeding or choosing appropriate electrosurgical settings and equipment.

Predictors within the sphincterotomy subgroup of ERCP cases are probably more relevant for case selection. In this group [11], coagulopathy (OR 3.3), resumption of anticoagulants within 3 days (OR 5.1), cholangitis (OR 2.6) (perhaps because of hypervascularity and congestion of tissue, or confounded by the difficulty of removing impacted stones), low case volume (OR 2.2), and bleeding during the procedure (OR 1.7) predict a significant bleeding event. It is not clear if appropriate treatment of intraprocedural bleeding can decrease delayed bleeding, or if more vigilance of these patients overnight is helpful.

Antiplatelet agents do not appear to substantially increase the risk of postsphincterotomy bleeding [9, 11], but the power of analyses involving nonaspirin antiplatelets (e.g., thienopyridines like clopidogrel) and ERCP is admittedly more limited. A case control study in ERCP specifically did not show an increased risk with either aspirin or nonaspirin antiplatelet drugs [9]. Extrapolating from colonoscopic polypectomy literature, it appears that dual antiplatelet therapy may account for the apparent or anecdotal higher risk of clopidogrel, and that monotherapy with either clopidogrel or aspirin may not increase risk [49]. The American College of Chest Physicians (ACCP) guidelines suggest continuing aspirin in moderate- to high-thrombosis-risk patients for noncardiac surgery [50].

Risk reduction tips here include withholding anticoagulation when safe (usually 5 days allows a therapeutic international normalized ratio (INR) to normalize), when sphincterotomy is anticipated, and waiting a few days before starting/restarting anticoagulation (mechanical valves and recent embolism may need more prompt restarting of anticoagulation). However, weighing risks of bleeding and risks of thrombosis is important and summarized in an algorithm in the American Society for Gastrointestinal Endoscopy (ASGE) 2009 guidelines [10]. In addition, the validated $CHADS_2$ (*C*ongestive heart failure, *H*ypertension, *A*ge ≥ 75 years, *D*iabetes, history of *S*troke or transient ischemic attack (2 points)) score, and its modified versions, is endorsed by the ACCP to quantitate stroke risk in atrial fibrillation, and is easy to use [51, 52]; a $CHADS_2$ score of <3 is considered to have $<5\%$ annual stroke risk [50, 53]. Considering balloon sphincteroplasty or temporary stenting in patients who cannot come off anticoagulation is reasonable.

Of note, cholestasis or jaundice, malnutrition, antibiotic therapy, and pancreatic insufficiency are all risk factors for (occult) vitamin K deficiency. Therefore, while a preprocedure INR for all-patients for ERCP is not suggested, selective preprocedural INR in these high-risk groups (ideally 1 day before, to allow time for vitamin K to be given and work), is important. Patients with concomitant liver disease should also get a platelet count and an INR, although the INR may not be predictive of their bleeding risk [54, 55]. In addition, however, patients with liver disease, due to increase portal pressures and duodenal venous congestion, may be at mildly higher risk for bleeding after sphincterotomy, independent of the INR.

Aspirin monotherapy does not need to be stopped, but dual therapy should likely be adjusted to monotherapy, when safe, extrapolating from the polypectomy literature. ASGE guidelines suggest discontinuing nonaspiring antiplatelet drugs in low-thrombotic-risk patients [10]. Thrombosis of a coronary stent after stopping antiplatelet drugs is recognized to occur after noncardiac surgery [9, 11, 48, 49], especially in patients with high-risk coronary anatomy, that is, within 6 weeks of placing a bare metal stent, and within 1 year with drug-eluting stents [48]. The type of stent and the time since insertion need to be included in risk assessment.

Guidelines regarding how long to hold antiplatelets are usually based on the fact that irreversible antiplatelet drugs generally require 7–10 days of cessation to allow full marrow replenishment with new normal platelets [10, 56]. However, even after 5 days, most platelet function has returned and this delay is generally considered good enough to allow even major surgery, based on bleeding outcomes being comparable after bypass surgery for aspirin–clopidogrel dual therapy (stopped 5 days prior) versus aspirin monotherapy (versus 1.5 times higher if clopidogrel is taken within 5 days of surgery) [57]. Since cardiac mortality can increase with as little as 7 days of antiplatelet cessation in the context of gastrointestinal (GI) bleeding [58], in my opinion, 5–7 days may be a better balance of risks and benefits. The ideal time to resume antiplatelet dual therapy after sphincterotomy is not known [10].

Maintaining an adequate endoscopist and team volume of cases and making sure the endoscopist and team are comfortable with what to do with intraprocedural bleeding are both important. Lastly, one must keep in mind that certain rescue techniques (precut) will not be available in patients left on anticoagulation or dual antiplatelet therapy; some patients not anticipated to "need" a sphincterotomy may end up having a difficult cannulation, and so withholding anticoagulation, when safe, may still be a consideration even in those patients.

Infection

Infection is rare after ERCP. It is reported to be more likely in liver transplant patients (OR 5.2) [4], hilar/intrahepatic strictures (e.g., Klatskin-type tumors or primary sclerosing cholangitis (PSC)) [5, 6], and in small-volume centers (OR 1.4) [7]. It also appears higher in (obstructive) jaundice (OR 1.4) [7], although it is still questionable whether this risk applies if the obstruction is relieved by the procedure. Increasing intraductal pressure should be avoided by aspirating bile and limiting the volume of injection. This is particularly a concern for patients who have already had colonization of their bile via prior manipulation of their ducts (stents/sphincterotomy).

Although contract agents are delivered sterile, they are injected through a catheter that touches the scope tip that has been through the patient's mouth. Therefore, even in patients without prior duct contamination or colonization, procedures that involve contrast entering nondrainable sterile body cavities (e.g., the peritoneum) have a higher risk of infection; this includes leaks or "fistulas" (both biliary and pancreatic).

Based on what has been discussed earlier, prophylactic antibiotics should be given to patients anticipated to have nondrainable (or difficult to drain) obstructed duct segments (PSC, hilar tumors, selected chronic pancreatitis stricture patients), pseudocyst and bile leak cases, and liver transplant patients. Unanticipated cases with infection risk (e.g., failed stone extraction) should get antibiotics as quickly as possible, preferably during the procedure. Antibiotics are not generally recommended before ERCP in all jaundiced patients, although some endoscopists still choose to do this.

Perforation

Perforation is rare. It comes in two forms—scope-induced luminal (big hole) or accessory-induced (small hole). In multivariate analyses, luminal perforation has been associated with surgically altered anatomy (OR 2.5), likely due to the long length of scope needed, tortuous anatomy, and adhesions [7, 8]. Sphincterotomy accounts for most accessory-type perforations, and precut (OR 2.0) has higher risk than conventional sphincterotomy [7]; if recognized during the procedure, a temporary stent may help. Intramural contrast injection (OR 1.9) was found to increase risk, although this may just be a marker of a difficult cannulation and considerable accessory manipulation of the duct and ampulla [7]. Rare ductal perforations have been associated with biopsies, ablations, or scopes within the ducts. Submucosal or transmural tracking of guide wires is technically a small perforation, but is generally well-tolerated (usually not reaching the "adverse event" definition threshold), with or without a stent or antibiotics.

Avoiding excessive manipulation, care in sphincterotomy technique (especially for precut), and appropriate consent of patients with altered anatomy undergoing ERCP (and knowing when to bail out in these cases when not progressing) are ways to integrate this information into practice, to reduce this risk.

Cardiopulmonary events

The role of risk factors and risk modification of cardiopulmonary events has been detailed elsewhere [2]. Briefly, much of the literature on preoperative evaluation has been done for surgical settings, not for endoscopy specifically. For many reasons, some of these do not apply very well to endoscopy.

Case context and comorbidity quantification

Age, [27] ASA score (American Society of Anesthesiologists physiological classification), [27, 28], type of anesthesia [28, 31–34], inpatient status [27], nonuniversity hospital [27], and trainee involvement [27, 35] are among the risk factors identified in the endoscopy literature (mostly colonoscopy), with ASA score being the most powerful predictor [27, 28, 42]. In addition, a number of scoring systems were developed to help adjust for confounding related to comorbidities, mainly in surgery [2]. Although the comorbidity scoring systems are not practical for daily use, the elements they identify give a perspective on the important factors.

APACHE II (Acute Physiology And Chronic Health Evaluation) scores, cardiopulmonary disease, and, recent myocardial infarction (MI) specifically, may also predict AEs [26, 30, 36–39]; APACHE II is a complex instrument, with dimensions that include a physiology score (12 inputs), an age score and organ failure points, with a number of elements (e.g. PaO_2 and arterial pH) that are not available for most endoscopies.

Sleep apnea and body mass index (BMI) may be important. However, for moderate sedation in left lateral position, unrecognized sleep apnea [59] did not appear to predict transient hypoxia or AEs in one routine endoscopy study [37]; another study found that BMI in ASA I–II patients predicted the number of hypoxemic episodes [43]. Increased BMI and obstructive sleep apnea can predict perioperative morbidity after surgery [60] and may increase risk and make airway maintenance more difficult in deep sedation [42], especially for the semiprone positioning that is standard for ERCP. Intubating a patient during ERCP, because of these upper airway issues, who is semiprone on an X-ray table is more cumbersome, generally requiring "flipping" the patient on to a stretcher in a supine position for intubation, and then rolling them back on to the X-ray table once intubated to complete the procedure. Despite this theoretical concern, deep sedation, without intubation, in ERCP has been shown to be safe in a meta-analysis of randomized trials [61].

A variety of other scoring systems exist. The Charlson comorbidity index [18] is simply a weighted list of 19 comorbidities created to predict life expectancy over months or years. It is not helpful in predicting events in the short term (e.g., 30 days). The POSSUM [25, 46, 47] (Physiologic and Operative Severity Score for the enUmeration of Mortality and Morbidity) score has both graded physiological and operative elements predicting surgical morbidity and mortality, but it is cumbersome to calculate a score manually (online calculator available), and most of the elements (peritoneal soiling, etc.) do not pertain to endoscopy. NSQIP (National Surgical Quality Improvement Program) is a registry of multiple preoperative risk factors, laboratory data, operative procedure details, ASA, Mallampati score, wound class, and postoperative events. The first section's data entry is quite labor-intensive, with > 30 yes/no questions. However, the 20 factors felt to be most important (in roughly decreasing predictive importance) might be helpful in assessing anesthesia risk in ERCP: functional status (i.e., dependence (partial/total), dyspnea (resting/exertional), altered sensorium, morbid obesity), prior cardiac intervention, current smoking, stroke, hypertension, diabetes, chronic obstructive pulmonary disease (COPD), age, and hypoalbuminemia.

Cardiac risk assessment

There are a few risk assessment tools for cardiac risk in noncardiac surgery, including Goldman's [40] and Detsky's [41]. The former had nine independent predictors of outcome: active heart failure and MI (within 6 months) were most powerful, followed by arrhythmias, age (>70), surgery type, and poor overall/"functional" status (hypoxia, hypercarbia, hypokalemia, low bicarbonate, creatinine > 2.5× normal, liver disease, or bedridden). A modified version, with male gender and propofol use, predicted cardiac AEs after endoscopy [62]. Detsky's score [41] is fairly simple and includes recent (inactive) heart failure, prior infarction, and the Canadian Cardiovascular Society Classification of Angina. Guidelines for perioperative cardiovascular evaluation for noncardiac surgery were updated in 2002 [63] and include many of these features, plus valvular disease, diabetes, stroke, and diastolic pressure > 100 mmHg, with recent infarction or active heart failure considered most important. Poor functional status was more precisely defined in metabolic equivalents [64] (METS) [63].

In the United States, the Joint Commission on Accreditation of Healthcare Organizations (JCAHO) emphasizes recording the continuation of beta-blockers for procedures involving an anesthesia team. However, this recommendation is based on a reduction in perioperative mortality in major abdominal, orthopedic, and vascular surgery, and not in endoscopy [65]. In addition, a larger meta-analysis of variable surgery types did not agree with the reduction in risk [66]. Patients are generally told to take their cardiac medicines with sips of water before ERCP anyway; however, the extrapolation of its importance to endoscopy does not seem evidence-based, yet required in the JCAHO "time-out" checklist and recorded as a NQF (National Quality Forum)-endorsed unit quality measure.

The factors that come up most often in the context of cardiopulmonary risk, and appear most important, include age, prior and recent MI, prior or current/recent heart failure, arrhythmia, diabetes, renal failure, uncontrolled hypertension, prior stroke or other neurological impairment, and the inability to do a 4–6 METS activity (walk up a flight of stairs, do yard work, golf without a cart, or walk >4 mph). Other factors such as sleep apnea, obesity, polypharmacy, severe COPD and use of home oxygen, procedure duration and depth of sedation also likely modify cardiopulmonary risk in endoscopy and deserve further study. These factors should be taken into consideration when considering ERCP, especially with weak indications in high-risk subjects. Although some of these factors are not modifiable, controlling hypertension, waiting 4–6 weeks after MI or heart failure admissions, correcting valve pathology, and improving functional status will likely decrease the cardiopulmonary risk after ERCP, and should all be considered when feasible.

Failure of cannulation

Failure of cannulation is not a traditional "risk" but is an important AE that may lead to downstream rescue procedures, with their attendant risks. In addition, endoscopists, units, or patient groups with higher failure rates generally have higher rates of other AEs because of cannulation difficulties. Recently, we used a subset of the multicenter ERCP quality network, comprising over 10,000 ERCPs performed by over 80 endoscopists, to assess for associations with cannulation failure [65]. Conventional (without precut assistance) success was more likely in outpatients (OR 1.21), but less likely in complex contexts (OR 0.59), sicker patients (ASA grade (II, III/V: OR 0.81, 0.77)), teaching cases (OR 0.53), and certain indications (strictures, active pancreatitis). Overall cannulation success (i.e., some precut-assisted) was more likely with higher-volume endoscopists (>239/year: OR 2.79), more efficient fluoroscopy practices (OR 1.72), and lower with moderate (versus deeper) sedation (OR 0.67) [26].

Radiation exposure and dye allergy

Using an eligible subset of the ERCP quality network database, comprising >9000 procedures performed by over 50 endoscopists, the 90th percentile for providers for fluoroscopy time was found to be 10 min (and 22% of total procedure time); 14 min (mean plus 2 SD) was defined as excessive [66]. Every sequential group of 50 cases entered in the registry was associated with lower fluoroscopy time (by 0.2 min; $p=0.001$) raising the possibility that simply tracking one's own times helps lower them. In addition, multivariate analysis revealed that lower lifetime (<1000) and annual (<100/year) volumes, higher difficulty grade, academics, trainee involvement, deep sedation, non-UK/non-US country, various therapeutics (sphincterotomy, balloon dilation, stent, stone removal), and failed cannulation were all independently associated with longer fluoroscopy times and/or higher chance of having excessive times. The experience of X-ray technicians may also help lower times.

Allergic reactions to contrast used at ERCP are very rare, even in high-risk groups who reported a prior significant reaction [67]. The radiology guidelines most commonly recommend those with a history of reaction or a history of severe atopy (foods, asthma, etc.) receive oral prednisone prophylaxis approximately 6, 12, and 1 h prior (three doses) prior to ERCP, with or without an antihistamine with their last dose. Giving steroids intravenously just prior to ERCP is likely ineffective [68].

These points emphasize the importance of experience, self-awareness of fluoroscopy time, and the goal of achieving lower failure rates in reducing radiation exposure. Dye allergy prophylaxis may be overused, but 12 h of repeated oral steroid is the standard.

Pregnancy

There are multiple harms associated with ERCP in pregnancy, including the anesthesia hemodynamics and drugs, the radiation exposure, and the scope and scope-related AEs themselves; other than in emergencies, the first trimester should be avoided [69]. Consultation with the obstetrics team for fetal monitoring should be sought. Appropriate patient selection, good use of non-invasive tests to avoid normal ERCPs, appropriate patient positioning, lead shielding, and using the absolute minimum fluoroscopy time needed should all reduce risk [69].

Adverse event outcome modifiers and specialized risks

Some factors do not increase the likelihood of a particular AE, but influence the risk of other outcomes like length of stay and mortality via their alteration in the consequences of the event. Advanced age and major comorbidities are examples of factors that may influence the outcome of a perforation even though the rate of perforation in these groups may not, itself, be higher. Obesity is likely another such factor; there is some belief that although a higher BMI does not likely increase the risk of pancreatitis, it may influence the severity, morbidity, and mortality when pancreatitis occurs.

Other related complex procedures like transmural pseudocyst drainage and endoscopic necrosectomy, transmural (endoscopic-ultrasound-guided) duct drainage or rendezvous procedures, ampullectomy, percutaneous chol-angioscopy, laser or electrohydraulic lithotripsy (e.g., duct perforation), intraductal ablation (e.g., photodynamic therapy), and probe-based endomi-croscopy each have unique risks. Data are limited on risk prediction within each group.

Key considerations in preparing patients for ERCP, to reduce the risk

In order to advise patients appropriately regarding the risk–benefit ratio of ERCP, and to perform ERCP as safely as possible, it is essential to understand the patient and procedural factors that contribute to risk, and to minimize their impact. This involves careful assessment of the precise clinical situation, consideration of whether ERCP is indeed the best method for addressing the problem at hand and worth the risk for the respective indication, referral to a specific ERCP endoscopist and support team that have adequate volumes and skills, and implementing appropriate risk-reducing pharmacological and/or procedural interventions.

References

1 Cotton PB, Lehman G, Vennes J, et al. Endoscopic sphincterotomy complications and their management: an attempt at consensus. Gastrointest Endosc. 1991;37(3):383–93.
2 Romagnuolo J, Cotton PB, Eisen G, et al. Identifying and reporting risk factors for adverse events in endoscopy. Part I: cardiopulmonary events. Gastrointest Endosc. 2011;73(3):579–85.
3 Romagnuolo J, Cotton PB, Eisen G, et al. Identifying and reporting risk factors for adverse events in endoscopy. Part II: noncardiopulmonary events. Gastrointest Endosc. 2011;73(3):586–97.
4 Cotton PB, Connor P, Rawls E, Romagnuolo J. Infection after ERCP, and antibiotic prophy-laxis: a sequential quality-improvement approach over 11 years. Gastrointest Endosc. 2008; 67(3):471–5.
5 Bangarulingam SY, Gossard AA, Petersen BT, et al. Complications of endoscopic retrograde cholangiopancreatography in primary sclerosing cholangitis. Am J Gastroenterol. 2009; 104(4):855–60.
6 Ertugrul I, Yuksel I, Parlak E, et al. Risk factors for endoscopic retrograde cholangiopancreatog-raphy-related cholangitis: a prospective study. Turk J Gastroenterol. 2009;20(2):116–21.
7 Loperfido S, Angelini G, Benedetti G, et al. Major early complications from diagnostic and therapeutic ERCP: a prospective multicenter study [see comment]. Gastrointest Endosc. 1998;48(1):1–10.

8 Cotton PB, Garrow DA, Gallagher J, Romagnuolo J. Risk factors for complications after ERCP: a multivariate analysis of 11,497 procedures over 12 years. Gastrointest Endosc. 2009;70(1):80–8.

9 Hussain N, Alsulaiman R, Burtin P, et al. The safety of endoscopic sphincterotomy in patients receiving antiplatelet agents: a case–control study. Aliment Pharmacol Ther. 2007;25(5):579–84.

10 Anderson MA, Ben-Menachem T, Gan SI, et al. Management of antithrombotic agents for endoscopic procedures. Gastrointest Endosc. 2009;70(6):1060–70.

11 Freeman ML, Nelson DB, Sherman S, et al. Complications of endoscopic biliary sphincterotomy. N Engl J Med. 1996;335(13):909–18.

12 Freeman ML, DiSario JA, Nelson DB, et al. Risk factors for post-ERCP pancreatitis: a prospective, multicenter study [see comment]. Gastrointest Endosc. 2001;54(4):425–34.

13 Cheng CL, Sherman S, Watkins JL, et al. Risk factors for post-ERCP pancreatitis: a prospective multicenter study. Am J Gastroenterol. 2006;101(1):139–47.

14 Bailey AA, Bourke MJ, Kaffes AJ, et al. Needle-knife sphincterotomy: factors predicting its use and the relationship with post-ERCP pancreatitis (with video). Gastrointest Endosc. 2010;71(2):266–71.

15 Williams EJ, Taylor S, Fairclough P, et al. Risk factors for complication following ERCP: results of a large-scale, prospective multicenter study. Endoscopy. 2007;39(9):793–801.

16 Wang P, Li ZS, Liu F, et al. Risk factors for ERCP-related complications: a prospective multicenter study. Am J Gastroenterol. 2009;104(1):31–40.

17 Cennamo V, Fuccio L, Zagari RM, et al. Can early precut implementation reduce endoscopic retrograde cholangiopancreatography-related complication risk? Meta-analysis of randomized controlled trials. Endoscopy. 2010;42(5):381–8.

18 Gong B, Hao L, Bie L, et al. Does precut technique improve selective bile duct cannulation or increase post-ERCP pancreatitis rate? A meta-analysis of randomized controlled trials. Surg Endosc. 2010;Nov;24(11):2670–80.

19 Romagnuolo J, Hilsden R, Sandha GS, et al. Allopurinol to prevent pancreatitis after endoscopic retrograde cholangiopancreatography (ERCP): a randomized placebo-controlled trial. Clin Gastroenterol Hepatol. 2008;6:465–71.

20 Ho KY, Montes H, Sossenheimer MJ, et al. Features that may predict hospital admission following outpatient therapeutic ERCP. Gastrointest Endosc. 1999;49(5):587–92.

21 Cheon YK, Cho KB, Watkins JL, et al. Frequency and severity of post-ERCP pancreatitis correlated with extent of pancreatic ductal opacification. Gastrointest Endosc. 2007; 65(3):385–93.

22 Andriulli A, Forlano R, Napolitano G, et al. Pancreatic duct stents in the prophylaxis of pancreatic damage after endoscopic retrograde cholangiopancreatography: a systematic analysis of benefits and associated risks. Digestion. 2007;75(2–3):156–63.

23 Fazel A, Quadri A, Catalano MF, et al. Does a pancreatic duct stent prevent post-ERCP pancreatitis? A prospective randomized study. Gastrointest Endosc. 2003;57(3):291–4.

24 Singh P, Das A, Isenberg G, et al. Does prophylactic pancreatic stent placement reduce the risk of post-ERCP acute pancreatitis? A meta-analysis of controlled trials. Gastrointest Endosc. 2004;60(4):544–50.

25 Weinberg BM, Shindy W, Lo S. Endoscopic balloon sphincter dilation (sphincteroplasty) versus sphincterotomy for common bile duct stones. Cochrane Database Syst Rev. 2006(4): CD004890.

26 Cappell MS, Iacovone FM, Jr. Safety and efficacy of esophagogastroduodenoscopy after myocardial infarction. Am J Med. 1999;106(1):29–35.

27 Sharma VK, Nguyen CC, Crowell MD, et al. A national study of cardiopulmonary unplanned events after GI endoscopy. Gastrointest Endosc. 2007;66(1):27–34.

28 Vargo JJ, Holub JL, Faigel DO, *et al*. Risk factors for cardiopulmonary events during propo-fol-mediated upper endoscopy and colonoscopy. Aliment Pharmacol Ther. 2006;24(6): 955–63.

29 Ko CW, Riffle S, Michaels L, *et al*. Serious complications within 30 days of screening and surveillance colonoscopy are uncommon. Clin Gastroenterol Hepatol. 2010;8(2):166–73.

30 Cappell MS. Safety and efficacy of colonoscopy after myocardial infarction: an analysis of 100 study patients and 100 control patients at two tertiary cardiac referral hospitals. Gastrointest Endosc. 2004;60(6):901–9.

31 Qadeer MA, Vargo JJ, Khandwala F, *et al*. Propofol versus traditional sedative agents for gastrointestinal endoscopy: a meta-analysis. Clin Gastroenterol Hepatol. 2005;3(11): 1049–56.

32 Singh H, Poluha W, Cheung M, *et al*. Propofol for sedation during colonoscopy. Cochrane Database Syst Rev. 2008;Oct 8(4):CD006268.

33 Rex DK, Deenadayalu VP, Eid E, *et al*. Endoscopist-directed administration of propofol: a worldwide safety experience. Gastroenterology. 2009;137(4):1229–37; quiz 518–9.

34 Horiuchi A, Nakayama Y, Hidaka N, *et al*. Low-dose propofol sedation for diag-nostic esophagogastroduodenoscopy: results in 10,662 adults. Am J Gastroenterol. 2009; 104(7):1650–5.

35 Bini EJ, Firoozi B, Choung RJ, *et al*. Systematic evaluation of complications related to endos-copy in a training setting: A prospective 30-day outcomes study. Gastrointest Endosc. 2003;57(1):8–16.

36 Steffes CP, Sugawa C, *et al*. Oxygen saturation monitoring during endoscopy. Surg Endosc. 1990;4(3):175–8.

37 Khiani VS, Salah W, Maimone S, *et al*. Sedation during endoscopy for patients at risk of obstructive sleep apnea. Gastrointest Endosc. 2009;70(6):1116–20.

38 Spier BJ, Said A, Moncher K, Pfau PR. Safety of endoscopy after myocardial infarction based on cardiovascular risk categories: a retrospective analysis of 135 patients at a tertiary referral medical center. J Clin Gastroenterol. 2007;41(5):462–7.

39 Cappell MS. Safety and clinical efficacy of flexible sigmoidoscopy and colonoscopy for gastro-intestinal bleeding after myocardial infarction. A six-year study of 18 consecutive lower endoscopies at two university teaching hospitals. Dig Dis Sci. 1994;39(3):473–80.

40 Goldman L, Caldera DL, Nussbaum SR, *et al*. Multifactorial index of cardiac risk in noncar-diac surgical procedures. N Engl J Med. 1977;297(16):845–50.

41 Detsky AS, Abrams HB, Forbath N, *et al*. Cardiac assessment for patients undergoing noncar-diac surgery. A multifactorial clinical risk index. Arch Intern Med. 1986;146(11):2131–4.

42 Cote GA, Hovis RM, Ansstas MA, *et al*. Incidence of sedation-related complications with propofol use during advanced endoscopic procedures. Clin Gastroenterol Hepatol. 2010; 8(2):137–42.

43 Qadeer MA, Rocio Lopez A, *et al*. Risk factors for hypoxemia during ambulatory gastrointes-tinal endoscopy in ASA I-II patients. Dig Dis Sci. 2009;54(5):1035–40.

44 Cotton PB, Eisen GM, Aabakken L, *et al*. A lexicon for endoscopic adverse events: report of an ASGE workshop. Gastrointest Endosc. 2010;71(3):446–54.

45 Elmunzer BJ, Scheiman JM, Lehman GA, *et al*. A randomized trial of rectal indomethacin to prevent post-ERCP pancreatitis. N Engl J Med. 2012;366(15):1414–22.

46 Liao WC, Tu YK, Wu MS, *et al*. Balloon dilation with adequate duration is safer than sphinc-terotomy for extracting bile duct stones: a systematic review and meta-analyses. Clin Gastroenterol Hepatol. 2012;10(10):1101–9.

47 Wang WL, Wu ZH, Sun Q, *et al*. Meta-analysis: the use of carbon dioxide insufflation vs. room air insufflation for gastrointestinal endoscopy. Aliment Pharmacol Ther. 2012;35(10):1145–54.

48 Borckardt JJ, Romagnuolo J, Reeves ST, *et al.* Feasibility, safety, and effectiveness of transcranial direct current stimulation for decreasing post-ERCP pain: a randomized, sham-controlled, pilot study. Gastrointestinal Endosc. 2011;Jun73(6):1158–64.

49 Singh M, Mehta N, Murthy UK, *et al.* Postpolypectomy bleeding in patients undergoing colonoscopy on uninterrupted clopidogrel therapy. Gastrointest Endosc. 2010; May;71(6): 998–1005.

50 Douketis JD, Spyropoulos AC, Spencer FA, *et al.* Perioperative management of antithrombotic therapy: Antithrombotic Therapy and Prevention of Thrombosis, 9th ed: American College of Chest Physicians Evidence-Based Clinical Practice Guidelines. Chest. 2012; 141(2 Suppl):e326S–50S.

51 Gage BF, Waterman AD, Shannon W, *et al.* Validation of clinical classification schemes for predicting stroke: results from the National Registry of Atrial Fibrillation. JAMA. 2001; 285(22):2864–70.

52 Lip GY, Nieuwlaat R, Pisters R, *et al.* Refining clinical risk stratification for predicting stroke and thromboembolism in atrial fibrillation using a novel risk factor-based approach: the euro heart survey on atrial fibrillation. Chest. 2010;137(2):263–72.

53 Nutescu EA. Oral anticoagulant therapies: balancing the risks. Am J Health Syst Pharm. 2013;70(10 Suppl 1):S3–11.

54 Townsend JC, Heard R, Powers ER, Reuben A. Usefulness of international normalized ratio to predict bleeding complications in patients with end-stage liver disease who undergo cardiac catheterization. Am J Cardiol. 2012;110(7):1062–5.

55 Giannini EG, Greco A, Marenco S, *et al.* Incidence of bleeding following invasive procedures in patients with thrombocytopenia and advanced liver disease. Clin Gastroenterol Hepatol. 2010;8(10):899–902; quiz e109.

56 Kwok A, Faigel DO. Management of anticoagulation before and after gastrointestinal endoscopy. Am J Gastroenterol. 2009;104(12):3085–97; quiz 98.

57 Plavix(R) Prescribing information. September 2013 ed. http://packageinserts.bms.com/pi/ pi_plavix.pdf: Bristol-Meyers Squibb (accessed on August 6, 2014).

58 Sung JJ, Lau JY, Ching JY, *et al.* Continuation of low-dose aspirin therapy in peptic ulcer bleeding: a randomized trial. Ann Intern Med. 2010;152(1):1–9.

59 Netzer NC, Stoohs RA, Netzer CM, *et al.* Using the Berlin Questionnaire to identify patients at risk for the sleep apnea syndrome. Ann Intern Med. 1999;131(7):485–91.

60 Hillman DR, Loadsman JA, *et al.* Obstructive sleep apnoea and anaesthesia. Sleep Med Rev. 2004;8(6):459–71.

61 Bo LL, Bai Y, Bian JJ, *et al.* Propofol vs traditional sedative agents for endoscopic retrograde cholangiopancreatography: a meta-analysis. World J Gastroenterol. 2011;17(30): 3538–43.

62 Gangi S, Saidi F, Patel K, *et al.* Cardiovascular complications after GI endoscopy: occurrence and risks in a large hospital system. Gastrointest Endosc. 2004;60(5):679–85.

63 Eagle KA, Berger PB, Calkins H, *et al.* ACC/AHA guideline update for perioperative cardiovascular evaluation for noncardiac surgery—executive summary: a report of the American College of Cardiology/American Heart Association Task Force on Practice Guidelines (Committee to Update the 1996 Guidelines on Perioperative Cardiovascular Evaluation for Noncardiac Surgery). J Am Coll Cardiol. 2002;39(3):542–53.

64 Hlatky MA, Boineau RE, Higginbotham MB, *et al.* A brief self-administered questionnaire to determine functional capacity (the Duke Activity Status Index). Am J Cardiol. 1989; 64(10):651–4.

65 Peng C, Nietert PJ, Cotton PB, *et al.* Predicting native papilla biliary cannulation success using a multinational Endoscopic Retrograde Cholangiopancreatography (ERCP) Quality Network. BMC Gastroenterol. 2013;13(1):147.

66 Romagnuolo J, Cotton PB. Recording ERCP fluoroscopy metrics using a multinational quality network: establishing benchmarks and examining time-related improvements. Am J Gastroenterol. 2013;108(8):1224–30.

67 Draganov PV, Forsmark CE. Prospective evaluation of adverse reactions to iodine-containing contrast media after ERCP. Gastrointest Endosc. 2008;68(6):1098–101.

68 Draganov P, Cotton PB. Iodinated contrast sensitivity in ERCP. Am J Gastroenterol. 2000;95(6):1398–401.

69 Chan CH, Enns RA. ERCP in the management of choledocholithiasis in pregnancy. Curr Gastroenterol Rep. 2012;14(6):504–10.

CHAPTER 6

Sedation, anesthesia, and medications

John J. Vargo, II

Department of Gastroenterology and Hepatology, Cleveland Clinic, Cleveland, USA

KEY POINTS

- The complexity of ERCP procedures demands great care in providing appropriate sedation/anesthesia.
- As for all endoscopic procedures, choices are determined by evaluation of the patient's health and infirmities, and the planned procedure.
- Careful intra- and postprocedure monitoring are essential.
- The trend is towards greater use of propofol anesthesia, without endotracheal intubation, in most cases.

The principles governing the optimal use of sedation/anesthesia for ERCP are no different from those for other gastrointestinal endoscopic procedures, but they tend to be more complex and often prolonged, so that optimal conditions are essential to maximize the chances of a successful outcome, and minimize the risks of adverse events.

A thorough understanding of the continuum of sedation and analgesia, which ranges from minimal sedation or anxiolysis through deep sedation in general anesthesia, is necessary [1]. Most patients undergoing ERCP will require deep sedation or general anesthesia. In this state, patients may respond only to painful stimuli. Additionally, the patients' protective airway reflexes and spontaneous ventilation may become compromised [1]. Hence, dedicated nursing or anesthesia personnel are necessary to provide continuous monitoring of the patient's vital signs and protective airway reflexes or the use of an anesthesia team is necessary in most cases. In a minority of cases, moderate sedation can be employed. In this state, the patient is able to give a purposeful response after verbal or tactile (not painful) sensation and there is no compromise to the patient's airway, ventilation, or cardiovascular function.

ERCP: The Fundamentals, Second Edition. Edited by Peter B. Cotton and Joseph Leung.
© 2015 John Wiley & Sons, Ltd. Published 2015 by John Wiley & Sons, Ltd.
Companion Website: www.wiley.com\go\cotton\ercp

Preprocedure preparation

The procedural team must take into account a thorough preprocedural assessment including history of present illness, past medical history, and a physical examination. Appropriate selection of patients for moderate or deep sedation/general anesthesia should be based on multiple factors including:
- The existence of significant comorbidities.
- Sedation and/or anesthesia history including intolerance or potential allergy to any of the planned drugs.
- Psychiatric history.
- History of illicit drug or alcohol use.
- Pharmacological profile including the use of sedatives, analgesics.
- Potential airway and other findings on physical examination, which may make the planned sedation problematic.

Sedation agents

Clearly, a thorough understanding of the pharmacokinetics and pharmacodynamics of different sedation agents including their potential interactions with other medications and other adverse reactions should be an important prerequisite to procedural sedation. This should include opioids such as meperidine and fentanyl, benzodiazepines such as midazolam and diazepam, propofol, pharyngeal anesthetic agents, and potential adjunctive agents such as ketamine, diphenhydramine, promethazine, and droperidol. Additionally, the use of reversal agents such as flumazenil and naloxone should be mastered (Table 6.1).

Patient monitoring

In addition to the traditional physiological monitoring avenues including pulse oximetry, blood pressure monitoring, and electrocardiography, capnography should be considered. The latter is important as deep sedation can be associated with apneic episodes, which can be missed by visual inspection and are only detected by pulse oximetry after significant alveolar hypoventilation has occurred. Additionally, the presence of fluoroscopic equipment may hinder the visual inspection of the patient's respiratory activity, which can further hinder the detection of respiratory compromise. In a prospective, randomized controlled, single-blinded study, the use of capnography was found to significantly reduce hypoxemic events and apnea when compared to standard monitoring, which included pulse oximetry and visual inspection in patients undergoing gastroenterologist-administered sedation for ERCP and endoscopic ultrasound (EUS) [2]. Bispectral index monitoring (BIS) is a complex evaluation of

Table 6.1 Pharmacological profile of drugs used for endoscopic sedation.

Drug	Onset of action (min)	Peak effect (min)	Duration of effect (min)	Initial dose	Pharmacological antagonist	Side effects
Dexemedetomidine (µg)	<5	15	Unknown	1 µg/kg	None	Bradycardia hypotension
Diazepam (mg)	2–3	3–5	360	5–10	Flumazenil	Chemical phlebitis, respiratory depression
Diphenhydramine (mg)	2–3	60–90	>240	25–50	None	Prolonged sedation, dizziness
Droperidol (mg)	3–10	30	120–240	1.5–2.5	None	QT interval prolongation, ventricular arrhythmia, extrapyramidal effects, dissociative reaction
Fentanyl (µg)	1–2	3–5	30–60	50–100	Naloxone	Respiratory depression, vomiting
Flumazenil (mg)	1–2	3	60	0.5–0.3		Agitation, withdrawal symptoms
Ketamine (mg)	<1	1	10–15	0.5/kg	None	Emergence reaction, apnea, laryngospasm
Meperidine (mg)	3–6	5–7	60–180	25–50	Naloxone	Respiratory depression, pruritus, vomiting, interaction with monoamine oxidase inhibitors
Midazolam (mg)	1–2	3–5	15–80	1–2	Flumazenil	Dysinhibition, respiratory depression
Naloxone (mg)	1–2	5	35–45	0.2–0.4		Narcotic withdrawal
Nitrous oxide	2–3	Dose dependent	15–30	Titrate to effect	None	Respiratory depression, headache
Promethazine (mg)	2–5	Unknown	>120	12.5–25	None	Respiratory depression, extrapyramidal effects, hypotension
Propofol (mg)	<1	1–2	4–8	10–40	None	Respiratory depression, cardiovascular instability

electroencephalographic measurements of frontal cortex activity that corresponds to varying levels of sedation. The BIS scale varies from 0 to 100 (0 no cortical activity or coma; 40–60 unconscious; 70–90 varying levels of conscious sedation; 100 fully awake). Unfortunately, there is patient to patient variability in the score, which limits it use in the endoscopy suite [3]. An exciting development for future monitoring may be automated responsiveness monitoring (ARM) [4]. This platform uses the response to auditory and vibratory stimuli to predict the transition from moderate to deep sedation. In 20 volunteers who received escalating doses of a propofol infusion, the loss of the ARM response reliably occurred prior to transitioning from moderate into deep sedation. ARM has been used successfully in a multicenter study using propofol-mediated sedation for upper endoscopy and colonoscopy that was targeting moderate sedation. It is hoped that such technology will be available in the future for patients who require deeper levels of sedation.

Cardiopulmonary risk assessment and consequences

Defining cardiopulmonary risk to patients undergoing ERCP may have an important influence on the type of sedation regimen that is utilized. The American Society of Anesthesiologists physiological classification (Table 6.2) has been found to be a useful predictor of unplanned cardiopulmonary events. In a study utilizing the clinical outcomes research initiative (CORI), the ASA physical classification was used to define the risk of the occurrence of unplanned cardiopulmonary events. For ERCP, the odds ratio for unplanned cardiopulmonary events was statistically increased in ASA class 4 and 5 patients (OR: 2.21; 95% CI: 1.18, 3.82). It should also be noted that the rate of serious adverse events such as hospital admission, emergency department referral, surgery, and cardiopulmonary resuscitation was quantitatively higher in patients undergoing ERCP at 1.84% when compared to much lower rates with esophagogastroduodenoscopy (0.33%),

Table 6.2 ASA physical classification (Adapted from the American Society of Anesthesiologist website http://education.asahq.org/find/?q=continuum+of+sedation&op=Go).

ASA classification	Description
I	A normal healthy patient
II	Patient with mild systemic disease
III	Patient with severe systemic disease
IV	Patient with severe systemic disease that is a constant threat to life
V	A moribund patient who is not expected to survive without intervention
VI	A declared brain-dead patient whose organs are being removed for donor purposes

colonoscopy (0.35%), and flexible sigmoidoscopy (0.12%). This study also found that increasing age was a risk factor for serious adverse events. Coté *et al.* also found that an ASA physical classification of 3 or greater was a risk factor for anesthesia personnel performing airway maneuvers such as a chin lift, nasal airway placement, or the use of modified facemask ventilation in a prospective cohort of 799 patients undergoing advanced endoscopic procedures such as ERCP and EUS [6]. Other independent predictors included increasing body mass index (BMI) and male gender. It is interesting to note that the Mallampati classification as well as the total propofol dose did not predict an increased risk for airway maneuvers. Overall, 14.4% of the patients required airway maneuvers. This study also emphasizes that even in the hands of an anesthesia team, when patients undergo advanced endoscopic procedures such as ERCP, airway maneuvers are sometimes necessary.

The use of a validated screening tool for obstructive sleep apnea known as the STOP-BANG score has also been shown to be predictive of the need for airway maneuvers during anesthesiologist-directed propofol sedation during advanced endoscopic procedures [7]. This instrument includes four questions and four clinical characteristics. Subjects with a STOP-BANG score ≥3 were associated with a significantly higher risk for airway maneuver intervention (OR: 1.81; 95% CI: 1.36, 2.42). Subjects with an elevated STOP-BANG score were also found to be at increased risk for apnea (OR: 1.63; 95% CI: 1.19, 2.25). Similarly, obesity defined as a BMI > 30 kg/m² was associated with an increased risk of sedation-related complications during anesthesiologist-directed propofol-mediated sedation for advanced endoscopic procedures [8].

Are ERCP outcomes influenced by the type of sedation/anesthesia utilized?

There is scant data to help answer this question. A case control study addressed the success of deep biliary cannulation in patients undergoing ERCP with either gastroenterologist-administered sedation with a combination of an opioid and benzodiazepine or anesthesiologist-directed sedation [9]. In this study, success was defined as deep biliary cannulation in patients with a native papilla. The study found that though anesthesia-directed sedation exhibited a trend for improvement in deep biliary cannulation (95.2% versus 94.4%); this did not reach statistical significance. Though this study is too small to address ERCP complications with a cohort size of 367, there was no discernible difference in post-ERCP pancreatitis or cholangitis. In a large systematic analysis, propofol-mediated sedation was compared to a combination of opioid and benzodiazepine. This included four randomized controlled trials involving a total of 510 patients [10–14]. Of note, in these trials all of the sedation was administered by a nonanesthesiologist provider. There was no mortality or significant cardiopulmonary events such as hypoxemia or hypotension. The recovery of patients who received propofol-mediated sedation was significantly improved.

Patient's position

ERCP is traditionally and conveniently (for the endoscopist) usually performed with the patient in the semiprone position. Sometimes, anesthesiologists prefer the supine position. Does patient positioning affect the outcome? A prospective, randomized trial utilizing gastroenterologist-administered midazolam-mediated sedation found no difference in ERCP success rates or subsequent complications when comparing prone versus supine positioning [15]. A much smaller randomized trial involving 34 patients did find a significantly lower technical difficulty in performing the ERCP in the prone position by utilizing the Freeman score [16]. There was also an increase in cardiorespiratory events in the supine position when compared to the prone position (41% versus 6%, $P = 0.039$). Despite this statistical significance, this study should be called into question due to its smaller sample size leading to the potential of a type 2 error. In a large case control study involving 649 patients, in which 143 were in the supine position, Ferreira and Baron found no difference between the positions for success or complication rates. However, the procedural degree of difficulty was significantly higher in the supine group [17]. In summary, it appears that the positioning for ERCP in the supine position may carry with it a more technically challenging milieu for the endoscopist but the data does not convincingly show any difference in success or complication rates.

Propofol for everyone? Endotracheal intubation?

Propofol-mediated sedation for ERCP is becoming the de facto standard of care, at least in referral centers performing more complex procedures, and there has also been an evolution away from elective endotracheal intubation during these cases. Important prerequisites for this type of approach include a dedicated anesthesia staff who engage in active airway management throughout the case as well as the use of monitoring including pulse oximetry, electrocardiogram, blood pressure, and either capnography or visual inspection to detect apnea. Many case series have found this approach to be quite effective [6–8, 18]. It also appears to have a very high safety profile but comparative numbers to propofol-mediated sedation with endotracheal intubation are not available to definitively answer the safety issue. Candidates for elective endotracheal intubation would include problematic airway anatomy that would render urgent intubation very difficult in achalasia, gastroparesis, and in cases where

ERCP is combined with endoscopic pseudocyst drainage [19]. There is also a propensity in the literature to provide elective endotracheal intubation for patients with obesity (BMI > 30 kg/m²) although no safety benefit has been realized. It has been our practice to consider elective intubation in patients who have a BMI > 35 kg/m².

Conclusion

There are many factors to consider when utilizing anesthesia assistance for ERCP. Aside from outcomes such as onset of appropriate sedation and recovery parameters, there may be many other factors that would lead a clinician to consider propofol-mediated sedation for ERCP. The multisociety sedation curriculum for gastrointestinal endoscopy lists an ASA physical status of 4 or greater as being associated with an increased risk for cardiopulmonary complications. Additionally, the use of analgesics, sedatives, and alcohol can also increase the sedation-related risk. Other guidelines for anesthesiology assistance are listed in Table 6.3.

In summary, propofol-mediated sedation targeting deep sedation or general anesthesia is superior to the combination of a benzodiazepine and opioid that targets moderate sedation in terms of rapidity of onset and recovery profile. Other parameters such as patient satisfaction, safety, and efficacy appear to be equivalent. Of note is that all of the randomized controlled studies comparing these two sedation regimens have involved non-anesthesiologist-administered routes for propofol. There is emerging evidence that the majority of cases receiving propofol do not require endotracheal intubation. In the future we hope to have further perspective randomized trials as well as the emergence of computer-assisted sedation platforms that may further improve the safety, efficacy, and patient satisfaction for procedural sedation for ERCP.

Table 6.3 Guidelines for anesthesiology assistance during ERCP.

Anticipated intolerance, allergy or paradoxical reaction to standard sedation regimens
Increased risk of complications because of severe comorbidity (ASA class 4 and higher)
Increased risk of airway obstruction
History of stridor
History of severe sleep apnea
Dysmorphic facial features (i.e., trisomy 21)
Oral abnormalities (i.e., <3 cm oral opening in adults)
Neck abnormalities (i.e., decreased hyoid–mental distance < 3 cm in adults)
Cervical spine disease (i.e., advanced rheumatoid arthritis or trauma)
Severe tracheal deviation
Jaw abnormalities (i.e., trismus, retrognathia, or micrognathia)

References

1 https://www.asahq.org/For-Members/Standards-Guidelines-and-Statements.aspx (accessed on February 22, 2014).

2 Qadeer MA, Vargo JJ, Dumot JA, *et al.* Capnographic monitoring of respiratory activity improves safety of sedation for endoscopic cholangiopancreatography and ultrasonography. Gastroenterology 2009;136:1568–1576.

3 Bower AL, Ripepi A, Dilger J, *et al.* Bispectral index monitoring of sedation during endoscopy. Gastrointest Endosc 2000;52:192–196.

4 Doufas AG, Moriorka N, Mahgoub AN, *et al.* Automated responsiveness monitor to titrate propofol sedation. Anesth Analg 2009;109(3):778–86.

5 Enestvedt BK, Eisen GM, Holub J, Lieberman DA. Is the American Society of Anesthesiologists classification useful in risk stratification for endoscopic procedures? Gastrointest Endosc 2013;77:464–471.

6 Coté GA, Hovis RM, Anastas MA, *et al.* Incidence of sedation-related complications with propofol use during advanced endoscopic procedures. Clin Gastroenterol Hepatol 2010;8:137–142.

7 Coté GA, Hovis CE, Hovis RM, *et al.* A screening instrument for sleep apnea predicts airway maneuvers in patients undergoing advanced endoscopic procedures. Clin Gastroenterol Hepatol 2010;8:660–665.

8 Wani S, Azar R, Hovis CE, *et al.* Obesity is a risk factor for sedation related complications during propofol mediated sedation for advanced endoscopic procedures. Gastrointest Endosc 2011;74:1238–1247.

9 Mehta P, Vargo JJ, Dumot JA, *et al.* Does anesthesiologist-directed sedation for ERCP improve deep cannulation and complication rates? Dig Dis Sci 2011;56:2185–2190.

10 Garewal D, Powell S, Milan SJ, *et al.* Sedative techniques for endoscopic retrograde cholangiopancreatography. The Cochrane Library 2012;6: http://www.thecochranelibrary.com (accessed on February 1, 2014).

11 Kongkam P, Rerknimitr R, Punyathavorn S, *et al.* Propofol infusion versus intermittent meperidine and midazolam injection for conscious sedation in ERCP. J Gastrointest Liv Dis 2008;17:291–297.

12 Riphaus A, Steriou N, Wehmann T. Sedation with propofol for routine ERCP in high risk octogenarians: a randomized controlled study. Am J Gastroenterol 2005;100:1957–1963.

13 Schilling D, Rosenbaum A, Schweizer S, *et al.* Sedation with propofol for interventional endoscopy by trained nurses in high-risk octogenarians. A prospective randomized controlled study. Endoscopy 2009;41:295–298.

14 Vargo JJ, Zuccaro G, Dumot JA, *et al.* Gastroenterologist-administered propofol versus midazolam/meperidine for advanced upper endoscopy: a prospective randomized trial. Gastroenterology 2002;123:8–16.

15 Tringali A, Mutignani M, Milano A, *et al.* No difference between supine and prone position for ERCP in conscious sedated patients: A prospective, randomized study. Endoscopy 2008;40: 93–97.

16 Terruzzi V, Radaelli F, Meucci G, Minoli G. Is the supine position as safe and effective as the prone position for endoscopic retrograde cholangiopancreatography? A prospective, randomized study. Endoscopy 2005;37:1211–1214.

17 Ferreira LE, Baron TH. Comparison of safety and efficacy of ERCP performed with the patient in supine position and prone positions. Gastrointest Endosc 2008;67:1037–1043.

18 Barnett SR, Berzin T, Sanaka S, *et al.* Deep sedation without intubation for ERCP is appropriate in healthier, non-obese patients. Dig Dis Sci 2013;58:3287–3292.

19 Vargo JJ, DeLegge MH, Feld AD, *et al.* Multisociety sedation curriculum for gastrointestinal endoscopy. Gastrointest Endosc 2012;76:e1–e25.

SECTION 2
Techniques

CHAPTER 7

Standard devices and techniques

Joseph Leung

Department of Gastroenterology and Hepatology, Davis School of Medicine, University of California, Sacramento, USA
Section of Gastroenterology, VA Northern California Health Care System, Sacramento VAMC, Mather, USA

KEY POINTS

- Up to 12 different maneuvers (14 if a sphincterotome is used) may be needed to control the scope tip and accessory/guide wire to achieve selective cannulation.

- Combining the endoscopy and fluoroscopy images provides a three-dimensional picture of the papilla and the axis of the respective ductal systems to facilitate selective cannulation.

- Shaping the sphincterotome to improve alignment of the cutting wire with the papilla and performing a stepwise controlled cut along the imaginary "perfect" bile duct axis will improve the clinical outcome of endoscopic retrograde cholangiopancreatography (ERCP)/sphincterotomy.

- It is important to compare the size of bile duct stone(s) with the distal common bile duct (CBD) and sphincterotomy to determine the ease of stone extraction.

- A significant discrepancy between stone size and exit passage will require lithotripsy to assist with stone extraction.

- Prolonged (5 min) balloon dilation improves the success of stone extraction and minimizes the risk of post-ERCP pancreatitis.

- A combination of different tissue/cytology sampling methods will improve the diagnostic yield for underlying pancreaticobiliary pathologies.

- A single stent is sufficient for drainage of mid or distal CBD obstruction. It is preferable to drain both intrahepatic ducts in hilar obstruction, using dual stents.

- Short wire system with intraductal release (IDR) of the guide wire above the obstruction facilitates multiple stenting for benign bile duct stricture.

Intubation and examination of the stomach

When the patient is adequately sedated, a self-retaining mouth guard is placed and the patient is positioned in a left lateral/semiprone position. This position facilitates intubation and examination of the upper gastrointestinal tract (GI) tract

---

ERCP: The Fundamentals, Second Edition. Edited by Peter B. Cotton and Joseph Leung.
© 2015 John Wiley & Sons, Ltd. Published 2015 by John Wiley & Sons, Ltd.
Companion Website: www.wiley.com\go\cotton\ercp

with a side-viewing duodenoscope. The scope is inserted with initial upward tip deflection to pass the back of the tongue and then the tip is deflected downward to enter the esophagus. Simultaneous swallowing by the (partially sedated) patient will assist with esophageal intubation. By gently deflecting the tip downward, and insufflating air, part of the esophageal lumen can be examined as the scope advances into the stomach. With the patient in the prone position, slight left wrist rotation helps to put the long axis of the scope in line with the gastric lumen. Once in the stomach, the residual gastric juice is suctioned to minimize the risk of aspiration. Unless the patient has not already had a formal upper endoscopy, and if there is suspicion of gastric pathology, the stomach is inflated only enough to allow a view of the lumen. Gentle downward tip deflection allows good visualization and reversing the deflection will facilitate advancement. The scope is advanced slowly, sliding along the greater curve to pass the incisura and into the antrum. The cardia can be examined by upangulation and withdrawal of the scope. If difficulty is encountered while advancing the scope, the patient can be held temporarily in a more lateral position (by lifting the right shoulder) to improve the orientation.

Once past the incisura, the tip of the scope is angled further downward and the pylorus is visualized. The scope is positioned so that the pylorus lies in the center of the endoscopy view. The tip of the endoscope is then returned to the neutral position as the scope is advanced and as the pylorus disappears from view, the so-called sun-setting sign. Fine adjustment of the scope tip position may be necessary. Gentle pushing will advance the scope into the first part of the duodenum. The resistance that is overcome at that point means that the tip may impact the far wall, so that it may be necessary to withdraw slowly to get a good view, at the same time angling the tip down, and insufflating air. Careful examination is performed to rule out any pathology such as ulcers or duodenitis. The scope is advanced further past the junction of the first and second part of the duodenum before scope shortening (by sideway angulation to the right (right-hand control) followed by upward angulation of the tip (left thumb control) and rotating the left wrist to the right while pulling back the scope gently). If necessary, the patient is then rotated to lie prone on the fluoroscopy table.

With the scope angled right and upward, and by rotating the (left wrist) scope to the right and withdrawing slowly, the tip of the scope is advanced further into the second part of the duodenum. This paradoxical movement shortens the scope using the pylorus as a pivot, bringing it into the usual "short scope" position. (Figure 7.1a–c). At this point, the markings on the duodenoscope should indicate 60–65 cm at the incisors. In patients with duodenal deformity, it may be necessary to advance the tip of the scope further into the third or fourth part of the duodenum before rotating the scope to the right and pulling back to shorten. Never lock the scope tip while performing the shortening maneuver to avoid accidental injury to the duodenum [1].

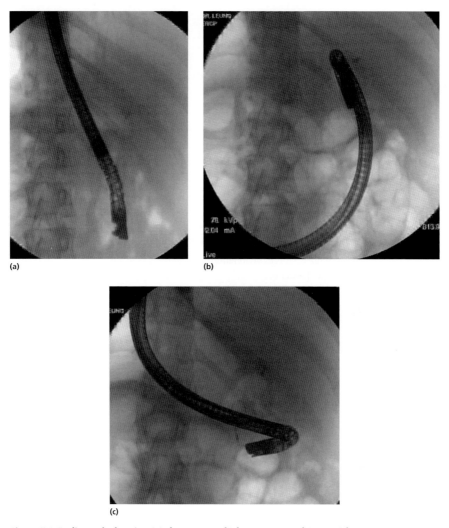

(a)   (b)

(c)

Figure 7.1 Radiograph showing (a) short scope, (b) long scope, and (c) semi-long scope positions for cannulation.

Approaching the main papilla

With the patient in the prone position, the scope is returned to a neutral position (by gentle rotation of the left wrist to the left or slight left angulation); and the papilla is usually well visualized on the posteromedial wall of the second portion of the duodenum. The anatomical landmark for locating the papilla is the junction of the horizontal fold meeting with the vertical fold (T-junction) (Figure 7.2). Duodenal diverticula may distort or displace the papilla to the edge or rarely inside, and can cause difficulty with cannulation (Figure 7.3a). Difficulties may also be encountered with other less common pathologies such as impacted stones (which can cause edema and displacement of the papillary orifice, usually downward) and

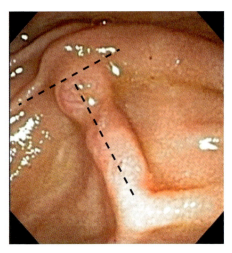

Figure 7.2 Location of papilla is where the longitudinal fold meets the vertical fold (T-junction) in the second portion of the duodenum.

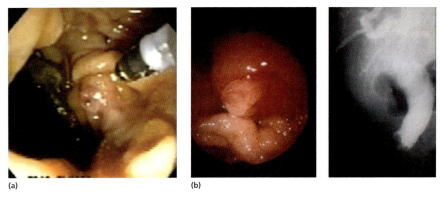

(a)   (b)

Figure 7.3 (a) Displaced papilla on edge of a duodenal diverticulum and (b) abnormal papilla due to ampullary tumor.

the presence of an (ulcerated) ampullary tumor (Figure 7.3b). Depending on the position of the endoscopy monitor and setup, some endoscopists perform the ERCP with the patient lying supine and this may require further rotation of the endoscopist's body to the right to compensate for a change in the axis to get better alignment with the papilla.

Before cannulating the papilla and injecting contrast, a control (plain) film of the right upper abdomen with the scope in place (short scope position) is taken to ensure there are no potential artifacts, and to look for diagnostic clues, such as pancreatic calcification, or air in the biliary system. Discussion of radiological findings is given in Chapter 12. There are basically two ways to display the image on the fluoroscopy monitor. Some endoscopists prefer to have the image displayed in the usual way of reading an X-ray film (i.e., the liver and bile duct is on the left side and the tail of the pancreas is on the right side of the screen). I prefer to orientate the fluoroscopy image similar to the anatomical position of the patient, that is, the right side of the screen represents the right side of the patient in a prone position. In a short scope position, the top right area above the scope represents the biliary area except for the distal bile duct, which is below the scope. The left side of the screen below the scope represents the pancreatic area. Cannulation in the short scope position allows better control of the scope tip angulations and deflection. In difficult cases with a distorted anatomy, or in attempted minor papilla cannulation, the long or semilong scope approach (with redundant looping of the scope in the body of the stomach) may be adopted (Figure 7.1c).

Excess bubbles around the papilla can be removed by infusing a dilute simethicone solution into the duodenum, and contractions may be reduced by using intravenous injections of glucagon or hyoscine butylbromide.

Cannulation principles

There are certain basic techniques and tricks of the trade in scope manipulation and handling of accessories that can improve the success of the procedure. An important aspect is to understand the need for proper access. Three key words that summarize the approach are **A**xis, **O**rientation, and **A**lignment or **AOA**.

Axis is the luminal direction of the distal bile duct or pancreas in relation to the papillary structure/prominence in the duodenum. This is an anatomical component and is not likely to change except with conditions that alter the anatomy including large periampullary diverticula or other abnormalities/pathologies such as ampullary or pancreatic tumors. The axis of a bile duct or pancreatic stricture is defined as the course of the luminal narrowing of respective ducts whether it is straight, tortuous, or distorted depending on the nature of the underlying pathology.

Orientation is the approach to the bile duct or pancreatic orifices using the duodenoscope. In general, orientation is affected by the scope position (short or long), sideway angulations, and duodenal anatomy. With a short scope position, the papilla can be seen in a proper en face position in about 95% of cases. When there is distortion of the duodenum or periampullary diverticula, adjustment of the scope position is necessary to maintain proper orientation with the papilla to facilitate cannulation. Similarly, when attempting to enter a biliary stricture, the orientation of the accessory or guide wire inside the bile duct and/or pancreatic duct (PD) can be optimized by moving the scope tip, and by advance or withdrawal of the accessory/catheter.

Alignment refers to the importance of positioning the accessory (exiting from the scope channel) in line with the axis of the respective ductal system. Whether contrast is injected or a guide wire is used to guide the cannulation process, further adjustment of this alignment can be achieved with fine adjustment of the scope tip or by changing the angle/curvature of the accessories such as a sphincterotome by insertion or withdrawal, or by traction on the cutting wire. In most cases, the tip of the guide wire is straight and the direction can be maintained/altered by movement of the tip of the accessory or by controlling how much wire is protruding from the tip of the accessory. Another way to change the alignment is by shaping the tip of the accessory (catheter or sphincterotome) being used to insert the guide wire (see later).

Use of guide wires

Most if not all ERCP procedures require the use of or are facilitated by an indwelling guide wire. Most conventional accessories, for example, catheters, sphincterotomes, balloons, and baskets, are 200–260 cm in length and are used with long guide wires (400–480 cm).

With the long wire system, exchange is performed over the full length of the wire, which requires active coordination with an assistant. Long wires tend to tangle, making this process rather cumbersome. It is preferable to loop the long wires and to form/unwind each loop during exchange (Figure 7.4), keeping the wire under control (and to prevent its end from dropping on the floor) (Video 1a and b, www.wiley.com\go\cotton\ercp). Some assistants prefer to leave the end of the wire in a sterile tray or clean plastic bag to minimize contamination. Holding the looped/coiled guide wire with a clip or wet gauze keeps the wire under control when not in use.

The earlier guide wires were made of stainless steel with a Teflon coating and kinked rather easily. Today, most are made of nitinol (nickel/titanium alloy), which is kink resistant. The hydrophilic tip is radio-opaque, but the shaft is less so. The surface coating has obvious color stripes or markings that help monitor and maintain the wire position by visual control during exchange, reducing the need for fluoroscopy.

Guide wires are used as path finders for selective and deep cannulation, and to help place larger accessories. They vary in properties to serve different purposes (Table 7.1). Wires with a more flexible tip are useful for cannulation, but rigidity is needed to provide stiffness during exchange of accessories, especially for

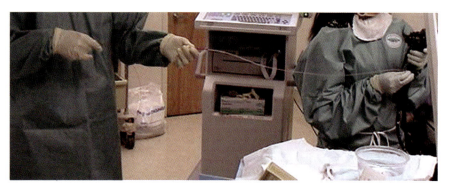

Figure 7.4 Keeping accessories relatively straight and looping a long guide wire helps in manipulation and exchange of accessories.

Table 7.1 A comparison of commonly used guide wires.

Guide wire	Examples	Path finder	Cannulation	Bridge	Exchange	Remarks
Hydrophilic tip, Teflon-coated Nitinol; regular (0.035")	Metro tracer (C), Dream (B), LinearGlideV (O)	Excellent	Excellent (MT tip can be shaped)	Good	Excellent(radio-opaque tip and visual markers)	All-purpose wires
Small caliber (0.025")	Tracer (C), JAG (B), VisiGlide (O)	Excellent	Excellent	Good	Fair (flimsy)	Smaller all-purpose wire
Small caliber (0.021")	0.021" wire (C)	Good	Good	No	Fair	Used with 021 Omni sphincterotome
Teflon-coated stainless steel	THSF (C)	No	Rarely used	Excellent	Fair	Stiff wire, for stenting of difficult stricture
Fully hydrophilic	Glidewire (T), Navipro(B), Delta (C)	Excellent	Excellent	Good	Good	Very slippery when wet, more difficult to control
Stainless steel wire 0.018"	Road runner (C), Pathfinder (B)	No	No	For small-caliber accessories	No	For manometry and 3 Fr pancreatic stent

B, Boston Scientific; C, Cook Endoscopy, O, Olympus, T, Terumo.

stent placement. Wires should also be insulated for sphincterotomy. Wires with a full hydrophilic coating are very slippery when wet and flexible but they are also more difficult to handle. Some wires only have a 3-cm flexible hydrophilic tip and the shaft has a Teflon sheath, which is less slippery and easier to handle during exchange. If necessary, wires can be changed to accomplish a specific individual task, for example, switching to a stiffer wire for stenting of the left hepatic duct.

A significant advance in the use of guide wires was the development of the "V-scopes" from Olympus. The wire can be trapped within a notch on the elevator and increased lift allows the wire to be anchored during exchanges (Figure 7.5a). The accessory can be removed quickly without coordinated exchange. However, the grip of the wire is lost temporarily when the accessory goes over the elevator. When long wires are used with the V scope, the assistant should maintain traction on the wire to prevent it from becoming kinked or looped inside the channel.

Short wire systems

The need for close cooperation between the assistant and endoscopist in handling long wire exchanges effectively has been obviated recently by the development of short wire platforms that give the endoscopists complete control. The short wire is anchored to the scope (at biopsy valve) or gripped at the elevator. Short wires range from 185 to 260 cm in length. Long accessories are often not compatible with short wires, but short wire accessories can be used with long wires. There are two main short wire systems

The RX System (Boston Scientific, Natik, MA) utilizes a special biopsy valve and a wire-lock strapped to the scope above the biopsy valve (Figure 7.5b), which can anchor up to two guide wires. Manipulation of accessories is controlled by the endoscopist. Exchange is facilitated by the C-channel on the accessory shaft that can be "split" to free the wire until the distal 9–20 cm where there is a complete lumen. The short length of the accessory is exchanged over the wire at the biopsy valve. There is a potential problem with leakage of air and bile at the biopsy valve. An extension wire is available to convert the short wire to a long wire for use with conventional accessories.

The Fusion system (Cook Endoscopy, Winston Salem, NC) involves a novel concept to exchange accessories by creating a side hole at 6 or 9 cm (2.5 cm for inner catheter of stenting system) from the distal tip of the accessories to facilitate exchanges.

A disposable biopsy valve with built-in wire-lock anchors the guide wire (Figure 7.5c). A double membrane within the valve helps prevent leakage. The guide wire is inserted through the side hole of the catheter and exits from the tip (i.e., only a short length of wire is within the catheter lumen). The wire is positioned flushed with the tip and held (jammed) in place by an inner stylet using a luer-lock. The rest of the wire stays alongside the catheter within the scope

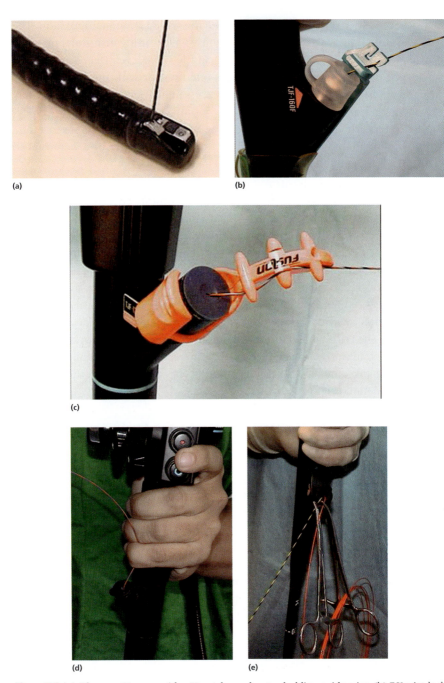

Figure 7.5 (a) Olympus V-scope with a V-notch on elevator holding guide wire, (b) RX wire lock and special biopsy valve attached to scope, (c) fusion biopsy valve with wire lock attached to scope, (d) anchoring guide wire with left little finger facilitate exchange of accessories, and (e) hemostat(s) used to clip and hold guide wire to/at the biopsy valve.

channel. The inner stylet is unlocked to free the wire during manipulation. The proximal end of the wire is locked at the biopsy valve during insertion and withdrawal of accessories with a short exchange at the valve level. Deep cannulation is achieved with the catheter and wire (as one unit) or with the wire alone by the endoscopist. Caution is taken to avoid excess pullback of the wire as this may dislodge the wire from the catheter. It is important to "free" the wire by unlocking the inner stylet and at the valve during manipulation. In the absence of a wire-lock, the guide wire can be held by the left little finger or a hemostat to anchor the wire and facilitate exchanges (Figure 7.5d and e).

Intraductal exchange

Upon deep cannulation, the wire is freed and inserted deep in the bile duct or to negotiate the stricture. The catheter is removed leaving the wire in place and the other accessory is exchanged over the proximal end of the wire in the usual manner. A unique feature of the Fusion system is the ability to free the wire within the bile duct or above the stricture (IDR or exchange) thus avoiding the need for repeat cannulation (Table 7.2). The wire is pulled back until it separates from the catheter within the bile duct or above a stricture at the side hole under fluoroscopy. The wire is then advanced further up the duct and locked in place at the biopsy valve. The accessory is then removed. This method allows repeat access to the bile duct, for example, multiple stenting without the need for repeat cannulation (Figure 7.6).

Using standard length accessories with the Fusion system

In situations where intervention requires the use of standard length accessories, a long guide wire can be inserted through the end of the catheter or sphincterotome after removing the inner stylet, and exchanged in the usual manner. Alternatively and if needed, a long guide wire can be cut short using a wire cutter to be used with the short wire accessories (Figure 7.7a–d).

Table 7.2 A comparison of different short wire system for biliary stenting.

	Rapid exchange	Fusion	V-system
Locking device for guide wire	Fixed to scope above biopsy valve	Modified biopsy valve with anchor	V-notch on elevator to grip guide wire
Short wire guide	Yes	Yes	Yes
Exchange outside scope	20-cm rapid exchange	6-cm zip exchange	Accessory over full length of wire
Intraductal release of guide wire	No	Yes	No
Multiple stents without recannulation	No	Yes	No

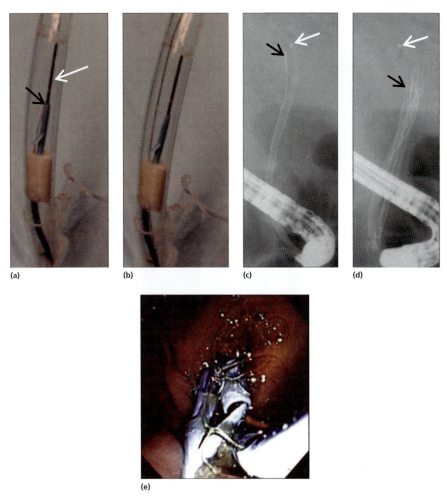

(a)   (b)   (c)   (d)

(e)

Figure 7.6 (a) Fusion OSAIS stenting system with guide wire, inner catheter and stent inserted through a simulated bile duct stricture (note that the stent is "caught" between the wire and inner catheter (black arrow)), (b) after intraductal release (IDR) of guide wire, guide wire and stent stay above bile duct stricture before final stent deployment, (c) radiograph showing IDR before deployment of first stent, guide wire tip (white arrow) is separated from inner catheter, (d) multiple stents placed across stricture in bile duct using IDR, and (e) multiple stents in duodenum.

Cannulation of the bile duct

Selective bile duct cannulation can be achieved by experts in close to 100% of cases (in the absence of major pathology or surgical diversion), but it is technically challenging. Success rates of 85–90% are often suggested as reasonable minimal standards (see chapters 1).

Cannulation is best performed from the en face position. Attention to the appropriate AXIS is key to successful access. The biliary axis is that of the intraduodenal

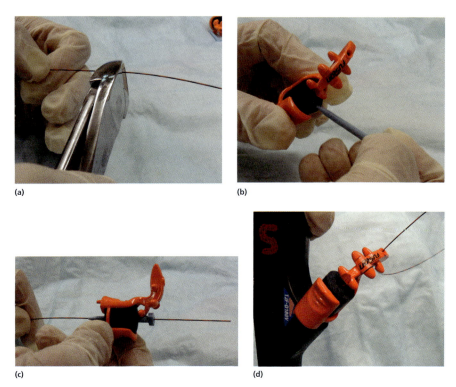

(a)   (b)

(c)   (d)

Figure 7.7 (a) Cutting a long guide wire, (b) inserting guide wire adaptor/introducer through Fusion wire lock valve, (c) guide wire inserted through the valve in retrograde fashion, and (d) final position of short wire anchored on wire lock.

and intrapapillary segment of the distal bile duct, and is represented visually by the prominence above the papilla along the 11–12 o'clock direction (Figure 7.8a). Likewise, the pancreatic axis is that of the intrapapillary and terminal part of the PD, and is usually in the 1–2 o'clock direction (Figure 7.8b).

Cannulation of the CBD is usually achieved by approaching the papilla orifice from below, and aligning the catheter with the correct axis. The tip of the catheter, or of a contained guide wire, is directed to the left upper corner of the papilla in the 11 o'clock position.

Cannulation is usually attempted initially with a catheter of 5 FG with a rounded or tapered (but not too sharp) tip. Double-lumen catheters are preferred, since they allow injection of contrast and advancement of a guide wire independently. For a single-lumen catheter, a special adaptor, for example, DSA (Cook Endoscopy) permits alternating injection of contrast or passage of a guide wire. When sphincterotomy is anticipated, it is often preferable to initiate cannulation with a sphincterotome (the bowing of which can facilitate access).

The catheter or sphincterotome should be flushed and primed with normal contrast to remove any air bubbles prior to insertion into the duodenoscope.

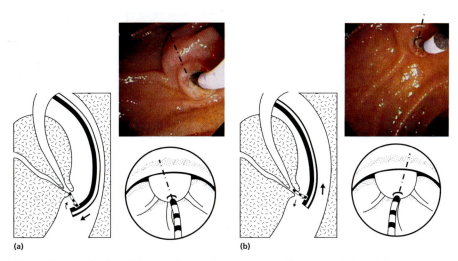

Figure 7.8 (a) Selective CBD cannulation. Stay close to papilla, approach from below, lift roof of papilla. Catheter directed at 11–12 o'clock position, (b) selective pancreatic duct cannulation. Catheter perpendicular to duodenal wall aiming at 1–2 o'clock position. 'Drop' the catheter by withdrawing tip of scope, relax up angulation or lower elevator. Use hydrophilic tip guide wire for cannulation.

Air mixed with contrast injected into the biliary system can mimic stones, and it can be more serious (due to overdistension) if air is injected into the pancreas. Flushing contrast into the duodenum to prime the catheter should be avoided since the hypertonic contrast stimulates duodenal motility.

Once an accessory is engaged in the papilla, further manipulation is guided partly by fluoroscopy, by observing the guide wire, or by injecting small amounts of contrast. This may show what maneuvers are needed to achieve deep cannulation. The combination of the fluoroscopy and endoscopy images can provide a three-dimensional image of the papilla and distal bile duct. Excess pressure of the catheter on or in the papilla should be avoided as it tends to distort the papilla and distal duct (so called J-shaped distal bile duct), thus increasing the difficulty of deep cannulation. When using a sphincterotome, the alignment of the tip and contained guide wire can be changed by tightening the cutting wire. However, excess traction will cause the tip to deviate to the right and makes cannulation more difficult.

It is daunting to realize that up to 12 different maneuvers of the scope can be used to position the tip of the catheter (or sphincterotome) in relation to the papillary orifice for cannulation (Figure 7.9). These include up/down and right/left sideway angulations, left wrist right and left rotation of the endoscope, advancing and withdrawing the scope, and up and down movement of the elevator. Suction collapses the duodenum and pulls the papilla closer to the tip of the scope, while air insufflation pushes it away [2].

During attempted cannulation, the control wheels should be locked to allow fine adjustment of the scope tip position and to avoid any recoil while adjusting

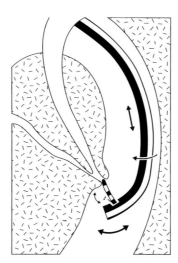

Figure 7.9 A combination of 12 different maneuvers (indicated by arrows) to control the scope tip position for selective cannulation.

the scope controls. However, the locks should be released if repositioning involves excess angulation and major adjustment of the endoscope position.

Guide wire cannulation

Testing the success of biliary cannulation with repeated injections of contrast risks overfilling the pancreas and increases the risk of pancreatitis. This is the rationale behind probing with the tip of a guide wire (0.035″ gauge) when initial attempts fail, or, indeed from the start. Using a guide wire tip protruding from a sphincterotome provides a variety of options in changing the axis [3]. Successful guide wire cannulation is obvious when the tip "jumps" up the duct. Sometimes, a wire will advance when it is forced to loop by applying pressure (carefully) when the tip is impacted.

Shaping the accessories

Changing the shape of the tip of the accessories may facilitate cannulation. Those with straight tips come out of the channel pointing "downward," and there may not be sufficient elevator "lift" to orientate them toward the correct axis. Curving the tip of a catheter (by running the thumb nail gently over the distal end) will create a curve, which, with the help of the elevator, can provide a better alignment. Hold the catheter close to the tip when inserting into the channel to avoid accidental buckling of the tip.

With most sphincterotomes, the tip tends to deviate to the right side when traction is applied to the cutting wire (this applies less with sphincterotomes with long (>25 mm) cutting wires). The tip tends to flip toward the pancreas making selective cannulation of the bile duct more difficult. It may be helpful to shape the sphincterotome to overcome this potential problem. It is performed by turning the straightened tip of the sphincterotome 70–90° so that the wire is on

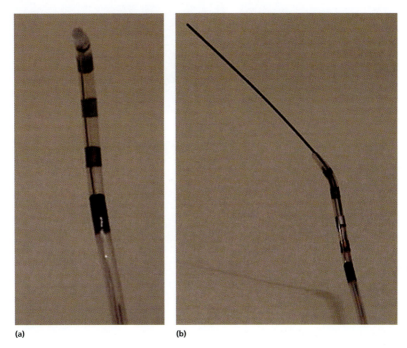

(a)   (b)

Figure 7.10 (a) Shaping the sphincterotome allows the cutting wire to stay on the left side of the catheter, (b) gentle bending of the tip of sphincterotome helps to deflect the guide wire towards the left side in line with the biliary axis.

the left side of the catheter, then curling the tip of the sphincterotome with the fingers to preform the tip and ensure that the wire stays on the left side of the catheter when the wire is tightened (Figure 7.10a and b).

Shaping the sphincterotome may be helpful for two reasons: First, it ensures that the cutting wire is on the left side of the catheter, so in the event of a deviation with traction, the cutting wire stays on the left side of the catheter (a more neutral position) to perform the biliary cut. Second, bending the tip of the sphincterotome gently toward the left side favors selective cannulation of the bile duct, especially when using a guide wire. Although the tip of the sphinc-terotome may appear to deviate to the left as it emerges from the scope channel, gentle traction of the cutting wire will deflect the tip upward, putting the tip back in line with the bile duct axis for selective cannulation (Video 2, www.wiley.com\go\cotton\ercp).

There may be circumstances where shaping the tip of a guide wire may also be helpful, especially when attempting to access tortuous strictures. Creating a single curve (C-shape) or a double curve (S-shape) on the flexible tip of the wire encourages it to bend when it encounters resistance to form a loop (Figure 7.11a–c). Advancing a guide wire with looping may be easier and certainly less trau-matic and increases the success of negotiating tight and angulated strictures (Video 3, www.wiley.com\go\cotton\ercp). The double curve or S-shape will

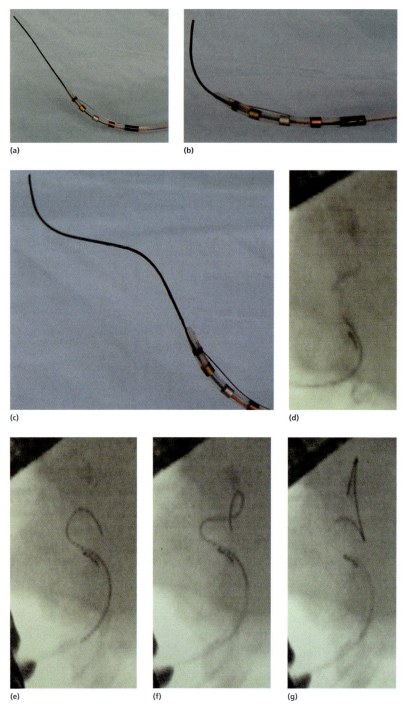

Figure 7.11 (a) Straight guide wire protruding from sphincterotome, (b) a gentle curve (C-curve) created at tip of guide wire, and (c) double (S) curve created at tip of guide wire, to facilitate looping and selective cannulation, and (d–g) radiographs showing cannulation of distal CBD stricture with guide wire and papillotome, note looping of tip of guide wire across a very tortuous stricture.

enable the wire tip to bend in opposite directions when resistance is encountered at the stricture. This technique is especially helpful when attempting selective cannulation of the right and left intrahepatic systems. This concept is different from the "loop-tip" guide wire (Cook Endoscopy). The small nylon loop at the tip of the guide wire is designed to facilitate deep cannulation of the PD and to prevent it from lodging in the papillary structure or side branches. However, this wire does not have the usual 3-cm flexible tip and it does not loop or negotiate tight strictures easily.

Slippery and floppy hydrophilic tip guide wires may facilitate cannulation of an angulated stricture.

Cholangiography

When cholangiography is intended, we start with full-strength contrast and consider switching over to dilute contrast when stones are suspected. In patients with cholangitis, after deep cannulation is successful, it is wise to aspirate bile before injecting contrast to avoid increasing the intrabiliary pressure, which can precipitate septicemia.

The CBD and common hepatic duct fill first. We emphasize the need for taking early filling films as this helps to define the presence or absence of ductal stones (which often show up initially as a meniscus sign). Multiple films are taken as more contrast is injected. It may be necessary to change the scope position to expose the part of the common duct obscured by the scope. The left hepatic ducts fill before the right because they are more dependent with the patient in the prone position. Further injection of contrast will fill the right system. The cystic duct and gallbladder are usually filled by the time the intrahepatic ducts are visualized, and cystic duct obstruction is suspected if they are not. If deep cannulation is achieved before contrast is injected, it is necessary to pull back the catheter to fill the distal duct to avoid missing a small stone. If deep cannulation is achieved with a guide wire, using a double-lumen catheter allows simultaneous injection of contrast. If a single-lumen catheter is used, it should be advanced deep into the duct, and the wire removed; bile is aspirated to remove the air in the catheter before injecting contrast. At the end of the procedure the endoscope is withdrawn and air/fluid is suctioned from the stomach (by rotating the scope to the left) to minimize discomfort and the risk of aspiration. If possible, the patient is turned to a supine position and more radiographs are taken in different projections as the right hepatic system and the tail of the pancreas are often better filled in the supine position. The cystic duct may be more obvious with the patient in the right oblique position as it often overlaps with the common duct.

In patients with a partially filled gallbladder, the diagnosis and exclusion of gallstones may be difficult due to the inadequate mixing of contrast with bile. Delayed films of the gallbladder, preferably with the patient upright, may reveal small stones after adequate mixing.

More details of radiographic technique are given in Chapter 12.

Cannulation of the pancreatic duct and pancreatography

Successful pancreatography and deep cannulation for therapeutics should be achieved in over 90% of standard cases, remembering that there are a few anomalies that make it difficult or impossible.

Most novice endoscopists find pancreatography easier to perform than cholangiography as the PD axis is more horizontal, and in line with the catheter as it emerges from the scope channel. PD cannulation is normally achieved by inserting the catheter (with or without a guide wire) in a direction perpendicular to the duodenal wall, along the 1–2 o'clock orientation in relation to the papillary orifice (Figure 7.8b). Success is assessed by small injections of contrast under fluoroscopy. If a guide wire is used it should not be advanced more than a 1 or 2 cm (unless looping) to prevent entering and damaging a branch duct (or disrupting the small ventral duct if the patient has pancreas divisum).

Full-strength contrast is injected under fluoroscopy to monitor filling of the main duct to the tail and side branches as clinically indicated. Care is taken to avoid overfilling the pancreas. Antegrade filling of the accessory or Santorini's duct is sometimes observed with contrast draining through the minor papilla. Sometimes a dominant branch duct is seen running parallel to the main PD, giving an image of a bifid pancreas. With the patient in a prone position, the tail of the pancreas may not be filled readily.

Cannulation of the minor papilla

The minor papilla is located proximally and to the right of the main papilla. It can be identified as a small protruding structure. It may not be obvious or may appear as a slightly pinkish nipple-like structure between the duodenal folds. When prominent, it can sometimes be mistaken for the main papilla; however, it does not have a distinct vertical fold and the small opening often resists cannulation.

Cannulation is indicated in patients with suspected or proven pancreas divisum on imaging or when cannulation of the main PD fails at the major papilla. It is usually best performed in a long or semilong scope position using a sharply tapered cannula with a 3 FG tip, or with an 0.018″ or 0.021″ protruding guide wire. Shaping the tip of the catheter (Figure 7.12a and b) may be helpful (Video 4, www.wiley.com\go\cotton\ercp), and sometimes cannulation is easier with a miniversion of the standard sphincterotome, for example, 021 Omni sphincterotome (Cook Endoscopy).

It is important to identify the correct location of the orifice before any attempt is made to inject contrast, as trauma from the catheter may result in edema and bleeding, which can obscure the opening. If the papilla or minor orifice is not obvious, it is useful to give an injection of secretin by slow IV infusion and wait 2 min to observe the flow of pancreatic juice. This flow is made more obvious by

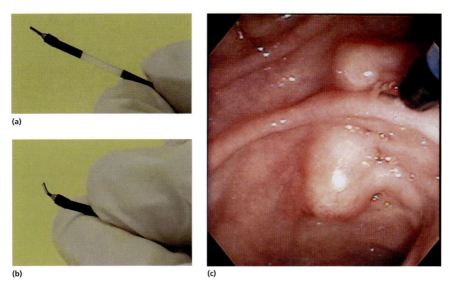

(a)

(b)   (c)

Figure 7.12 (a) Needle tip catheter with a straight tip, (b) gentle bend at needle tip improves the approach to minor papilla, and (c) cannulation of the minor papilla in pancreas divisum.

flushing the area with a diluted indigo carmine or methylene blue solution, which helps to highlight the flow of clear pancreatic juice and shows the opening.

During contrast injection, it is important to monitor the PD filling by fluoroscopy as the tip of the catheter is often obscured by the endoscope in a long scope position.

The success rate for minor papilla cannulation is very operator-dependent, and is certainly lower than that for the main duct.

Techniques of sphincterotomy; biliary, pancreatic, minor

Endoscopic sphincterotomy was first described in 1973. It is designed to allow access to the pancreaticobiliary system for removal of stones and facilitate passage of large or multiple accessories, such as stents. Sphincterotomy is considered the most dangerous part of ERCP procedures as serious complications can occur as a result of an uncontrolled or deviated cut.

Standard biliary sphincterotomy

Most sphincterotomes are either double or triple lumen with a cutting wire exposed for 2–3 cm close to the tip. The other end of the cutting wire is insulated and connected via an adaptor to the diathermy or electrosurgical unit. Triple-lumen sphincterotomes allow injection of contrast and passage of a guide wire

independently through separate channels. Double-lumen varieties sphincterotomes (e.g., DASH system, Cook Endoscopy) have a side-arm adaptor that allows
contrast injection and insertion of a (0.025″ or 0.035″) guide wire at the same
time. The adaptor can be tightened to close an O-ring around the guide wire to
prevent spillage of contrast. The O-ring can be loosened to allow free passage of a
guide wire through the sphincterotome. Rotatable or reverse types are available
for patients with altered anatomy following gastric surgery (e.g., Billroth II gastrectomy). The advantage of double- or triple-lumen sphincterotomes is that they
can be inserted over a guide wire already placed in the ductal system. The wire
anchors and stabilizes the sphincterotome during the cut and ensures that it is
within the confines of the duct. Most of the commonly used guide wires are insulated and can be left in place during sphincterotomy. Most sphincterotome cutting
wires tend to deviate to the right when traction is applied (bowed or tightened),
potentially resulting in a deviated cut and increased risk of complications (i.e.,
bleeding, perforation, and pancreatitis). Shaping the wire as described earlier may
be necessary to ensure that it stays in the correct position when bowed.

After cholangiography, the guide wire is inserted deeply, into the intrahepatic system, to stabilize the sphincterotome. The sphincterotome is then
withdrawn until only one-third of the cutting wire lies within the papilla.
Traction is applied gently to tighten the cutting wire so that it is in firm contact
with the roof of the papilla. Excess bowing should be avoided to prevent an
uncontrolled or "zipper" cut. The position of the wire and contact with the
papillary tissue is adjusted and maintained by the elevator and up/down
control of the endoscope tip.

A blended (cutting and coagulation) current is passed in short bursts to cut
the roof of the papilla in a stepwise manner in the 11–12 o'clock direction.
Whitening of the tissue upon passage of current is indicative of the beginning of
the cut. If the tissue does not blanch within a few seconds, it is necessary to pull
back the sphincterotome wire to reduce the length of wire in contact with the
tissue, thus increasing the current density. It is important to avoid simply
increasing the power setting on the diathermy unit without adjusting or repositioning the cutting wire when the sphincterotomy fails to cut. Too little contact
may generate only smoke and not effective cutting. Excess tension on the cutting
wire may result in a rapid splitting of the tissue upon passage of the electrical
current and an uncontrolled cut.

Axis of a sphincterotomy

In performing a biliary sphincterotomy, it is important to recognize the "perfect" axis, which is the long axis of the distal bile duct and the intraduodenal
portion of the papilla [4]. This is usually denoted by the 11–12 o'clock
direction in relation to the prominence of the papilla and papillary orifice
(Figure 7.13). The sphincterotome and cutting wire should be orientated
along this axis and in a controlled stepwise manner, which allows fine

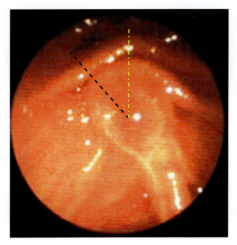

Figure 7.13 Perfect biliary axis along 11–12 o'clock direction (blacked dotted line) in relation to prominence of papilla and papillary orifice and NOT 12 o'clock direction (yellow dotted line) as seen on endoscopy view.

adjustment. The axis that represents the anatomy will not change but the orientation of the papilla can change with the scope position (Video 5, www. wiley.com\go\cotton\ercp). Therefore, it is more important to recognize this imaginary axis and be able to cut along it than to manipulate the scope to put this (biliary) axis in the 12 o'clock position as some endoscopists have suggested.

Adequacy of sphincterotomy

The size (length of cut) needed to perform a complete sphincterotomy depends on the configuration of the distal bile duct and the shape of the papilla. Since these structures can vary greatly, it is important to recognize the limits of a sphincterotomy. It should not go beyond the impression (reflection) of the common duct on the duodenal wall in order to avoid a perforation. The size of the sphincterotomy can be adjusted relative to the intraduodenal segment and not just by an absolute measurement of the cut itself, which we arbitrarily define as small = 1/3, medium = 1/2, and large = 2/3 of the cuttable length (Figure 7.14a and b). A gush of bile is usually seen flowing from the bile duct when the sphincter is cut completely. The size (or adequacy) of a sphincterotomy can be gauged by pulling a fully tightened (bowed) sphincterotome from within the distal bile duct and assessing any resistance to its passage. An alternative method is to pull an inflated stone extraction balloon through the opening. Any deformity of the balloon or resistance to passage indicates the sphincterotomy is smaller than the balloon size, which may predict the ease of extracting a stone. The intended size of the sphincterotomy will depend on the indication (access, stenting, or stone extraction), any prior attempted sphincterotomy, the configuration of the distal

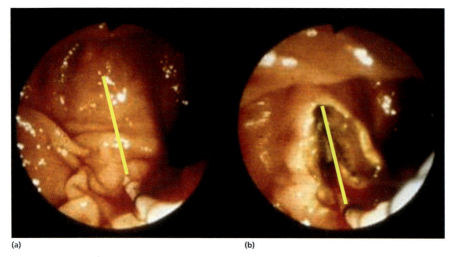

(a)   (b)

Figure 7.14 (a) Intraduodenal papilla and distal bile duct determines the extent of a sphincterotomy cut (black dotted line), (b) a relatively large biliary sphincterotomy (yellow dotted line).

bile duct, and size and shape of the papilla as well as the axis. With large stones, it may be necessary to consider the use of adjuvant therapy such as balloon dilation and lithotripsy to avoid the risks involved in creating too large a sphincterotomy.

Sphincterotomy with periampullary diverticula
Selective cannulation may be technically more difficult if the papilla is on the edge or within a diverticulum, and the risk of perforation may be increased as a result of a deviated cut. It is important to try to appreciate potential changes in the biliary axis before attempting the sphincterotomy, and adjunctive balloon dilation may be needed to minimize the risk of bleeding and perforation (see later).

Sphincterotomy with altered anatomy (Billroth II) cases
A previous Billroth II gastrectomy or hepaticojejunostomy following gastric bypass greatly increases the technical difficulty of ERCP and sphincterotomy. Although a forward-viewing scope (e.g., pediatric colonoscope) may facilitate entry into the afferent loop, most experts prefer to use the side-viewing duode-noscope because of the elevator control. The papilla is seen upside-down when approached from below through the afferent loop. Most of the conventional accessories, including standard sphincterotomes, tend to point away from the bile duct orifice and axis when tightened. This increases the risk of failure as well as complications. The use of a "reverse" sphincterotome, in which the tip of the sphincterotome and wire is shaped such that it points in the correct direction of the bile duct axis, may be helpful. Most experts prefer to place a stent into the distal bile duct, and then to use a needle knife to cut down onto the stent in its

axis. Patients with altered anatomy as a result of gastric bypass operation will require additional devices including single- or double-balloon enteroscopy to access the afferent limb and the papilla (see Chapter 8).

Precut sphincterotomy for impacted stone

The use of precutting to gain access when standard techniques fail is described in detail in Chapter 8. One relatively common and clinically important situation is when cannulation is hindered by a stone impacted at the papilla. The biliary orifice is often displaced more distally because of the bulging papilla, and regular cannulation may still be successful by pushing the scope further into the duodenum or using a semilong position to approach the papilla from below. Use of traction on the sphincterotome to "hook" the biliary orifice is possible with or without a guide wire. Alternatively, a precut sphincterotomy can be performed. This uses a "needle knife," which is basically a bare wire that protrudes for 4–5 mm at the tip of a Teflon catheter. It is effective and relatively safe to cut directly on to the bulging intraduodenal portion of the papilla [5]. The needle knife is placed a little above the biliary orifice (to avoid injury to the pancreatic orifice) and the cut is made upward by lifting the knife with the elevator or with slight upward angulation, to create a fistula. Alternatively, the knife can be used to cut downward onto the bulging papilla by dropping the elevator. The risk of pancreatitis is minimal because the impacted stone pushes the bile duct wall away from the pancreatic orifice. It is not necessary to adjust the diathermy setting although some endoscopists prefer to use a lower power setting on the diathermy unit when considering precut sphincterotomy. Once access to the bile duct is achieved, the sphincterotomy can be extended stepwise either by using the needle knife or by switching to a standard sphincterotome (Figure 7.15 and Video 6, www.wiley.com\go\cotton\ercp). The impacted stone often passes spontaneously into the duodenum after an adequate sphincterotomy is performed.

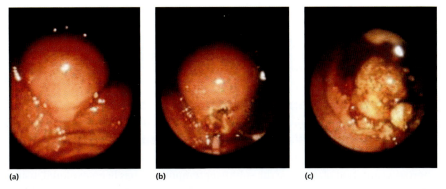

(a)   (b)   (c)

Figure 7.15 (a) Bulging papilla from impacted stone, (b) standard sphincterotome inserted (after needle knife precut) to extend sphincterotomy, and (c) spontaneous passage of impacted stone.

Pancreatic sphincterotomy

Pancreatic sphincterotomy is done to allow access to the PD for removal of ductal stones, dilation and stenting of pancreatic strictures, and much less commonly for the management of pancreatic sphincter of Oddi dysfunction.

The technique of pancreatic sphincterotomy is similar to that for biliary sphincterotomy except that the pancreatic axis is more in the 1–2 o'clock direction, and the duct in general is much smaller. Sphincterotomy is best performed using a smaller-diameter sphincterotome over a guide wire (0.018″ or 0.021″) placed in the midportion of the pancreas, and to cut in a stepwise manner (Video 7, www.wiley.com\go\cotton\ercp). When to stop cutting is easier to judge when there has been a prior biliary sphincterotomy, which exposes the septum (and some experts will do one for that reason). Pancreatic sphincterotomy can also be performed by cutting down onto the septum after placing a stent in the PD. Another useful end point is when a slightly bowed sphincterotome can be pulled and pushed through the orifice with little resistance. Some authorities recommend using only cutting current to reduce the amount of coagulation and possible late stenosis.

It is advisable to leave a 3 Fr or 5 Fr stent in the duct to ensure drainage and to reduce the risk of pancreatitis. These stents usually fall out after a 1 or 2-week but it is necessary to do an X-ray of the abdomen to check.

Minor sphincterotomy

Sphincterotomy of the minor papilla is performed in pancreas divisum to improve drainage of the dorsal duct, and occasionally in patients with normal anatomy and pathology in the head of the pancreas. If cannulation can be achieved using a small pull-type sphincterotome, the minor papilla can be cut in the usual fashion, limiting the extent of the cut to within the duodenal wall (Video 8, www.wiley.com\go\cotton\ercp). The long axis of the dorsal duct is along the 10 o'clock direction so the cut should be directed slightly to the left. Alternatively, a small stent can be placed initially over a guide wire. Sphincterotomy is performed using a needle knife to cut along the axis (Video 9, www.wiley.com\go\cotton\ercp). In all cases it is wise to leave a stent temporarily to prevent pancreatitis, and perhaps to reduce the chance of restenosis.

Dilation of the papillary orifice and strictures

Dilation of the papillary orifice—balloon sphincteroplasty

Because of the known and potential complications of sphincterotomy, an alternative method of opening the sphincter temporarily has been explored, using balloon dilation (so-called balloon sphincteroplasty). The approach is used widely in Eastern countries (see Chapter 14), but not in the United States because of a randomized trial showing a higher incidence of pancreatitis, indeed two deaths. However, it is certainly worth considering in patients at increased risk of bleeding (underlying liver disease, anticoagulation, or antiplatelet therapy).

Balloon sphincteroplasty can be performed easily once a guide wire is inserted deep into the bile duct. Over the guide wire, pneumatic balloons, a fixed diameter (4, 6, 8, or 10 mm) for example, Quantum balloons or Fusion balloons (Cook Endoscopy), or the CRE balloons (Boston Scientific) with a maximum diameter no larger than 15 mm can be used (Figure 7.16a–d). The choice of balloon size depends on the diameter of the distal bile duct and any stone. It appears advantageous to keep the balloon inflated for 5 min [6]. Too short (<1 min) a dilation interval may result in inadequate stretching of the sphincter muscle and the resultant edema may compress the pancreatic orifice increasing the risk of post-dilation pancreatitis. Some experts place a small pancreatic stent before dilation, to reduce this risk. Subsequent stone extraction can be performed with the guide

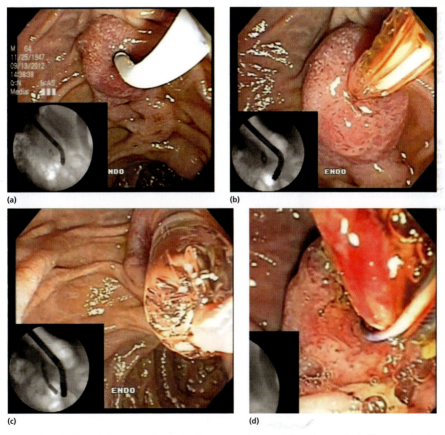

(a)   (b)   (c)   (d)

Figure 7.16 Balloon sphincteroplasty, (a) deep cannulation with catheter, (b) balloon inserted into distal CBD, cholangiogram showed small stone in distal duct, (c) balloon fully inflated, and (d) stone extracted with basket.

wire left *in situ* in case subsequent edema requires the placement of a biliary stent for decompression. In cases where a very large (20 mm) balloon sphincteroplasty is used for extraction of CBD stone, the duration of balloon inflation is still being debated. Some would favor a shorter duration based on the observation that complete obliteration of the waist is indicative of a successful sphincteroplasty and this avoids excess compression of the pancreatic sphincter.

Balloon dilation can be used also to treat a stenosed choledochoduodeostomy and as part of managing pancreatic pseudocysts (see Chapter 22).

Combined sphincterotomy and balloon sphincteroplasty

There is a growing trend in favor of combining a small- to medium-size sphincterotomy with balloon sphincteroplasty for the removal of large CBD stones. This combination reduces, but does not eliminate, the inherent risks of bleeding and perforation. Balloons of up to 20-mm diameter have been used, but it probably wise not to go above 15 mm. Because of a potential change in the axis of the balloon within the sphincter following the sphincterotomy, there may be less compression on the pancreatic orifice and less risk of pancreatitis.

Dilation of ductal strictures

The possible indications for endoscopic management of biliary and PD strictures are discussed in other chapters. Dilation can be achieved (always over a guide wire) with tapered or stepped bougies, or with balloons.

Biliary strictures

Dilation is best performed with a large channel scope using pneumatic noncompliant polyethylene balloons. Balloons come in different sizes and lengths: 4, 6, 8, or 10 mm in diameter and vary from 2 to 6 cm long.

A prior sphincterotomy is not necessary but may facilitate the introduction of large catheters and for exchange of accessories. The balloon is positioned over the guide wire so that the stricture lies at the midpoint, as judged by radio-opaque markers. The balloon is inflated with dilute (10–20%) contrast and the pressure adjusted according to the type of balloon and the manufacturer's recommendation. Effective dilation is achieved when the waist in the balloon disappears (Figure 7.17). The patient may experience pain during balloon distension and additional medication may be needed. The balloon is usually kept inflated for 1–2 min. It is helpful to reinflate the balloon and note the opening pressure when the waist disappears on the balloon. After successful dilation, the opening pressure should be less with repeat dilation.

Repeat dilation at regular (3 months) intervals coupled with placement of multiple plastic stents or fully covered SEMS for up to a year may be necessary to keep benign strictures open (see Chapter 18).

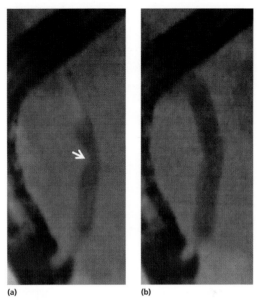

(a)   (b)

Figure 7.17 Distal CBD stricture (see Figure 7.11d), (a) partially inflated balloon showing waist (white arrow) at stricture level, and (b) obliteration of waist on dilation balloon upon full inflation.

Intrahepatic bile duct stones have been successfully removed following balloon dilation of intrahepatic strictures.

Pancreatic strictures

It is essential, but sometimes difficult, to first place a guide wire across the stricture. We use hydrophilic wires or shape the tip of a standard wire to facilitate loop formation (see earlier). Dilation can be performed using graded dilators or balloons. Graded Teflon dilating catheters with tapered tips (e.g., 5, 7, 10 Fr) are often preferred initially with tight strictures, followed by balloon dilation (Figure 7.18a–d). The balloon is kept inflated for 2–3 min. Persistence of the waist and resistance to moving a fully inflated balloon indicates persistence of a tight stricture. Choice of balloon size (usually 4- or 6-mm diameter) depends on the size of the normal part of the duct usually downstream from the obstruction. Larger balloons may be used sometimes in patients with chronic pancreatitis and large ducts.

When very tight strictures fail to admit even the smallest graded dilators, it may be useful to consider using the Soehendra stent retriever (a metal sheath with a screw tip for retrieval of biliary stent). The device is inserted over the guide wire and pushed against the stricture while being rotated slowly in order to "screw" through it (Figure 7.19a–c). This also facilitates subsequent passage of dilation balloons. It is important to align the stent retriever with the long axis of the guide wire when trying to drill through a tight stricture.

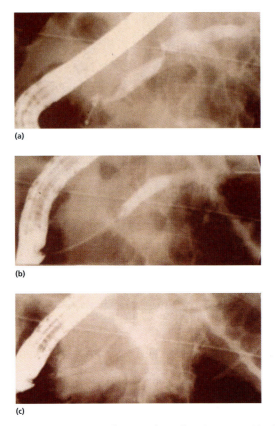

Figure 7.18 (a) Stricture in mid pancreatic duct (PD) from chronic pancreatitis, (b) dilation balloon inflated across the PD stricture, and (c) PD stent in position.

Following dilation, it is usually necessary to place a stent to ensure drainage and decompression of the ductal system. Several small-diameter stents (3–5 FG) of different lengths may function as well as one large stent, and are less likely to cause damage to the duct at the distal tip. Pancreatic stents block as quickly, or more quickly, than biliary stents, so it is common practice to remove or exchange them after a few weeks or months. Indeed, this provides an opportunity to repeat the dilation with a larger balloon.

Bile duct stone extraction

With an adequate biliary sphincterotomy, most small bile duct stones will pass spontaneously. However, this expectant policy carries a risk of stone impaction and subsequent cholangitis. The current recommendation/practice is to remove all the stones at the time of sphincterotomy, and to place a temporary stent if

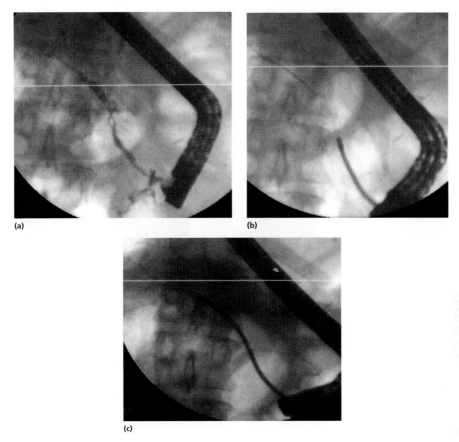

Figure 7.19 (a) Tight PD stricture in mid body, (b) dilation with Soehendra stent retriever over guide wire, and (c) successful stricture dilation with Soehendra stent retriever.

that cannot be achieved. Accessories commonly used for stone extraction include balloons, baskets, and mechanical lithotripters.

Balloon stone extraction

We usually choose an 8 Fr double-lumen catheter with a balloon at the tip. The size of the balloon can be varied depending on the amount of air inflated (8-, 12-, or 15-mm diameter). The stiff tip of the catheter may make cannulation difficult and is best done over an established guide wire. It may be helpful to gently curl the tip of the catheter to facilitate cannulation. When there are several stones, they are best removed one at a time starting with those nearest the papilla (Figure 7.20) (Video 10, www.wiley.com\go\cotton\ercp).

With an adequate sphincterotomy, the stone can be pulled down and expelled from the CBD using downward tip deflection of the scope. Care is taken to avoid pulling the balloon too hard against the stone as excess resistance may rupture the balloon, or it may deform and slip past the stone.

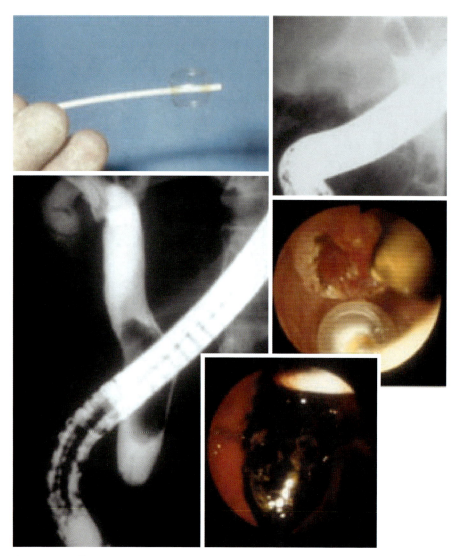

Figure 7.20 Balloon stone extraction. Extraction of small stones with balloon and stones expelled by retracting balloon catheter. Similarly large stone can be removed with balloon if axis is correct.

The possibility of resulting distal stone impaction is defused by maintaining the indwelling guide wire. When resistance is felt, rather than simply pulling harder on the balloon, it is often better to use a downward deflection of the endoscope tip (and right rotation), which keeps the catheter in the correct axis. Complete clearance can be checked by several sweeps of the duct with the balloon, and by an occlusion cholangiogram, that is, by injecting contrast above an inflated balloon.

Basket stone extraction

Stone extraction baskets consist of braided stainless-steel or nitinol wires that can be exposed to open to form a trap. The basket is inserted and opened above the stone and withdrawn in a fully opened position. The basket is moved gently up and down or jiggled around the stone to trap it. When the stone is engaged the basket is closed gently (but not necessarily completely) and pulled back to the level of the papilla. The tip of the endoscope is angled up against the papillary orifice and tension is applied to the basket. The stone is extracted by downward tip deflection and if necessary right rotation of the endoscope (Figure 7.21). The maneuver may

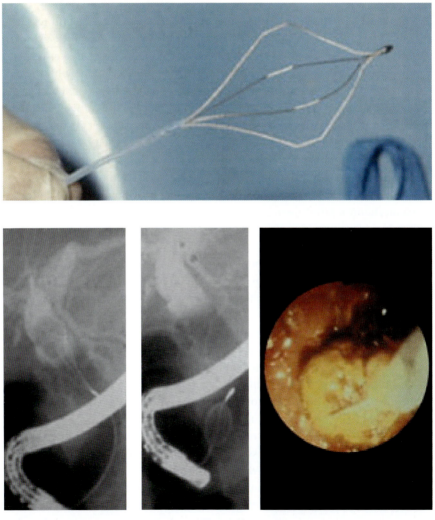

Figure 7.21 Dormia basket stone extraction, basket opened above stone and trawled back to engage stone, stone removed with traction on the basket and (downward) scope tip deflection.

need to be repeated. Again, it is important to start with the lowest stones and to avoid trapping too many at the same time.

It is also important to avoid getting the basket impacted and trapped when these methods fail. Never close the basket tightly around the stone unless one is committed to pull (hard) to remove the stone. Excess tension on the wires may cause them to cut into the stone making it difficult to release. A trapped stone can usually be ejected from the basket by pushing the stone and basket up the duct against the bifurcation, preferably at an angle so that the basket wires tend to buckle. Further advancement of the basket wires will cause them to loop and the stone is dropped. Then close the basket above the stone by advancing the basket sheath. Caution is taken to avoid pushing the stone into the intrahepatic ducts.

In special situations such as intrahepatic stones, it may be helpful to shape the tip of the catheter. If so, do it when the basket is fully opened, so as not to distort the wires. The gently curved (single- or double-curve) basket catheter can be used to deflect the tip of the partially opened basket in line with the axis (usually the left side) of the intrahepatic ducts. The partially opened basket can function like a guide wire, facilitating the advancement of the catheter sheath by opening and closing the basket while advancing the catheter in the selected direction. Alternatively, a wire-guided basket can be inserted over a wire into the respective intrahepatic system.

When these methods for stone extraction fail, a decision must then be made whether to enlarge the sphincterotomy by cutting or balloon dilation and/or to use a mechanical lithotripter.

Mechanical lithotripsy

Large stones (say >10-mm diameter, or bigger than the endoscope on fluoroscopy) are more difficult to remove, especially if there is a discrepancy between the size of the stone and the exit, that is, a relatively small sphincterotomy or balloon sphincteroplasty.

There are several different devices that can be used endoscopically to crush duct stones. The earliest iteration was designed to manage stone and basket impaction. The basket is cut at the handle, and the scope is removed, leaving the basket and stone in place. It is helpful to retain the Teflon sheath. The "Soehendra lithotripter" (Cook Endoscopy) consists of a 14 Fr metal sheath and a self-locking crank handle. The metal sheath is railroaded over the basket wires. Some tape can be used to round off the tip of the sheath to prevent injury to the posterior pharynx and to prevent the wires from being caught at the tip of the sheath. The metal sheath is advanced all the way to the level of the stone under fluoroscopic control. The proximal ends of the wires are then connected to the crank handle and tightened slowly using the self-locking mechanism to crush the stone against the metal sheath (Figure 7.22) [7]. It is important to remember that standard baskets are not designed for lithotripsy. If traction is applied too quickly,

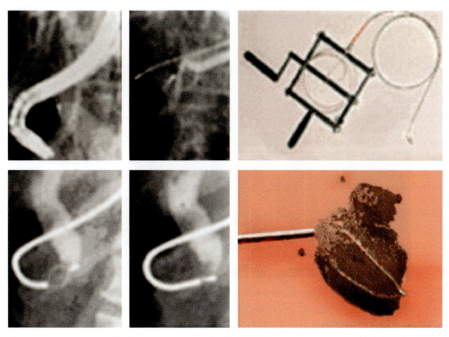

Figure 7.22 Mechanical lithotripsy (Soehendra lithotripter) or "life-saver," metal sheath inserted over basket wires. Stone crushed with a crank handle, this method is used for unexpected stone and basket impaction.

the wires of the basket may break but not the stone. A variant of this technique employs a smaller- (10 Fr) diameter metal sheath that goes through the 4.2-mm channel of a therapeutic scope (over the basket wires). The presence of the scope helps with the manipulation of the basket and in positioning the sheath for proper lithotripsy. In either case, the stone will be fragmented or the basket broken to free the impacted stone. Further procedures may be required to complete the lithotripsy.

Rather than rely on using the Soehendra method to resolve an impaction situation, it is perhaps wiser to use lithotripsy devices designed to go through the scope when difficulty is anticipated. One advantage is that these baskets are designed to break (when needed) in ways that mean that they can be retrieved, rather than get stuck in the patient (which can happen when applying the Soehendra method to standard baskets).

There are several variants of mechanical lithotripsy. Most, such as the BML lithotripter (Olympus Optical Co., Tokyo, Japan), come in three layers, consisting of a large and strong four-wire basket, a Teflon catheter, and an overlying metal sheath (Figure 7.23) [8]. Those whose diameter requires a therapeutic scope channel are more effective, and contrast injection is easier. Cannulation is achieved with the catheter, and the metal sheath is advanced over it when lithotripsy is required. Stone engagement may require complex

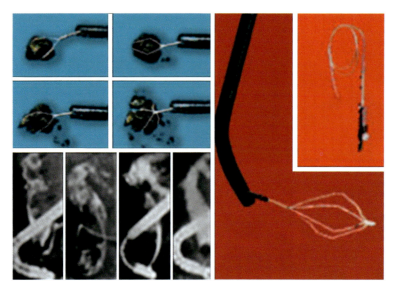

Figure 7.23 Through-the-scope mechanical lithotripter (BML, Olympus). Three layers system with strong wire basket, Teflon sheath and metal sheath connected to crank handle. Large CBD stone(s) are engaged in basket and crushed by traction on wire. Repeat stone crushing may be necessary before complete duct clearance.

maneuvers, such as shaking and rotating the basket. Traction is then applied to the wires by turning the control handle in to crush the stone against the metal sheath. With very hard stones, the basket wires may become deformed. The basket should be removed and the wires reshaped. Repeated stone crushing may be needed.

There are reusable and disposable variants of the standard device, and newer versions in which the metal sheath is covered with a plastic coating that carries a separate channel to accommodate a guide wire, for example, Trapezoid basket (Boston Scientific) or Hercules basket (Cook Endoscopy). Because they are relatively stiff, these baskets are best inserted over the preplaced wire (Figure 7.24a and b).

These lithotripsy baskets can be used for simple stone extraction, but when lithotripsy is needed, the handle of the basket can be connected to a special handle and traction applied to crush the stone against the sheath.

Mechanical lithotripsy is usually effective, and safe, but there have been instances of perforation of the bile duct, and excessive force in removing a basket and stone may bruise the pancreatic orifice and cause pancreatitis. Stents should be placed if extraction fails. In general the straight stent, for example, Cotton-Leung stent can be used (Figure 7.25) but sometimes we prefer those with double pigtails to avoid the risk of stent migration with the straight stents.

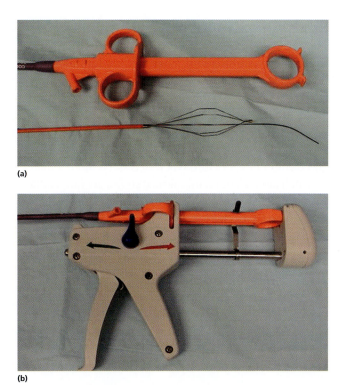

(a)

(b)

Figure 7.24 (a) Newly designed lithotripsy compatible basket and (b) Basket handle connected to cranking device for stone fragmentation.

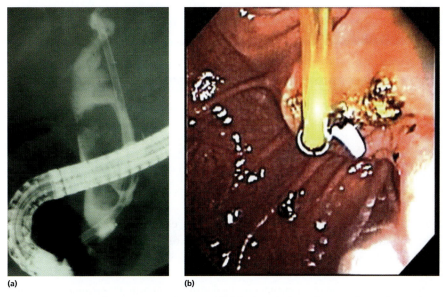

(a)   (b)

Figure 7.25 (a) Straight stent inserted to provide bile duct drainage bypass a large obstructing stone and (b) pus draining from stent.

Pancreatic stone extraction

Pancreatic stones vary considerably from soft sludgy material to diamond-hard calcified stones. Both can be visualized by contract injection during ERCP, and calcified stones show up well on a plain X-ray or computed tomography (CT) scan. Depending on their size and position, they may cause PD obstruction and dilation upstream.

Pancreatic stones can be extracted from the main duct after a pancreatic sphincterototomy and dilation of a stricture when necessary. Sludgy material is easy to remove (even with balloons), but hard calcified stones are often difficult, especially if they track into a branch duct. Baskets and mechanical lithotripters should be used only with great caution, since there is a serious risk of impaction (Figure 7.26a–d). In most cases, a PD stent should be placed after these procedures.

An effective adjunctive method is to use extracorporeal shockwave lithotripsy (ESWL) to fragment the hard stones. ERCP is usually repeated after ESWL to clear the duct, but may not be necessary, since fragments can pass spontaneously.

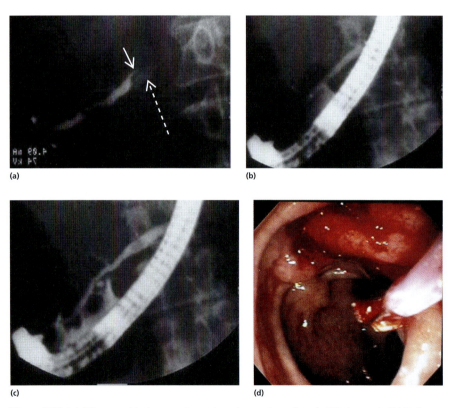

(a)

(b)

(c)

(d)

Figure 7.26 (a) PD stone (dash arrow) causing obstruction of main PD (arrow), (b) balloon dilation of PD obstruction, (c) PD stone visualized in head/neck region, (d) stone removed with Dormia basket.

Tissue sampling from the bile duct

Tissue sampling from the bile duct at the time of ERCP is often indicated to investigate the possibility of malignancy [9]. There are several methods, the advantages and disadvantages of which are discussed in Chapter 19.

Bile can be aspirated after deep CBD cannulation but simple bile cytology has a very low diagnostic yield (at best 25%).

Brush cytology is the most popular technique, using a double-lumen catheter; the brush is held in one lumen, while the other is used to slide the device over a guide wire, which has been placed thought the stricture. With the help of radio-opaque markers, the cytology brush is advanced from the catheter into the dilated proximal duct. The brush is then pulled back to the level of the stricture, and samples are obtained by back and forth movement of the brush through the stricture. An X-ray is taken to document contact of the bare brush with the stricture (Figure 7.27). The brush is then retracted back into the lumen to avoid losing the cells, and the device is removed. The tip of the brush is pushed out and cut off and saved in cytology solution. It may be useful to remove the stylet for the brush and to flush air or cytology solution through the brush channel to collect any retained fluid inside (which may increase the yield for cytology).

A single-lumen system with a thinner catheter can be used if there is a very tight stricture. A guide wire is placed through the obstruction and the catheter sheath of the cytology brush is inserted over it. After the brush has been pushed and pulled through the stricture several times, the catheter sheath is advanced above the stricture, the brush is removed through the sheath, and the tip is prepared for cytology. Bile is aspirated from the catheter (salvage cytology) to improve

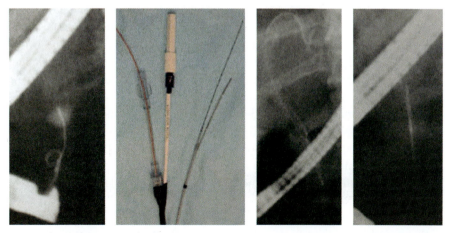

Figure 7.27 Brush cytology of distal bile duct stricture. Double lumen cytology brush, guide wire to negotiate stricture. Brush pushed out above stricture and withdrawn back through the stricture for cytology, X-ray documentation to show (bare) brush in contact with stricture.

the diagnostic yield. The guide wire is then replaced and the cytology sheath is exchanged for the inner catheter of a stenting system.

Several different brush-type devices have been developed, including one with a scoop-like tip with tends to traumatize the stricture and similarly yield more cells. With all methods, the cytological yield may be greater if the stricture is dilated before brushing.

Other methods for obtaining ductal tissue include using small forceps or needle aspiration under fluoroscopic control, or during choledochoscopy (see Chapter 9). Individually, these modalities are not very sensitive, but the accuracy improves if a combination is used (Chapter 19).

Tissue sampling from the pancreatic duct

Brush cytology can be performed in the PD using the double- or single-lumen cytology systems as described earlier. The technique is often difficult because of duct tortuosity and endoscopic ultrasound fine-needle aspiration is nowadays preferred when pancreatic tissue is needed. In patients with suspected main duct or side branch intraductal papillary mucinous neoplasm (IPMN), pancreatic juice can be collected by aspiration after deep PD cannulation, for analysis of tumor markers such as carcino embryonic antigen (CEA).

Nasobiliary catheter drainage for bile duct obstruction

Placing a nasobiliary drain is an alternative to stenting when drainage is required, for example, in patients with acute suppurative cholangitis [10]. The nasobiliary (NB) catheter is relatively easy to insert and is usually well tolerated for a few days (Table 7.3). It allows sequential cholangiography, bile culture, and irrigation [11]. The only disadvantage is that it may become displaced. Naso-gallbladder drains have also been inserted using flexible tip guide wires for drainage of acute cholecystitis.

Following a diagnostic ERCP, deep cannulation of the bile duct is achieved using a 0.035″ or 0.025″ guide wire. A NB catheter is a 6.5–7 Fr polyethylene tube (260 cm in length) with a preformed tip (angled or pigtail) and multiple side holes in the distal 10 cm. It can be inserted into the biliary system over a guide wire with or without a prior sphincterotomy. Direct cannulation is sometimes possible using a NB catheter with a right-angled tip (Figure 7.28). Once the NB catheter is in place, the endoscope is withdrawn slowly while advancing the catheter and guide wire leaving them in the bile duct. This exchange is performed under fluoroscopic control to avoid excess looping of the catheter in the duodenum. A nasopharyngeal or nasogastric suction tube (rerouting tube) is

Table 7.3 Comparison of nasobiliary catheter versus plastic stent for biliary drainage.

	NB catheter (7 Fr)	Stent (10 Fr)
Scope (channel size)	Regular scope (3.2 mm)	Therapeutic scope (4.2 mm)
Drainage	Active decompression (suction)	Passive drainage
Monitoring	Drainage/bile culture	No
Irrigation/dissolution	Yes	No
Complications	Dislodgement and external bile loss	Blockage and failed drainage
Potential risks	Injury to nares	Migration
Patient selection	Cooperative patient	For elderly or confused patients

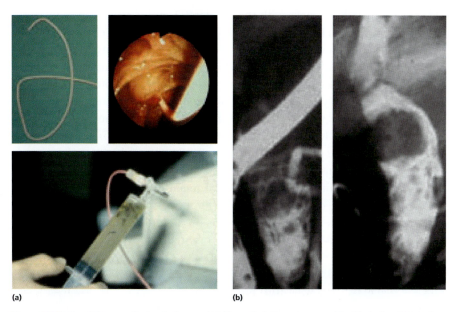

(a)   (b)

Figure 7.28 Nasobiliary catheter drainage. 6.5 Fr angled tip catheter with side holes. NB drain can be inserted with/without a prior sphincterotomy, bile aspirated for decompression via NB drain. NB drainage useful for unstable patients, multiple large stones and coagulopathy.

inserted through a nostril and brought out through the mouth. The end of the NB catheter is inserted through this tube until the proximal end of the catheter appears in the nasopharyngeal tube. The rerouting tube together with the NB catheter are pulled back through the nose. Care is taken to avoid looping and kinking of the NB catheter in the posterior pharynx. The NB catheter is then connected to a three-way adaptor and the bile ducts are decompressed by aspirating bile. A bile sample is sent for culture. The final position of the NB catheter is checked and confirmed under fluoroscopy and the catheter is anchored by taping it to the nose and face. Care is taken to avoid local pressure effect on the nares. The catheter is then connected to a drainage bag.

Biliary stenting

The technique of endoscopic insertion of biliary stents was first described in 1979, and is now an established method for the palliation of malignant obstructive jaundice. It is particularly useful in patients with carcinoma of the pancreas as fewer than 20% of patients are appropriate for surgical resection, and the 5-year survival is very low. While the design of plastic stents has changed little over three decades, there have been important developments in expandable metal stents. Stents are also used in patients with benign strictures.

Plastic stent insertion for malignant biliary obstruction

Side-viewing duodenoscopes with the smaller 3.2-mm channel can only accept 7–8.5 Fr stents, which block rather quickly. The larger 4.2-mm channel duodenscopes allows insertion of 10 or 11.5 Fr stents as well as the larger self-expandable metal stents (SEMS). The most commonly used plastic stents are the straight stents with side flaps anchorage system, for example, the Cotton-Leung stent (Cook Endoscopy) (Figure 7.29). Stents are made of 7, 8.5, 10, or 11.5 Fr radioopaque polyethylene tubes. They vary in length between the two anchoring flaps (5, 7, 8, 9, 10, 11, 12, and 15 cm). The standard applicator system consists of a 0.035″ guide wire (480 cm) with a 3-cm flexible tip, and a 6 Fr radio-opaque Teflon (260 cm in length) guiding catheter with a tapered tip to facilitate cannulation. Some guiding catheters have two metal rings (placed 7 cm apart) at the distal end for ease of identification and for measuring the length of the stricture. The outer pusher tube is made of Teflon and is used for positioning the stent during deployment; 7 Fr stents are inserted directly over a guide wire.

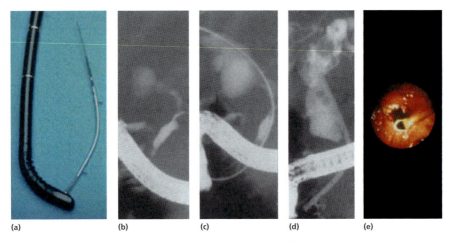

(a)   (b)   (c)   (d)   (e)

Figure 7.29 (a) Biliary stenting system with large channel duodenoscope, 0.035″ guide wire, 6Fr inner catheter, 10 Fr Cotton-Leung stent and 10 Fr pusher, (b) cholangiogram showing distal CBD stricture, (c) contrast filled dilated proximal bile duct with inner catheter and guide wire in position, (d) 10 Fr stent deployed across CBD stricture, and (e) bile draining from stent.

Stents with double pigtails to anchor the stent are useful for patients with stones and in treatment of pseudocysts; a straight stent with side flaps is preferred in malignant disease.

A sphincterotomy is not necessary for placement of a single stent but is useful to facilitate insertion of multiple stents, and may help prevent post-ERCP pancreatitis following stenting for hilar strictures, due to pressure of the distal end of the stents pressing against the pancreatic orifice.

Initial cannulation and insertion of the guide wire past the stricture can be performed using standard accessories. Using a hydrophilic wire or shaping the wire tip may facilitate insertion through angulated strictures. The guiding catheter is then passed over the guide wire beyond the obstruction. The guide wire can be removed to aspirate bile samples for culture and cytology. The length of the stricture is determined on cholangiography with the help of radio-opaque ring markers. A suitable-length stent is chosen so that the proximal flap of the stent lies about 1 cm above the obstruction while the distal flap is placed just outside the papilla.

The optimal length of the stent can be determined by measuring the separation between the proximal obstruction and the level of the papilla on the radiographs. If measurement is made from a radiograph, the correct length is adjusted after correcting for the magnification factor inherent in the fluoroscopy unit. It can also be estimated with reference to the number of scope diameters or by using the radio-opaque markers on the inner catheter. The stent length can also be determined by retracting a guide wire between the two points (i.e., upper level of the obstruction and the papilla) and measuring the distance traveled by the guide wire on the outside at the catheter port. Alternatively, a catheter can be pulled back over an indwelling guide wire from the upper level of obstruction (under fluoroscopy) to the papilla level (as seen on endoscopy) and measuring the distance traveled by the catheter at the biopsy valve (Figure 7.30). The stricture may be dilated (if tight) prior to stent insertion using graded dilators or pneumatic balloon dilators (4, 6, 8 mm) inserted over the guide wire.

The stent is loaded onto the guiding catheter and then advanced through the obstruction with the pusher tube. The stent is deployed by removing the inner catheter and guide wire. Bile is usually seen draining through the stent into the duodenum. The pusher is then removed.

An alternative "one-step" method is to have a suitable length stent (as described earlier) preloaded onto the introducer system and guide wire (Figure 7.31).

Self-expandable metal stents

Multiple types of metal stents have been developed in recent years. Their main advantage is that they expand to a much larger lumen (6, 8, or 10 mm) than plastic stents and block less quickly. They are made of either a continuous woven metal (nitinol) wires or interlaces of multiple (stainless-steel) wires or special

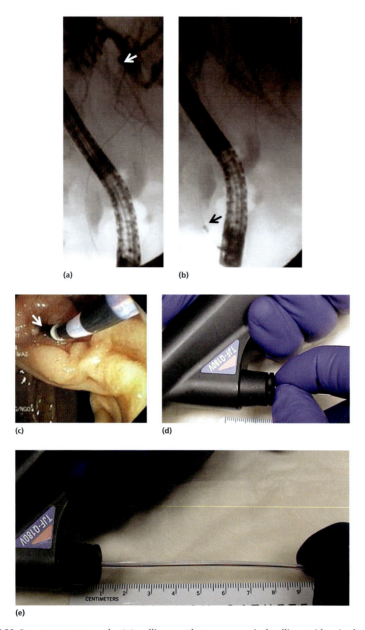

Figure 7.30 Stent measurement by (a) pulling a catheter over an indwelling guide wire back from the level of obstruction (white arrow) to (b) level of papilla (black arrow) under fluoroscopy or (c) seen under endoscopy (white arrow), and (d and e) measuring distance travel by catheter at the biopsy valve.

laser cut wire mesh from a cylindrical tube. In general, nitinol is less radio-opaque than stainless steel and additional radio-opaque (gold or platinum) markers are put on either end of the stents to improve the radio-opacity to facilitate proper positioning during deployment. There are basically two designs of

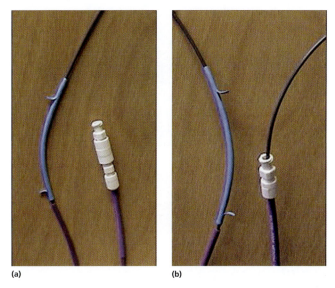

(a) (b)

Figure 7.31 (a) OASIS stenting system by combining inner catheter and pusher as a single unit using a luer lock and (b) unlocking and separating the inner catheter and pusher allows deployment of stent.

SEMS, those that foreshorten upon deployment and those where the length remain unchanged (Figure 7.32a and b). The earlier versions have open mesh designs but partially covered and fully covered (and retrievable) SEMS are now available and their application for biliary drainage will depend on the location of the obstruction and if the intrahepatic bile ducts are involved. The cover membrane is designed to prevent tumor ingrowth and to prolong stent patency. There are stents with a distal antireflux mechanism, and some fully covered SEMS have a retrieval nylon thread that can be used to collapse the stent to facilitate its removal. Other designs are only available in the Asian market, like the Y-stent (Taewoong, Seoul, Korea) for use in hilar lesions. This has a differential cell size in the midportion that allows easy passage of a guide wire through the first stent to facilitate the deployment of a second stent into the opposite side, resulting in a Y-configuration for bilateral drainage.

Introducer system

In general, the wire mesh metal stents are collapsed within a 6–6.5 Fr introducer catheter and restrained by an 8–8.5 Fr overlying plastic sheath. Smaller 6 Fr introducer systems are also available. Sterile water or saline is initially injected to flush the system to minimize friction between the stent and the restraining sheath and to facilitate stent deployment. The whole system is placed over a guide wire and advanced through the obstruction. With the stent correctly positioned across the stricture, the overlying/restraining sheath is pulled back while the applicator handle and introducer catheter is held steady. The stent is deployed slowly in a stepwise manner. Stent deployment can be

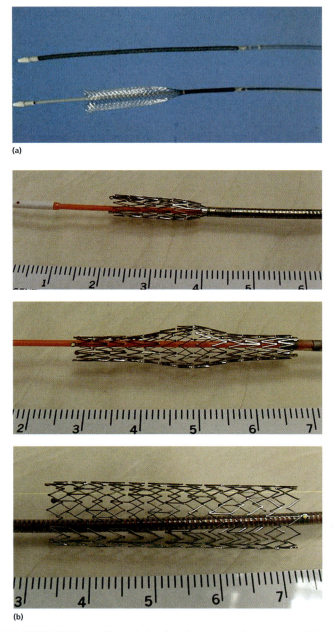

Figure 7.32 (a) SEMS (Wallstent, Boston) that foreshortens on deployment, (b) (top, middle, bottom panels) SEMS (Zilver stent, Cook) that does not foreshorten on deployment.

monitored under fluoroscopy using the radio-opaque markers or endoscopically by observing the distal end of the stent in the duodenum.

For stents that foreshorten, for example, the Wallflex stent (Boston Scientific) or the Evolution stent (Cook Endoscopy), adjustment of the stent position may be necessary before complete/final deployment. The stent can be recaptured in the deployment sheath and the position adjusted before redeployment. It is also easier to pull back than to advance a partially deployed stent through the stricture or obstruction. Newer designs utilize a gun handle design for a more controlled slow release or recapture of the stent during deployment.

For stents that do not foreshorten, for example, Zilver stent (Cook Endoscopy), the deployment is easier based on the position of the radio-opaque markers in relation to the stricture/obstruction. However, for these stents, because of friction between the restraining sheath and the stent, it may be necessary to push ("jerk") and open up the stent before subsequent gentle deployment. This type of stent cannot be recaptured to adjust the position so care should be taken to monitor the position of the radio-opaque markers during deployment (see Chapter 19).

For distal CBD obstruction, most SEMS are placed with the distal tip in the duodenum. Due to the limited lengths available, the stent may be placed completely inside the CBD for mid CBD obstruction or in intrahepatic ducts for hilar strictures. It is important to avoid leaving the tip of the stent just at the level of the papilla as this can cause discomfort.

Stenting for hilar obstruction

Hilar obstruction secondary to cholangiocarcinoma or lymphadenopathy from metastatic disease poses technical challenges to stenting. Whether it is necessary or desirable to drain all of the obstructed ducts remains controversial. The extent of ductal involvement is based on the Bismuth classification depending on the level of obstruction. Type I is cancer involving the common hepatic duct within 2 cm of the bifurcation but with communication between the right and left hepatic ducts. Type II is obstruction at the hilum with involvement of the right and left hepatic ducts but without involvement of the tertiary branch ducts. Type III is involvement of tertiary branch ducts limited to the right (IIIA) or left (IIIB) duct system. Type IV is involvement of tertiary branch ducts bilaterally. Type I and II are potentially resectable but type III and IV lesions are usually not.

Magnetic resonance cholangiopancreatography (MRCP) is the best noninvasive diagnostic imaging for initial assessment of the extent of ductal obstruction and underlying pathology as discussed in Chapter 19. In patients with multiple-segment involvement, contrast injection may outline the obstructed system but carries the risk of sepsis if drainage is inadequate. Indeed, preselection of the intrahepatic system for drainage with selective cannulation using a guide wire without injection of contrast is feasible, thus keeping the risk of infection to a minimum.

If endoscopic drainage fails, percutaneous transhepatic drainage of the obstructed system may be considered or the combined percutaneous and endoscopic approach (rendezvous procedure).

Prior studies have suggested that the recovery of liver function is proportional to the amount of liver volume/tissue successfully drained. Patients' survival is improved if >50% of the liver is drained. Ideally, more than one intrahepatic segment should be drained to achieve maximal benefits and we need to consider placement of one or more stents for bilateral biliary drainage using either plastic or SEMS.

Single-stent placement

Single stent placement is good enough for patients with type I obstruction because there is still communication between the right and left hepatic system. Plastic stents should be used if the patient is deemed resectable to avoid problems related to SEMS at the time of surgery. Because the right hepatic duct branches off after 1 cm whereas the left hepatic duct branches off after 2 cm, it would be more beneficial to consider selective cannulation of the left hepatic duct in the hope of prolonging drainage of two or more segments of the liver in the left lobe even when growth and extension of the tumor involve the bifurcation. Selective cannulation can be achieved with shaping of the guide wire for more easy deflection into the left hepatic system. Subsequent balloon dilation and brush cytology can be performed. The usual straight stent is good for the right hepatic system but a straight plastic stent may kink if it is placed in the left hepatic duct. This may require some preshaping or modification before the stent is inserted.

Placement of a SEMS is preferred in patients who are unlikely to proceed to surgery, and, because of the available lengths, stents are usually placed entirely inside the biliary system.

Multiple stents

In patients with type II or more extensive hilar involvement, and especially when contrast has entered more than one segment, it is necessary to consider placing two or more stents. This will require the initial placement of two guide wires, one each into the right and left hepatic system, respectively. The guide wires can be anchored using wire-locks or hemostats at the biopsy valve level. Most hilar strictures are tight and will require dilating with stepped dilators or balloons (6–8 mm). Brush cytology can be applied also. Either plastic or metal stents can be used. For bilateral stenting, placement of plastic stents is done in a parallel configuration (Figure 7.33). In most cases, it is preferable to consider stenting the left side first (using a modified stent), which is more difficult because of the anatomy and axis. The first plastic stent is placed with the distal tip a little further out in the duodenum. This is followed by insertion of the stent into the right side, which is technically easier. The second stent tends to drag the first stent further up the duct during insertion.

Bilateral SEMS

Bilateral SEMS can be deployed after placing appropriate guide wires and balloon dilation (Figure 7.34). Parallel SEMS placement is technically difficult if the stents are inserted one after another. Advancement of the second applicator

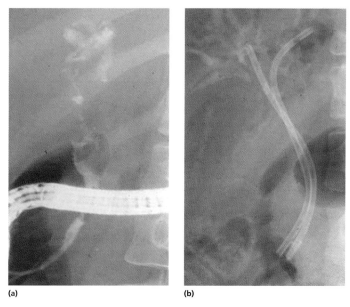

(a)   (b)

Figure 7.33 Bilateral plastic stents for hilar obstruction (a) extensive tumor obstruction of CBD/CHD and right and left hepatic ducts, (b) two 10 Fr plastic stents inserted into the right and left hepatic ducts.

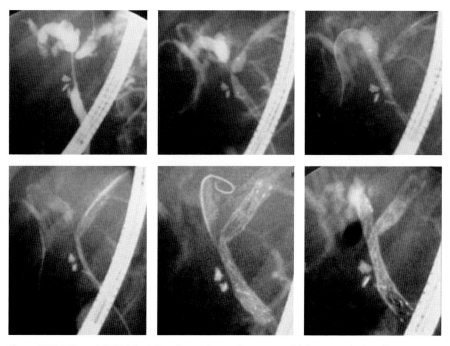

Figure 7.34 Bilateral SEMS for hilar obstruction, using stents with large mesh size allows passage of guide wire easily. Initial placement of two guide wires followed by balloon dilation of both right and left hepatic strictures, a SEMS is deployed in the left system followed by passage of guide wire through the mesh into right system and final deployment of SEMS in right hepatic duct giving a Y-configuration for the dual stenting.

system can be difficult because of the expansion of the distal end of the first SEMS inside the duct. The introduction of the 6 Fr delivery system allows two smaller stents (635 Zilver stents, Cook Endoscopy) to be placed simultaneously through a large channel (4.2 mm) duodenoscope. Lubrication is required to minimize friction, and the deployment is performed slowly while monitoring for the gradual expansion of the stents under fluoroscopy (Video 11, www.wiley.com\go\cotton\ercp). The stent-in-stent or Y-stent system allows placement of two stents. The first stent is placed into the right intrahepatic duct. A second guide wire is passed through the large mesh opening of the first stent into the right system, and a second stent deployed, resulting in a Y-configuration. Retrospective and randomized control studies showed that the Y-configuration or the smaller 6 Fr stenting systems both increase the success of bilateral stenting for hilar obstruction.

Multiple biliary stents for benign strictures

In patients with benign biliary strictures, placement of multiple stents to attain a maximum lumen diameter is preferable to gain long-term patency (see Chapter 18). This can be technically challenging because of the need for repeat cannulation and insertion of guide wires. The process is easier with the newer short wire systems. The concept of intraductal exchange and/or release of the guide wire has revolutionized therapeutic procedures by allowing and maintaining continuous access to the bile duct (or across a stricture) with minimal exchange conducted over a short guide wire. If necessary, a long guide wire can be cut short to turn it into a short wire system for use with the Fusion accessories. It is easy to exchange the wire-lock mechanism by inserting the wire guide adaptor through the special biopsy valve and introduce the wire retrogradely through the adaptor to traverse the valve, which can then be anchored onto the scope (Figure 7.7a–d). Finally, in situations where intervention requires use of standard-length accessories or when control over the guide wire is difficult, a standard-length guide wire can be inserted through the end of the accessory and exchange performed in the usual manner.

With this system, the guide wire is left across the stricture or papilla to facilitate deployment of subsequent stents without the concerns of losing access (Figure 7.6a and b). In addition, because the stent is "caught" between the inner catheter and pusher by the guide wire entering the side hole, repositioning especially in pulling back a malpositioned stent can be performed easily to adjust the stent position before final deployment. Stent deployment requires disengagement (release) of the guide wire from the inner catheter within the bile duct lumen. This is achieved by advancing the inner catheter further above the tip of the guide wire to free the guide wire. The stent is then deployed by pulling back the inner catheter while holding it in position with the pusher. Alternatively, the proximal end of the guide wire is unlocked from the valve and pulled back gently to free the distal tip. The free wire is then locked until the stent is deployed and the introducer system removed before readjusting the wire position further up into the bile duct. Because of the friction within the scope channel, advancing the guide wire with the stenting system in place can result in looping of the guide wire in the duodenum and losing its access across the stricture. The inner catheter and pusher of the Fusion system are smaller than the regular OASIS stenting system, but it is reinforced by a stainless-steel stylet wire that provides the mechanical force for stent insertion. Since the guide wire is now outside of the stenting system and does not offer any mechanical advantage to the pushing of the stent, fixing the distal tip of the inner catheter with the guide wire in position helps advancing the stent, and the guide wire should be released as late as possible before final stent deployment (Video 12, www.wiley.com\go\cotton\ercp).

Results of biliary stenting

The technical success rates for biliary stenting vary depending on the level of obstruction. Successful drainage for mid or distal CBD obstruction can exceed 90% but is much lower for hilar obstruction. Failure may be secondary to tumor compression and/or distortion of the duodenum, marked displacement of the papilla, or failure to insert a guide wire through a very tight stricture. Clinical success is usually easy to assess. With a jaundiced patient, pruritus usually disappears within days; the serum bilirubin declines by a mean of 2–3 mg/dl per day and may return to normal after 1–2 weeks. Incomplete or slow recovery of liver function may be related to prolonged obstruction, which affects hepatocyte function, or may be due to inadequate or incomplete drainage because of poor stent position, or involvement of multiple segments as in the case with hilar obstruction. When in doubt, the presence of air in the ducts on a plain film is reassuring. Patency can also be assessed by an isotope scan.

Early complications of stenting include pancreatitis, bleeding if a sphincterotomy is performed, cholangitis in patients with bifurcation obstruction, and early stent blockage by blood clots. Guide wire perforation (penetration) through a soft and necrotic tumor has been reported. Distal stent migration and traumatic ulceration of the duodenum by the distal tip of the stent (and rarely duodenal perforation) have been reported. Acute cholecystitis secondary to stenting is a rare complication.

Recurrent jaundice is the major late complication of endoscopic stenting. Tumor extension may account for a few cases, but most are due to clogging by biliary sludge. Sludge consists largely of calcium bilirubinate and small amounts of calcium palmitate, cholesterol, mucoprotein, and bacteria. The bacteria are mostly large bowel flora, which can ascend from the duodenum. Larger-lumen stents delay the onset of clogging, but antibacterial plastics and prophylactic antibiotics have not produced any clinically significant benefits [12]. The stent blockage problem is currently managed by exchanging (plastic) stents at regular intervals or by using SEMS. Covered metal stents reduces the risk of tumor ingrowth, but does not prevent clogging, and covered stents have a tendency to migrate.

Biliary stent migration

Distal stent migration—Depending on stent design, bile duct stricture, and size of stones/sphincterotomy (for stone extraction), plastic stents are at risk of distal migration. The commonly used plastic stents are straight stents with an angle in the distal shaft (e.g., Boston Scientific) or a C-curve in the midshaft (Cotton-Leung stent, Cook Endoscopy) and flaps anchorage system. The C-curve on the shaft (which can be molded using hot water) conforms to the bile duct anatomy, and this spring-like effect helps to resist downward stent migration [13]. However, without a tight stricture or large bile duct stone, most stents tend to migrate. The distally migrated stent can cause irritation/ulceration on the opposite duodenal wall and very rarely perforation of the duodenum. This problem can be overcome with the use of double-pigtail stents.

Proximal stent migration—Upward/inward migration of plastic stent is possible if a large sphincterotomy is performed or the distal anchoring flap is collapsed. The migrated stent can be removed using rat tooth forceps, basket, or stone extraction balloon to pull the stent back into the duodenum. A sphincterotomy may facilitate stent removal. Difficulty arises if the distal end of the stent is embedded in the distal bile duct wall. If the end of the stent is still in line with the distal bile duct axis and below the stricture, we try to cannulate the stent using a wire guide sphincterotome or balloon catheter. If successful, the wire is advanced through the stent into the intrahepatic duct followed by the sphincterotome. Traction is applied to the cutting wire to create friction inside of the stent. The stent is dragged out of the bile duct using the sphincterotome and removed with a snare (Video 13, www.wiley.com\go\cotton\ercp). Alternatively, a stone extraction balloon is inserted into the stent and inflated to create friction to pull the stent (Video 14, www.wiley.com\go\cotton\ercp). We did not find the Soehendra stent retriever useful as the relatively stiff retriever tends to jerk the stent further up the bile duct during engagement. In difficult cases, we have used a Dormia basket inserted deep into the bile duct to engage the top end of the stent and dragging it out of the bile duct. This maneuver is traumatic and may result in tissue injury and bleeding. In the unlikely situation that the stent migrated above the stricture, dilation of the stricture may be necessary to facilitate retrieval [14].

Plastic stents in the pancreas

Stents are placed in the pancreas temporarily to reduce the risk of postprocedure pancreatitis (Chapters 5 and 24), and to treat obstruction due to strictures or stones. The commonly used pancreatic stents are smaller than biliary stents, varying from 3 Fr to 7 Fr in diameter; 10 Fr stents are sometimes used in chronic pancreatitis. The lengths vary from 3 to 12 cm. The stents may have anchoring systems with double side flaps (Geenen stents, Cook Endoscopy) or an external pigtail to prevent migration into the duct. There are multiple side holes in the shaft of the

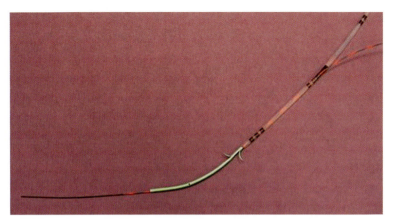

Figure 7.35 Pancreatic stent placement using a Fusion (short wire) catheter system to minimize exchanges.

stents to allow better drainage of pancreatic juice from the side branches. The technique is similar to biliary stenting, except that stents are placed directly over a guide wire without a guiding catheter system. With the long wire system, the pancreatic stent is loaded directly on the guide wire and inserted into position using a similar-size pusher tube. The guide wire is then removed to release the stent. The exchange process involved with stent placement can be simplified by the use of the short wire system. The guide wire is inserted into the pancreas and locked at the biopsy valve. A suitable-length stent is chosen and inserted over the guide wire followed by the use of the Fusion catheter, which has a side port placed at 6 cm. The guide wire emerges from the side port and is then locked in place. The stent is pushed into position by advancing the catheter (Figure 7.35). Since the guide wire is held steady by the wire lock, there will be little movement of the wire, minimizing the risk of the guide wire irritating the PD or side branches.

Small stents (3, 4, or 5 Fr) are used to prevent pancreatitis after ERCP. Some experts use short stents (4–5 cm), others prefer to cross the genu (8–12 cm). The stents have no internal flaps and are designed to pass spontaneously. This usually happens within 1–3 weeks, and a plain X-ray is taken to monitor migration. Retained stents can cause serious problems in the pancreas, so repeat endoscopy may be necessary to extract them.

Endoscopic management of bile leaks

The problem of postsurgical bile leaks is discussed in Chapter 15. They can usually be treated effectively by endoscopic stenting, sphincterotomy, or stenting, or combinations. Sphincterotomy can usually be avoided (with its attendant risks), since small leaks from the cystic duct usually resolve with placement of a NB catheter or stenting (with a short stent just across the papilla) for a few days. A leak associated with a duct injury may require placement of a stent across the leak for up to 4–6 weeks, and it is important to check for residual damage duct after removal of the stent, which may require further treatment.

Conclusion

In this section, we have discussed the different techniques and equipment used for ERCP in the management of patients with many underlying pancreatic and biliary pathologies. The most important issue is to recognize the respective axis of the ductal systems, and understand the limitations with each technique to ensure a safe procedure. When these various techniques are best used (and avoided) is discussed in the relevant clinical chapters.

References

1 Cotton PB, Williams C. Practical Gastrointestinal Endoscopy. 4th Edition, Oxford: Blackwell Science; 1996.
2 Leung JWC. Fundamentals of ERCP, in Cotton L., Ed. Advanced Digestive Endoscopy: ERCP. Malden, MA: Blackwell Publishing; 2005, pp. 17–81.
3 Lim B, Leung J. Wire for hire: the impact of wire-guided cannulation in ERCP. Gastrointest Endosc 2009;69:450–452.
4 Leung JWC, Leung FW. Papillotomy performance scoring scale—a pilot validation study focused on the cut axis. Aliment Pharmac Ther 2006;24:308–312.
5 Leung JWC, Banez VP, Chung SCS. Precut (needle knife) papillotomy for impacted common bile duct stone at the ampulla. Am J Gastroenterol 1990;85:991–993.
6 Liao WC, Lee CT, Chang CY, et al. Randomized trial of 1-minute versus 5-minute endoscopic balloon dilation for extraction of bile duct stones. Gastrointest Endosc 2010;72:1154–1162.
7 Ngo C, Leung JWC. Stone extraction, in Baron K and Carr-Locke DL, Eds. ERCP. 2nd Edition. Philadelphia, PA: Elsevier; 2013, 152–165.
8 Leung JWC, Neuhaus H, Chopita N. Mechanical lithotripsy in the common bile duct. Endoscopy 2001;33(9):800–804.
9 Lee JG, Leung JWC. Tissue sampling at ERCP in suspected pancreatic cancer. Gastrointest Endosc Clin N Am 1998;8:221–235.
10 Leung JWC, Cotton PB. Endoscopic nasobiliary catheter drainage in biliary and pancreatic disease. Am J Gastroenterol 1991;86:389–394.
11 Leung JWC, Chung SCS, Sung JY, et al. Urgent endoscopic drainage for acute suppurative cholangitis. Lancet 1989;1:1307–1309.
12 Libby E, Leung JWC. Prevention of biliary stent clogging: a clinical review. Am J Gastroenterol 1996;91:1301–1308.
13 Leung JWC. Whenever I place a stent for a stone impacted bile duct or for bile leak, the stent always seem to shift position distally, should I use a shorter stent or a pigtail stent? Is there a trick to keep these stent in place?, in Leung JWC and Lo S, Eds. Curbside Consultation in Endoscopy. Thorofare, NJ: Slack Inc.; 2008, 139–141.
14 Tarnasky PR, Cotton PB, Baillie J, et al. Proximal migration of biliary stents: attempted endoscopic retrieval in forty-one patients. Gastrointestinal Endoscopy 1995;42:513–519.

CHAPTER 8

When standard cannulation approaches fail

Sundeep Lakhtakia[1], Bronte A. Holt[2], & Shyam Varadarajulu[2]

[1] Asian Institute of Gastroenterology, Hyderabad, India
[2] Center for Interventional Endoscopy, Florida Hospital, Orlando, USA

KEY POINTS

- Selective cannulation is almost always achievable by experts using standard methods in patients with normal anatomy and no major pathology in the region of the papilla.

- When difficulties arise, deep biliary cannulation is best attempted using double guide wire and needle-knife techniques (best over a pancreatic stent).

- Rendezvous approaches allow endoscopic retrograde cholangiopancreatography (ERCP) after a guide wire has been passed antegradely through the papilla via the transhepatic route, or with endoscopic ultrasound (EUS).

- Patients with surgically altered biliary anatomy are increasingly common and pose the greatest challenges.

- These advanced techniques carry significant risks.

Principles of biliary access

The principle of selective biliary cannulation is akin to a skilled firefighter (endoscopist) who has to enter a building (bile duct) to evacuate trapped residents (obstructive pathology). Unlocking the latches at the entry gate (standard cannulation) should be the first attempt to enter the building without bothering the neighbor (pancreas). Trying to break in (traumatic cannulation attempts) or repeated knocking at the neighbor's door (pancreatic injections) can complicate the situation (post-ERCP pancreatitis (PEP)). If the neighbor's (pancreas) gate opens first, it is prudent to evacuate him (prophylactic pancreatic duct (PD) stent) to limit damage. Once successful entry is gained into the building (selective bile duct cannulation) the doors can be opened (sphincterotomy) to enable entry of fire extinguishers (accessories) to facilitate the exit of trapped residents (obstructed bile). If entry from the main gate to the building is not possible, a drill can be used

---

ERCP: The Fundamentals, Second Edition. Edited by Peter B. Cotton and Joseph Leung.
© 2015 John Wiley & Sons, Ltd. Published 2015 by John Wiley & Sons, Ltd.
Companion Website: www.wiley.com\go\cotton\ercp

to make a window (precut or EUS-guided common bile duct (CBD) access). If this fails, attempts to enter from the rear (percutaneous or EUS-guided transhepatic rendezvous) to help open the main gate (major papilla) or exit from rear gate itself (hepaticogastrostomy, choledochoduodenostomy, or percutaneous drainage catheter) may be required.

KEY POINTS

- Planning the cannulation technique: If it appears that standard biliary cannulation will be difficult, have a plan for the next method to use to gain access.

- Cannulation hierarchy is guided by papillary and duodenal anatomy, proceduralist skill set, and availability of ERCP accessories. As a general rule, the lowest risk and most familiar cannulation technique should be used first.

- When ERCP cannulation fails: Consider rescheduling the procedure for a second attempt after 24–48 h to allow time for the ampullary edema to subside, which can help identify the ampullary and ductal tissue planes. Consider asking a colleague for assistance during the initial or subsequent procedure. Consider a combined procedure with EUS or PTC guidance.

Placement of double guide wire or pancreatic stent to facilitate biliary access

Inadvertent and repeated cannulation of the PD can be frustrating if the duct of choice is the CBD. In such situations, passing a pancreatic guide wire or placing a pancreatic stent may facilitate biliary wire-guided cannulation [1]. The double guide wire technique involves placing a wire in the PD, then passing the cannula or sphincterotome with the biliary guide wire down the working channel, beside the pancreatic wire. The tip of the cannula or sphincterotome is aimed toward the superior lip of the papillary orifice, directing toward 11 o'clock. The pancreatic guide wire stabilizes and lifts the papilla toward the working channel, straightens the PD, and orients the biliary opening for selective access. It can also be used to place a prophylactic pancreatic stent, either before or after successful biliary cannulation. This technique is particularly useful in patients with surgically altered anatomy or a tortuous common channel. Negotiating the pancreatic guide wire through to the pancreatic body or tail can be challenging, as it may repeatedly enter the ductal side branches, with a resultant risk of PD perforation and pancreatitis. Anatomical variations such as a tortuous duct, complete or incomplete pancreas divisum, and ansa pancreatica can increase the difficulty. In these cases, using a thinner (0.018 in.) or nitinol-tipped wire may assist. Flipping the tip over may facilitate deep penetration.

Precut or access sphincterotomy

> ### KEY POINTS
>
> - Precut technique allows biliary access after failed initial cannulation.
> - The margin for error is much smaller when performing precut sphincterotomy than for standard sphincterotomy. Training should begin with the observation of multiple precut procedures, and progress to hands-on training when proficient at standard cannulation.
> - Precut is associated with a higher risk of complications [2, 3].
> - Precut is most commonly performed with a needle knife in a "below upward" direction, starting from the papillary orifice and cutting upward in layer-by-layer fashion.
> - Fistulotomy or "above downward" NKS is another useful access technique.
> - If a precut is performed, placement of a prophylactic PD stent reduces the chances of PEP.

Precut sphincterotomy or papillotomy technique refers to gaining access to the bile duct by deroofing the duodenal portion of the ampulla and incising the terminal bile duct. Precut is the most commonly used technique after conventional methods fail [4]. Precut is usually followed by conventional sphincterotomy to complete planned therapy such as stone extraction or stent placement. The decision to perform a precut depends on the indication for ERCP, "comfort level" of the endoscopist, and anatomical orientation of the papilla. Precut sphincterotomy is usually performed using a needle-knife catheter or occasionally with a traction papillotome.

Procedural techniques

Free-hand needle-knife sphincterotomy: The papilla can be incised either from "below upward" (Video 1, www.wiley.com\go\cotton\ercp), starting from the papillary orifice and cutting up toward the 11 o'clock direction, or approaching "above downward" (Video 2, www.wiley.com\go\cotton\ercp), starting from the junction of the upper one-third and lower two-third of the ampullary mound and cutting down toward the papilla. Most ERCP experts prefer the "below upward" approach. The needle knife is opened to expose 2–4 mm of the cutting segment. The needle-knife movements have to be precise, cutting in 1–2-mm longitudinal increments, with the intention of cutting the papilla down to the bile duct layer by layer.

- "Below upward" free-hand NKS

The needle-knife tip is placed at the superior aspect of the papillary orifice in the 11–12 o'clock position and the tissue is slightly tented in the direction of the planned cut. The cut extends upward along the ampullary mound in the 11–12 o'clock direction. The direction is controlled by either an upward motion with the large wheel and gentle leftward torsion or an upward sweeping motion of the elevator. The aim is to deroof the papillary mound in a controlled, stepwise fashion within one to three passes. The depth of the incision should be periodically checked by separating the cut edges with air or carbon dioxide insufflation, by saline irrigation through the needle-knife catheter, or by using the blunt end of the closed catheter. The proximal extent of the cut is determined by the intraduodenal bile duct, and must stop short of the upper margin of the ampullary mound. The intramural bile duct is seen as yellowish-white longitudinal muscular tissue. On further incision of the bile duct wall and with gentle suction, a speck of yellow-tinged bile is often visualized, especially if the proximal bile duct is not tightly obstructed. The bile duct is then selectively cannulated using a soft guide wire either through the needle knife or with a standard sphincterotome. Direct contrast injection from a distally impacted cannula should be avoided due to the risk of intramural extravasation within the divided tissue planes. Once the guide wire is passed into the biliary system, the sphincterotomy can be undertaken in the standard manner.

• "Above downward" free-hand NKS

The needle is positioned at the junction of upper third and the lower two-thirds of the ampullary mound. The incision generally starts in the 11 o'clock position, and extends down toward 5 o'clock, stopping short of the papillary orifice. The technique of incising the ampullary mound and not extending to the papillary orifice is also termed a fistulotomy (Video 3, www.wiley.com\go\cotton\ercp). Maintaining an inward thrust on the needle-knife catheter while cutting exerts enough pressure on the surface of the ampulla to stretch it and achieve an appropriate depth of incision. A downward motion with the large wheel of the duodenoscope and scope torsion controls the direction and the depth of cut. The correct tissue plane is generally entered with two to three incisions. The potential advantages of this method are reduction in the perforation risk as the upper extent of the cut is predefined, and reduction in the risk of pancreatitis because the pancreatic orifice remains untouched. This technique is useful in cases with an impacted ampullary stone or any papillary orifice obstruction with bulging infundibulum of intramural CBD.

Suprapapillary fistulotomy/infundibulotomy: This technique is only used in patients with a dilated bile duct causing a distinct impression upon the duodenal wall, and is generally above the occluded papillary orifice. A small opening is made into the intraduodenal segment of CBD, using a few "stabs" of short duration with a needle knife, in the endocut or blended current mode. The point of entry is 3–5 mm superior to the papillary orifice measured visually on the vertical axis. A spot of bile is often seen after incising the mucosa, and the opening is then probed with a cannula and guide wire to create a choledochoduodenal fistula. This technique should be avoided in patients with altered anatomy.

Over-the-stent NKS: Over-the-stent NKS is a technique where the needle-knife precut is performed after prophylactic PD stent placement, typically after repeated inadvertent PD cannulation. The PD stent protects the pancreatic orifice and reduces the chance of PEP [5], as well as straightens the intramural ampullary segment to facilitate passage of a guide wire into the CBD. The PD orifice is generally oriented in the 5 o'clock position, and the stent also serves as a landmark to help localize the biliary orifice, which is generally in the 11 o'clock position.

Less common precut techniques

- *Traction papillotome technique*: This technique (also referred to as "papillary roof incision") was originally described using a specialized short-nosed papillotome. The papillotome is wedged into the common channel, and the incision is made in the direction of the bile duct without wire guidance [6].
- *Transpancreatic precut sphincterotomy*: The tip of a standard sphincterotome is intentionally inserted into the PD. Incision is made in the direction of the bile duct, through the septum dividing the biliary and PD [7]. If feasible, a prophylactic pancreatic stent should be placed as there is a significant risk of PEP. There are also potential long-term consequences of a pancreatic sphincterotomy, such as pancreatic orifice stenosis [8].
- *Intramural incision technique*: This technique utilizes the false tract that can be created by the guide wire during biliary cannulation attempts. The sphincterotome is positioned in the false track at the intramural portion of the papilla and the biliary orifice is unroofed from the inside to out [9].
- *Endoscopic ampullectomy*: This has been reported as a technique for biliary access when other methods have failed in a very select group of patients [10].

Precut complications

The main complications include pancreatitis, perforation, and bleeding. It is often argued whether complications of precut are due to the precut itself or the preceding multiple failed cannulation attempts. A prospective, randomized multicenter study showed the pancreatitis risk was lower with early precut compared to persisting with cannulation attempts than performing a late precut [11]. A meta-analysis showed that conventional precut sphincterotomy without a pancreatic stent was a significant risk for PEP even after adjusting for other variables [12]. Prophylactic PD stent placement should always be considered.

Precut learning curve

Three studies [13–15] involving 603 patients have evaluated the learning curve for performing precut sphincterotomy (Table 8.1). While two studies did not demonstrate a learning curve to achieve proficiency [13, 14], in one study the success rates improved from 88 to 98% with time [15]. Also, while there was no difference in rates of complications in two studies [14, 15], in one study the complication rate decreased from 28 to 7% with time [13].

Table 8.1 Precut sphincterotomy learning curve.

Author	No.	Initial success (%)	Final success (%)	Complications	Learning curve
Akaraviputh et al. [13]	200	88	82	2 to 7%	Tech: No Complications: Yes
Robison et al. [14]	150	84	92	7%	No (after 200)
Harewood and Baron [15]	253	88	98	12-14%	Tech: Yes Complications: No

Intradiverticular papilla

Cannulation of the ampulla inside a diverticulum can be challenging (Video 4, www.wiley.com\go\cotton\ercp). The ampulla is most commonly on the rim of the diverticulum, but can be located anywhere within. The duodenoscope and sphincterotome should be aligned with the direction of the intradiverticular ampullary mound, which may require significant "right–left" movements with the small wheel and scope torsion. Often the ampulla can be exposed by "pulling" the surrounding tissue out from the diverticulum and into the duodenal lumen using the tip of the sphincterotome. The sphincterotome can be reshaped so it exits the working channel at a different angle, or a rotatable sphincterotome can be used. Other methods to improve access to the papilla include using a pediatric biopsy forceps alongside the sphincterotome, injection of saline inside the diverticulum, or endoscopically clipping the redundant mucosa along the rim (Figure 8.1a–c).

Altered surgical anatomy

KEY POINTS

- Commonly encountered altered surgical anatomy includes Billroth II gastrectomy, Roux-en-Y gastrojejunostomy (RYGJ), and Roux-en-Y gastric bypass (RYGB).
- Challenges are both in reaching the papilla and in subsequent biliary cannulation.
- Due to the retrograde approach, the orientation of major papilla is rotated by 180°.
- In Billroth II anatomy, either a forward-viewing endoscope or a duodenoscope can be used to reach the papilla. In RYGJ or hepaticojejunostomy, a pediatric colonoscope or balloon-assisted enteroscope may be used.
- In Roux-en-Y gastric bypass with long Roux and afferent limbs with intact antroduodenal path, laparoscope-assisted ERCP or ERCP through gastrostomy tube are options.

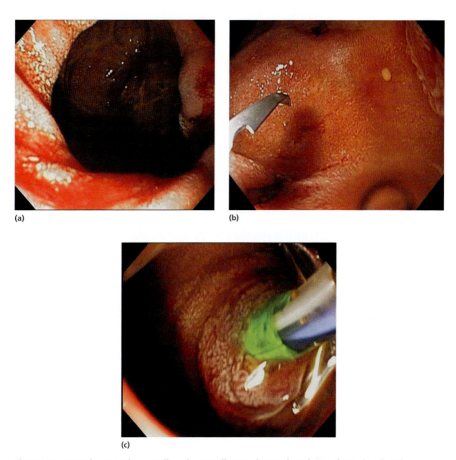

(a)   (b)

(c)

Figure 8.1 Intradiverticular papilla: The papilla was located within a deep duodenal diverticulum (a). Mucosa was "pulled" from the diverticulum and clipped with a hemostatic clip to improve access to the papilla (b). This allowed deep biliary cannulation with a sphincterotome (c) and successful endotherapy.

Patients with altered surgical anatomy pose a challenge at ERCP, firstly due to gaining endoscopic access to the papilla and secondly due to the challenge of biliary cannulation. After reaching the papilla, the cannulation success rate approaches that seen in patients with normal anatomy [16]. Billroth II procedures are becoming less common as the effectiveness of medical treatment for peptic ulcer disease has increased. In contrast, Roux-en-Y anatomy is becoming more common, due to its increased use as a bariatric surgery technique [17]. One of the main complications seen when performing ERCP in patients with altered surgical anatomy is luminal perforation. This usually occurs at surgical anastomoses or tight luminal angulations during scope insertion.

Reaching the papilla

Billroth II anatomy: The papilla can be reached using a duodenoscope or entero-scope in most cases as the afferent limb is relatively short. The afferent limb typi-cally is located along the lesser curve, whilst the efferent limb is along the greater curve. If the scope is looping within the stomach, abdominal compression, supine positioning, or placing a polypectomy snare in the endoscope working channel to serve as a stiffening device can assist. If the papilla cannot be initially reached with the duodenoscope, a forward-viewing scope can be passed first to mark the correct limb by taking a biopsy or to place a stiff guide wire in the afferent limb for subsequent "backloading" and duodenoscope advancement. Once the papilla is reached, the duodenoscope assumes a "hockey stick" configuration on fluoros-copy (Figure 8.2).

Roux-en-Y anatomy: Whilst a duodenoscope is advantageous for biliary can-nulation, a pediatric colonoscope, enteroscope, or balloon-assisted enteroscope is generally preferred for Roux-en-Y anatomy. In patients with RYGJ or Roux-en-Y hepaticojejunostomy (RYHJ) anatomy, a duodenoscope typically lacks the length and maneuverability needed to navigate the Roux limb to reach the papilla or hepaticojejunostomy. In gastroenterostomies with Roux-en-Y reconstruction, at the Roux anastomosis, the Roux limb is usually identified as the more proximal lumen with sharp angle of entry. Careful negotiation with gentle scope torque, slight scope withdrawal, and use of the wheels is required, as this is usually the

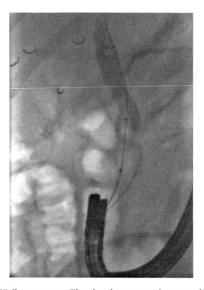

Figure 8.2 Billroth II ERCP fluoroscopy: The duodenoscope forms a "hockey stick" configuration on fluoroscopy in Billroth II anatomy. A pancreatic stent was placed after initial pancreatic duct cannulation. A biliary balloon sphincteroplasty was performed after biliary cannulation and a small needle-knife sphincterotomy.

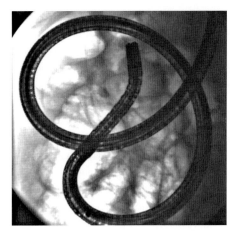

Figure 8.3 Roux-en-Y ERCP fluoroscopy: The pediatric colonoscope has a looped appearance with a Roux-en-Y ERCP, and typically passes from the left lower quadrant or midline to the right upper quadrant.

most challenging point of intubation, and has the highest risk of luminal perforation. On fluoroscopy, as the scope is advanced up the Roux limb toward the papilla, it approaches from the left abdomen or midline and moves toward the right upper quadrant (Figure 8.3). Movement away from the right upper quadrant on fluoroscopy indicates the Roux limb may not have been selected.

Cannulation

Because the papilla is approached in a retrograde direction, the major papilla is located more proximally and to the right of the minor papilla. Orientation of the bile duct and PD is reversed, with the pancreatic and biliary orifices usually found in the 11 o'clock and 5 o'clock positions, respectively.

Biliary cannulation with a forward-viewing endoscope is challenging with a success rate of only 70–80% [16]. Long accessories are required if a pediatric colonoscope or enteroscope is used. Selective biliary cannulation can be achieved by using a straight cannula, wire-guided Billroth II papillotomes (which has the cutting wire in the convex direction downwards), or rotatable papillotomes [18] in conjunction with guide wires. If sphincterotomy is required, it is usually performed with a needle-knife catheter over a biliary or pancreatic stent (Video 5, www.wiley.com\go\cotton\ercp). Free-hand NKS can be performed; however, it is challenging due to reduced scope tip control with altered anatomy, the lack of an elevator with colonoscopes and enteroscopes, and the altered papillary orientation. An increasingly popular method is to perform a small free-hand NKS followed by a balloon sphincteroplasty. This is technically easier than sphincterotomy, and has a similar complication rate [19].

Patients with RYGB differ from RYGJ and RYHJ reconstructions in two regards that are clinically relevant to the performance of biliary endoscopy. Firstly, the Roux jejunojejunostomy is often at a greater distance from the stomach, resulting in both longer alimentary (Roux) and biliopancreatic limbs, both adding to the degree of difficulty in reaching the biliary orifice. There are mixed opinions on whether RYGB anatomy is associated with a lower rate of successful access to the biliary orifice compared to RYGJ or RYHJ, when balloon-assisted enteroscopy is used. Secondly, the intact antroduodenal pathway to the biliary tree makes transgastric endoscopic approaches possible in RYGB patients, which are not options in RYGJ and RYHJ. An option is the creation of a surgical or radiological gastrostomy into the excluded stomach and subsequent access and dilation of the gastrostomy tract after allowing 3–4 weeks for tract maturation. Alternatively, laparoscopy-assisted ERCP involves the creation of a laparoscopic gastrostomy and intraoperative passage of a duodeno-scope via the newly created gastrostomy. The latter method has been associated with high (90–100%) success rates [12]. A gastrostomy tube can be placed after ERCP if repeat intervention is anticipated. Significant complications (up to 15%) have been reported with this technique, including perforation, leak, and wound infection at the gastrostomy site. Performing ERCP in patients with altered anatomy is categorized as the highest complexity procedure [20].

Combined procedures

KEY POINTS

- Combined procedures can be performed when ERCP fails, under PTC or EUS guidance.
- Should the need arise, a PTC can be converted to percutaneous biliary drainage.
- EUS-guided biliary access can be performed via the transhepatic or transduodenal route.
- EUS-guided antegrade drainage can be performed if the guide wire fails to pass across the papilla.
- Both PTC- and EUS-guided drainage procedures are associated with significant complications.

Biliary cannulation fails at ERCP in a small percentage of patients even in expert hands. In such instances, "combined" or "rendezvous" procedures can be employed where a guide wire is routed antegrade through the biliary tract across the papilla into duodenum. The duodenoscope is then advanced and the CBD is cannulated retrograde using the projecting guide wire. An important prerequisite for combined procedures is a dilated biliary ductal system.

Percutaneous approach

Traditionally, the percutaneous needle puncture is made into the peripheral right or left biliary system under transabdominal ultrasound and fluoroscopy guidance. After aspirating bile, a cholangiogram is obtained to provide a road map for guide wire passage. The guide wire is then passed via the PTC needle and negotiated across the papilla for subsequent ERCP. The current standard of care is to deploy an internal–external catheter that is followed several days later by a therapeutic ERCP. At ERCP, a guide wire is passed through the PTC-placed internal–external catheter into the duodenal lumen. The guide wire tip is captured with a snare or forceps and gently retracted out of the duodenoscope, in synchrony with external feeding of the guide wire from the percutaneous site. The PTC catheter is removed, leaving the wire passing from the PTC site, through the biliary system and out through the duodenoscope working channel. The most common complications encountered at PTC are sepsis, bile leak, and bleeding. In cases where the papilla is still not accessible at ERCP, therapeutic interventions such as metal stent placement or biliary stone extraction are undertaken via the percutaneous route. If temporary drainage is required, a pigtail catheter can be deployed over the guide wire (percutaneous transhepatic biliary drainage, PTBD) after dilating the percutaneous tract. In rare instances, combined procedures can be performed with a trans-papillary guide wire passed via prior surgically placed T-tubes or via the cystic duct during cholecystectomy to facilitate subsequent biliary ERCP.

EUS-guided approach

EUS is being increasingly used as an alternative to percutaneous techniques for accessing the biliary tract for combined procedures [21]. The major advantage of EUS-guided biliary approach is that both guide wire passage and ERCP can be undertaken in the same session (Figure 8.4a–d). EUS can also be used for antegrade drainage if the guide wire fails to cross the papilla or if the papilla is endoscopically inaccessible (Figure 8.5a–c). EUS usually provides more than one option for biliary access, such as via the left lobe of the liver or the distal CBD.

Whether the point of access is extra- or intrahepatic, there are three approaches to establishing biliary drainage. When the native papilla is endoscopically accessible, the preferred mode of drainage is by using the rendezvous technique. When the papilla is inaccessible, either antegrade stent placement or transluminal drainage (hepaticogastrostomy or choledochoduodenostomy) is undertaken.

EUS-guided procedural technique

EUS-guided biliary access is performed with the patient in the supine or prone position (not in lateral position) to adequately interpret the cholangiogram. It is mandatory to use carbon dioxide insufflation instead of air, since perforation can occur during biliary puncture or tract dilation. Adequate and prolonged sedation along with a patient endoscopist and staff is imperative to achieve technical success. The EUS-guided approach is a multistep process: guide wire manipulation across the distal stricture and toward the ampulla, a need to exchange the echoendoscope for a duodenoscope, guide wire retraction followed by subsequent retrograde biliary cannulation, and finally undertaking the therapeutic intervention. Only

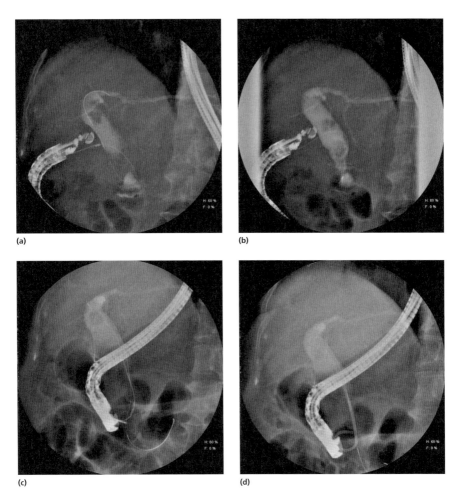

(a)   (b)

(c)   (d)

Figure 8.4 (a–d) EUS-guided rendezvous: EUS-guided rendezvous is performed by inserting a 19G FNA needle into the extrahepatic biliary system, through which a wire is passed and cholangiogram obtained (a). The wire is manipulated across the ampulla (b) and into the duodenum. The scope is then exchanged for a duodenoscope, and the wire at the ampulla is pulled through the working channel using forceps or a snare (c). The ERCP then proceeds in a standard manner (d).

endoscopists with skills in both EUS and ERCP should perform EUS-guided biliary rendezvous or drainage procedures. EUS-guided drainage should not be used to compensate for a lack of ERCP skills.

The biliary tree is usually accessed via the proximal stomach (trans-gastric intrahepatic route) (Video 6, www.wiley.com\go\cotton\ercp) or the first part of the duodenum (transduodenal extrahepatic route) (Video 7, www.wiley.com\go\cotton\ercp). The guide wire is manipulated antegrade through the native papilla for subsequent rendezvous ERCP.

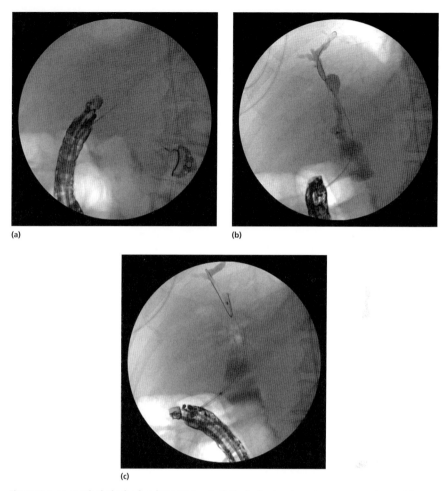

Figure 8.5 (a–c) Choledochoduodenostomy: A choledochoduodenostomy was performed in a patient with a distally obstructing pancreatic tumor. A 19G needle gained transduodenal biliary access (a) and a cholangiogram was obtained (b). The transmural tract was dilated, and a fully covered self-expanding metal stent inserted for biliary drainage (c).

The accessory used for EUS-guided bile duct puncture can be either a cautery-based flexible device (6–10 Fr cystotome), which has a round cutting tip and a stable diathermic sheath, or the more commonly used 19G FNA needle. Doppler is employed to avoid puncturing intervening vessels. After ductal access, bile is aspirated to confirm position, and contrast is injected through the needle to obtain an adequate biliary "road map." Whilst a 0.035-in. guide wire can be passed via a 19G needle, only a 0.018-in. guide wire can be passed if a 22G needle is used to access the biliary system.

Transduodenal drainage: The CBD is punctured with the echoendoscope in a long position and the needle has a natural tendency to eject toward the liver hilum, the preferential direction for guide wire passage. Manipulating the guide wire within a stiff needle to negotiate its passage across the papilla is one of the most challenging maneuvers in EUS-guided biliary drainage. There is a genuine risk for "shearing" the guide wire coating by the sharp beveled edge of the needle. To avoid shearing, newer 19G access needles with a blunt end and sharp stylet have been developed. Use of hydrophilic angle-tipped guide wire, sometimes of shorter length, helps to more accurately transmit the torque movement to the tip to negotiate the bends and strictures inside the bile duct. If this maneuver fails, the transmural tract can be minimally dilated with a tapered tip bougie (cannula) or by using a thin-caliber over-the-wire "fistulotome" (6 Fr) to enter the bile duct. Manipulating the guide wire with such an accessory inside the bile duct makes the further procedure comparatively easy.

Transhepatic drainage: The intrahepatic radicle of the left lobe of the liver is punctured with the echoendoscope in a relatively straight position in the stomach. However, compared to transduodenal drainage, the guide wire has to traverse a longer and more tortuous intra- and extrahepatic course to exit the papilla. Hilar and proximal biliary strictures are particularly challenging to pass, but can usually be achieved by dilating the puncture site by exchanging the EUS needle, over the wire, for a tapered bougie, wire-guided needle knife, or coaxial fistulotome. The aim is to drain the bile physiologically through the papilla into the duodenum, so all efforts must be made to negotiate the wire through the papilla. As a note of caution, if the transhepatic drainage is not completed, the patient is highly likely to develop a peritoneal bile leak. Furthermore, the dilated intrahepatic bile duct can rapidly collapse on initial puncture, and the subsequent contrast or bile extravasation can impair the endosonographic view making repeat puncture difficult. If the guide wire cannot be negotiated across the papilla or is obstructed proximally by a tight biliary stricture, a fully covered self-expanding metal stent (FCSEMS) should be deployed transmurally (Videos 8, www.wiley.com\go\cotton\ercp and 9, www.wiley.com\go\cotton\ercp).

The EUS rendezvous approach is preferred over EUS-guided transmural drainage as it drains the bile physiologically, and avoids the need for a permanent bilioenteric fistula that may require repeat dilations. It is prudent not to dilate the transluminal tract until satisfactory guide wire positioning has been obtained for stent placement.

Procedure-related complications include bile leak, peritonitis, cholecystitis, cholangitis, pancreatitis, fever, liver laceration, subcapsular liver hematoma, intraperitoneal stent migration, and retained sheared wire. Some of these complications can be avoided with the use of carbon dioxide insufflation and larger covered metal stents to seal the iatrogenic bilioenteric tracts to prevent bile leakage [22].

How to reduce adverse events in patients undergoing EUS-guided biliary drainage?

i. Transmural fistula should not be created unless the guide wire is placed at a desired angle in the preferred ducts. Avoid aggressive balloon dilation of the fistulous tract.

ii. Transmural fistula must preferentially be created with the aid of graded-dilation catheters or small-caliber balloons. Use of electrocautery must be minimized if possible.

iii. Avoid the temptation to view the puncture endoscopically: the puncture must be undertaken under EUS guidance and with the aid of fluoroscopy to ensure that the needle knife or cystotome is not "jammed" into the soft tissue but is in line with the axis of the guide wire as it enters the bile duct.

iv. Use FCSEMS for choledochoduodenostomies or hepaticogastrostomies instead of uncovered metals stents or plastic stents, to minimize the chances of bile leakage and perforation. However, there is a small but real risk of causing cholecystitis by occluding the cystic duct with the FCSEMS, as well as a risk of stent migration.

EUS-guided pancreatic duct access

Similar techniques can be used to access the PD by EUS-guided puncture from the stomach. A guide wire can then be passed through into the duodenum, unless there is complete obstruction. There are few indications for this approach, which involve risk of leak and pancreatitis.

Conclusion

Experienced endoscopists achieve cannulation using standard approaches in most routine cases. Needle-knife access and rendezvous techniques may be required when these prove difficult. Patients with surgically altered biliary anatomy and long limbs are the most challenging. Whilst almost all difficulties can be overcome by experts, there are significant risks involved. Fighting fires can be dangerous.

References

1 Cote GA, Mullady DK, Jonnalagadda SS, *et al.* Use of a pancreatic duct stent or guidewire facilitates bile duct access with low rates of precut sphincterotomy: a randomized clinical trial. Dig Dis Sci 2012; 57 (12): 3271–3278.

2 Glomsaker T, Hoff G, Kvaløy JT, *et al*. Patterns and predictive factors after endoscopic retrograde cholangiopancreatography. Brit J Surg 2013; 100 (3): 373–380.

3 Freeman ML, Nelson DB, Sherman S, *et al*. Complications of endoscopic biliary sphincterotomy. N Eng J Med 1996; 335 (13): 909–918.

4 Palm J, Saarela A, Mäkelä J. Safety of Erlangen precut papillotomy: an analysis of 1044 consecutive ERCP examinations in a single institution. J Clin Gastroenterol 2007; 41: 528–533.

5 Tarnasky PR, Palesch YY, Cunningham JT, *et al*. Pancreatic stenting prevents pancreatitis after biliary sphincterotomy in patients with sphincter of Oddi dysfunction. Gastroenterology. 1998; 115: 1518–1524.

6 Binmoeller KF, Seifert H, Gerke H, *et al*. Papillary roof incision using the Erlangen-type precut papillotome to achieve selective bile duct cannulation. Gastrointest Endosc 1996;44: 689–695.

7 Catalano MF, Linder JD, Geenen JE. Endoscopic transpancreatic papillary septotomy for inaccessible obstructed bile ducts: Comparison with standard pre-cut papillotomy. Gastrointest Endosc 2004; 60 (4): 57–561.

8 Katsinelos P, Gkagkalis S, Chatzimavroudis G, *et al*. Comparison of three types of precut technique to achieve common bile duct cannulation: a retrospective analysis of 274 cases. Dig Dis Sci 2012; 57: 3286–3292.

9 Misra SP, Dwivedi M. Intramural incision technique: a useful and safe procedure for obtaining ductal access during ERCP. Gastrointest Endosc 2008; 67: 629–633.

10 Farrell RJ, Khan MI, Noonan N, *et al*. Endoscopic papillectomy: a novel approach to difficult cannulation. Gut 1996; 39: 36–38.

11 Manes G, Di Giorgio P, Repici A, *et al*. An analysis of the factors associated with the development of complications in patients undergoing precut sphincterotomy: a prospective, controlled, randomized, multicenter study. Am J Gastroenterol 2009; 104 (10): 2412–2417.

12 Singh P, Das A, Isenberg G, *et al*. Does prophylactic pancreatic stent placement reduce the risk of post-ERCP acute pancreatitis? A meta-analysis of controlled trials. Gastrointest Endosc 2004; 60: 544–550.

13 Akaraviputh T, Lohsiriwat V, Swangsri J, *et al*. The learning curve for safety and success of precut sphincterotomy for therapeutic ERCP: a single endoscopist's experience. Endoscopy 2008; 40 (6): 513–516.

14 Robison LS, Varadarajulu S, Wilcox CM. Safety and success of precut biliary sphincterotomy: Is it linked to experience or expertise? World J Gastroenterol 2007; 13: 2183–2186.

15 Harewood GC, Baron TH. An assessment of the learning curve for precut biliary sphincterotomy. Am J Gastroenterol 2002; 97:1708–1712.

16 Lin LF, Siauw CP, Ho KS, Tung JC. ERCP in post-Billroth II gastrectomy patients: emphasis on technique. Am J Gastroenterol 1999; 94: 144–148.

17 Lopes TL, Clements RH, Wilcox CM. Laparoscopy-assisted ERCP: experience of a high-volume bariatric surgery center (with video). Gastrointest Endosc 2009; 70: 1254–1259.

18 Kim GH, Kang DH, Song CS, *et al*. Endoscopic removal or bile-duct stones by using a rotatable papillotome and a large-balloon dilator in patients with a Billroth II gastrectomy (with video). Gastrointest Endosc 2008; 67 (7): 1134–1138.

19 Maydeo A, Bhandari S. Balloon sphincteroplasty for removing difficult bile duct stones. Endoscopy 2007; 39: 958–961.

20 ASGE Committee on Training. ERCP core curriculum. Gastrointest Endosc 2006; 63: 361–376.

21 Dhir V, Bhandari S, Bapat M, Maydeo A. Comparison or EUS-guided rendezvous and precut papillotomy techniques for biliary access (with videos). Gastrointest Endosc 2012; 75 (2): 354–359.

22 Khashab MA, Valeshabad AK, Modayil R, *et al.* EUS-guided biliary drainage by using a standardized approach for malignant biliary obstruction: rendezvous versus direct transluminal techniques (with videos). Gastrointest Endosc 2013; 78: 734–741.

CHAPTER 9

Intraductal therapies

Mohan Ramchandani & D. Nageshwar Reddy

Department of Gastroenterology, Asian Institute of Gastroenterology, Hyderabad, India

KEY POINTS

- Peroral cholangioscopy (POCS) and pancreatoscopy can be achieved using "mother and baby" endoscope systems, small visual catheters passed through standard endoscopes, or with small endoscopes directly (after sphincterotomy).

- Direct vision of the ductal structures improves diagnostic accuracy in cases with indeterminate strictures, can show the extent of **intrapapillary mucinous neoplasms** (IPMN) changes in the pancreatic duct (PD), and can clarify whether all stone fragments have been removed.

- The main emerging roles for these techniques are therapeutic, that is, guided lithotripsy, photodynamic therapy (PDT), radiofrequency ablation (RFA), and brachytherapy.

- These methods are technically challenging and not without potential serious hazards.

Introduction and background

Over the last three decades endoscopic retrograde cholangiopancreatography (ERCP) has evolved from a diagnostic procedure to a therapeutic one [1]. Diagnostic ERCP has largely been replaced by noninvasive techniques like MRCP [2, 3] and endoscopic ultrasound (EUS) [4].

A major drawback of diagnostic ERCP is not only the potential for complications but also inadequate visualization of the interior of the common bile duct (CBD) and PD. Diagnosis remains a challenge in patients with pancreatobiliary disorders, even after extensive evaluation; with these modalities a diagnosis remain unclear in as many as 50% of the patients [5].

In recent years technological advances in POCS and peroral pancreatoscopy (POPS) have given us the ability to visualize the bile duct and PD more accurately. For example, with the advent of Peroralcholangiopancreatoscopy (POCPS) large biliary calculi and difficult PD calculi can be broken under direct vision. POCPS may use a fiberoptic or a video scope. In addition to peroral

ERCP: The Fundamentals, Second Edition. Edited by Peter B. Cotton and Joseph Leung.
© 2015 John Wiley & Sons, Ltd. Published 2015 by John Wiley & Sons, Ltd.
Companion Website: www.wiley.com\go\cotton\ercp

Table 9.1 Peroral cholangioscopic equipment.

	Fiber-optic cholangioscopes	Video (electronic) cholangioscopes	SpyGlass direct visualization system	"Ultraslim" electronic gastroscope system
Number of operators	Two	Two	One	One
Tip maneuverability	Two-way (up–down)	Two-way (up–down)	Four-way (up–down, left–right)	Four-way (up–down, left–right)
Irrigation channel	Nil	Nil	Separate	Nil
Exchangeable optics	No	No	Yes	No
Reusable endoscope	Yes	Yes	No	Yes
Image quality	Moderate to good	Excellent	Average	Excellent
Fragility	Yes	Yes	No	No

access, cholangiopancreatoscopy can be performed percutaneously or intraoperatively, for example, via a choledocholithotomy or the cystic duct [6–8].

Similarly to POCPS other ERCP-guided intraductal therapies like PDT, RFA, and brachytherapy are emerging to name just a few. This chapter discusses some of the advances in intraductal imaging and therapy of pancreatobiliary disease (Table 9.1).

Equipment and techniques

Mother and baby POCPS

POCPS can be performed with a single-operator or a two-operator system. Table 9.2 summarizes the currently available POCPS methods.

In the two-operator procedure, also known as "mother and baby" cholangioscopy, a cholangioscope is passed through the accessory channel of a duodenoscope (Figure 9.1) and then through the papilla for visualization of biliary or pancreatic ductal structures. Two operators are required to handle the cholangioscope (baby scope) and the duodenoscope (motherscope) seperately [9]. The initial prototype cholangioscope had inferior image quality, had no separated irrigation or accessory channel, and had no tip deflection. In the 1980s second-generation cholanigoscopes were introduced. These scopes had additional advantages of tip deflection and of a working channel that could be utilized for irrigation or therapeutic procedures. In the late 1990s videoendoscopes were introduced that improved the optical resolution significantly. The videocholangiopancreatoscopes [10–12] have charge-coupled device (CCD) technology at the distal end of the endoscope. The

Table 9.2 Endoscopic guided intraductal diagnostic and therapeutic procedures.

Diagnostic	Therapeutic

Cholangiopancreatoscopy
  Dual operator
  Single operator
    SpyGlass
    cholangiopancreatoscopy
Direct cholangioscopy
 	
Probe-based confocal endoscopic
microscopy
Image-enhanced
cholangiopancreatoscopy
	Cholangioscopy-guided
	  Laser lithotripsy
	  Electrohydrolic lithotripsy
	Photodynamic therapy
	Radiofrequency ablation
	Brachytherapy

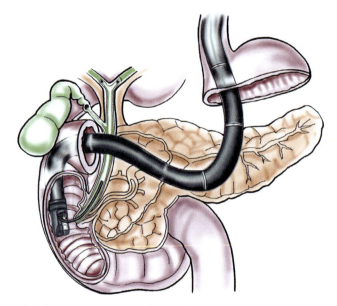

Figure 9.1 Graphical representation of mother and baby cholangioscopy.

baby scopes today have image-enhancing capabilities like narrow band imaging (NBI) [13, 14] and thus provide improved ability to detect abnormal vascularization of biliary mucosa, which is of importance for diagnosis of certain biliary malignancies. These cholangioscopes are still in prototype form and are not commercially available at present.

A channel diameter of 0.75 mm is available in smaller cholangioscopes allowing passage of a 0.025-in. guidewire. Larger cholangioscopes with a 3.1- and 3.4-mm diameter have a 1.2-mm channel. This allows the passage of a 1.9F to 3F electrohydraulic lithotripsy (EHL) fiber, a 0.035-in. guide wire, and biopsy forceps. Advantage of these cholangioscopes is that they allow tissue biopsy and can be used for various therapeutic procedures including lithotripsy. The disadvantage of mother and baby cholangioscopy is that it allows only single-plane tip deflection (up–down) of approximately 90° and that it does not have a separate irrigation channel. Moreover, two processors along with light sources, video monitors, a fluoroscopy unit, and an irrigation pump are required. These scopes are fragile and can potentially be damaged by the elevator of duodenoscope.

SpyGlass Direct Visualization System

The SpyGlass access and delivery system is a recent addition in the field of POCPS. The major advantage of this system is four-way tip deflection and separate irrigation channels (Table 9.2). This advancement in maneuverability of the SpyGlass system allows for four quadrant biopsies [15, 16]. The SpyGlass Direct Visualization System (Microvasive Endoscopy, Boston Scientific Corp., Natick, MA) consists of capital equipment, including a pump, a light source, and a monitor, and of three disposable devices (Figure 9.2):

1 Optical probe (SpyGlass)
2 Access and delivery catheter (SpyScope)
3 Biopsy forceps (SpyBite)

The SpyGlass probe is a 6000-pixel fiberoptic bundle and is designed to acquire and transmit endoscopic images and conduct light into the biliary anatomy, providing a 70° field of view. The SpyScope access and delivery catheter provides a pathway into the biliary anatomy for diagnostic and therapeutic devices and is 10 F in diameter. This four-lumen catheter has an optic channel through which the SpyGlass optical probe can be passed, a 1.2-mm accessory channel, and two independent irrigation channels. The delivery catheter has a handle with two knobs controlling four-way steering of the catheter. It can be attached to the handle of the duodenoscope for single-operator use. The SpyBite biopsy forceps is a single-use device, which passes through the biopsy channel of the SpyScope catheter. Its jaws open to 4.1 mm allowing tissue, which is adequate in a majority of cases. The drawback of this system is its average image quality, which requires further improvement.

Image-enhanced cholangioscopy

Image enhancement of the visualized mucosa can be performed with dye, autofluorescence, or NBI. Using methylene blue dye solution, malignant lesions can be differentiated from benign lesions as malignant lesions show irregular mucosa with dark-blue staining patterns while benign lesions have a smooth surface with uniform staining [17, 18].

Ultraslim endoscopes

An ultrathin gastroscope (5 mm) routinely used for transnasal endoscopy can be used as a cholangioscope and can be passed directly through the papilla. This is a single-operator system for POCS and has advantages of better image quality,

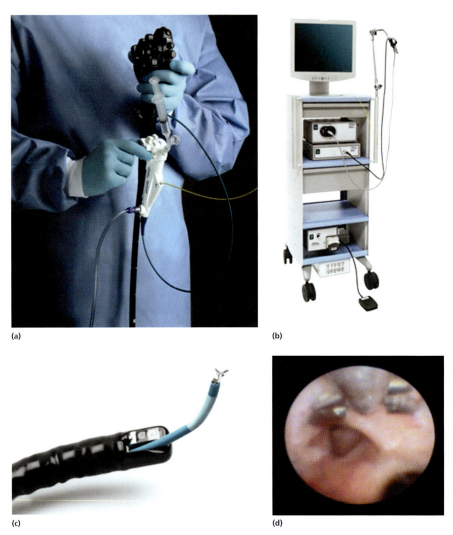

(a)

(b)

(c)

(d)

Figure 9.2 (a) SpyScope setup showing access and delivery catheter attached to a duodenoscope. (b) SpyScope and SpyBite at the distal end of the duodenoscope. (c) Full capital system including a pump, a light source, and a monitor. (d) Chlolangioscopic view showing intraductal SpyBite. Source: Boston Scientific Corporation. Reproduced with permission.

larger accessory channel, and excellent maneuverability [19, 20]. Addition of NBI allows better visualization and allows better characterization of biliary lesions. Direct POCS has been reported using a free cannulation technique but a major drawback of this procedure is that it is technically demanding, as it requires expertise to maneuver the acute angle between the duodenum and the bile duct. Specialized accessories are required to assist the scope insertion into the bile duct including a stiff guide wire, a balloon catheter, or an overtube. The guide wire is easy to use but the disadvantage is that it can dislodge leading to slippage of the direct POCS. The cholangioscope can be anchored by a balloon as follows. A superstiff guide wire is passed in the biliary system after ERCP and biliary sphincterotomy. An ultraslim endoscope is rail-roaded over a 5 F balloon catheter on the guide wire. The balloon catheter is then advanced into an intra-hepatic duct over the guide wire and inflated to anchor it. The endoscope is pushed forward over the balloon, which is already anchored. A feasibility study of balloon-guided direct POC was carried out by Moon *et al.* [21]. Eleven patients underwent the wire-guided POC while balloon-guided direct POC was carried out in 21 patients. Wire-guided direct POC was successful in 45.5% of patients and balloon-guided direct POC in 95.2%. Overtube-assisted cholangioscopy has been described and may be useful to perform therapeutic intervention. In a study overtube balloon–assisted direct cholangioscopy was performed success-fully in 10 of the 12 patients (83.3%). In another series of 14 patients, Tsou *et al.* demonstrated successful introduction of the ultraslim endoscope into the bile ducts of all the patients using the overtube balloon–assisted technique [22, 23]. A number of ultraslim endoscopes with a 2-mm accessory channel are commer-cially available.

Peroral pancreatoscopy

Pancreatoscopy can be performed by introducing a pancreatoscope through the accessory channel of a duodenoscope or by using a SpyGlass system [5]. A pancreatoscope with a larger diameter (3.3 or 4.5 mm) has advantage that tip maneuverability is possible and there is a working channel to assist in therapeutic procedures. However, it requires pancreatic sphincterotomy, carries a risk of instrumentation trauma to PD, and is suitable only for patients with dilated PD. On the other hand, an ultrathin pancreatoscope with a diameter of less than 1 mm, which can be inserted via an ordinary ERCP cannula, is available [24]. This scope has the advantage that it is easier to insert but the drawbacks are a restricted field of view due to lack of tip movement and poor image quality. An electronic pancreatoscope was developed, which has a 50,000-pixel interline CCD. The system has a 2.1-mm external diameter and a forward-viewing optical system with a field of view of 80°. It has no accessory channel but the tip of the scope can be moved bidirectionally [24].

Probe-based confocal laser endomicroscopy

Endoscopic real-time histological evaluation of the lesion can be performed by probe-based confocal laser endomicroscopy (pCLE) [25, 26]. pCLE is based upon the principle of illuminating a tissue with a low-power laser and then detecting fluorescent light reflected from the tissue. During ERCP, intraductal CLE is per-formed by a especially designed probe (CholangioFlex probe, Maunakea Tech, Paris, France), which has an external diameter of 0.94 mm, a field of view 325 μm wide, a lateral resolution of 3.5 μm, and an optical slice thickness of 30, 40–70 μm below the tissue surface. Since pCLE is based on tissue fluorescence, intravenous and/or topically applied contrast agents are required. Different dyes, such as fluorescein or cresyl violet, have been used for contrast enhancement.

pCLE can be performed under either cholangioscopic or fluoroscopic guidance. The probe can be inserted as a standard ERCP accessory device. The radiopaque tip of this probe helps in targeting the area of interest under fluoroscopic guidance. The probe can be easily passed through the working channel (1.2 mm) of a cholangioscope. The optical penetration of the confocal plane provides subsurface information with no interference from bile or solid residues.

Diagnostic applications

The major advantage of POCPS is that it enables direct endoscopic examination of indeterminate biliary strictures or filling defects and also allows biopsy under vision of the area of interest. Modern cholangioscopes have the additional advantage of using NBI, which further enhances diagnostic ability. Moreover, POCPS can further help in delineating longitudinal spread of biliary or PD malignancy prior to surgical resection, in examining posttransplant strictures, in collecting biliary fluid for cytology or culture, and in assessing intraductal extension of an ampullary adenoma.

Indeterminate biliary strictures and filling defects

Traditionally, ERCP is used as initial investigation for evaluation of patients with obstructive jaundice and imaging suggestive of a biliary stricture and intrahepatic ductal dilatation. However, cholagiographic images are only suggestive but not diagnostic of the disease. The inability to differentiate benign from malignant strictures is the major limitation of radiological studies. During ERCP endobiliary brush cytology is the most commonly used method for tissue acquisition. Diagnostic yield of brush cytology is low ranging from 18 to 60% in most studies. The low sensitivity is due to low cellularity and desmoplastic reaction of these tumors. The modification in brush design and stricture manipulation by dilatation has not shown to significantly increase the diagnostic yield [27–30].

Cholangioscopy has been shown to increase diagnostic yield in patients with indeterminate strictures. Various cholangioscopic features have been reported to be associated with malignancy including dilated tortuous tumor vessels [31, 32], intraductal nodules or masses, infiltrative or ulcerated strictures, and papillary or villous mucosal projections. The features that suggest benign lesions include smooth mucosa without neovascularization or homogenous granular mucosa without a mass. Direct correlation between such findings and a firm diagnosis are not perfect.

In a study by Fukuda *et al.* [33], POCS was performed in addition to ERCP for evaluation of biliary strictures or filling defects. Diagnostic accuracy was improved from 78 to 93% and sensitivity from 58 to 100% with additional use of cholangioscopy.

An international multicenter registry studying the role of SpyGlass cholangioscopy included 297 patients with various biliary disorders [34].Overall success rate was reported to be 89% with a sensitivity of SpyGlass visual impression in diagnosing malignancy of 88%.

Ramchandani *et al.* [35] reported their data of 36 patients with indeterminate biliary strictures/filling defects who were evaluated by using SpyGlass cholangioscopy. The overall accuracy of SpyGlass visual impression for differentiating malignant from benign ductal lesions was 89%. The accuracy of SpyBite biopsies for differentiating malignant from benign ductal lesions that were inconclusive on ERCP-guided brushing or biopsy was 82%.

Image-enhanced cholangioscopy can be of help in differentiating benign from malignant interterminate strictures, particularly using dye or NBI to improve visualization of vessels and improve the ability to delineate proximal and distal margin of malignant lesions.

pCLE can provide useful additional information to the assessment of indeterminate strictures or lesions. In a study by Meining *et al.* [25] patients with biliary strictures underwent pCLE examination via cholangioscopy. They reported that the presence of irregular, dilated, or "angiogenic" vessels were the best predictor of malignancy, with an accuracy of 86%, sensitivity of 83%, and specificity of 88%. In a multicenter registry, a total of 102 patients undergoing ERCP with pCLE to evaluate indeterminate pancreaticobiliary strictures were enrolled. In this study the authors concluded that combination of two or more pCLE image criteria have better sensitivity and specificity in predicting malignancy than one image criteria. The characteristics on imaging that suggest malignancy include thick white bands (>20 μm), or thick dark bands (>40 μm), or dark clumps, or epithelial structures. These provided sensitivity and specificity of 97 and 33%, respectively, in predicting malignancy [26].

Extent of intrapapillary mucinous neoplasms

Similar to biliary lesions, direct visualization of an indeterminate stricture or filling defect by pancreatoscopy is helpful in discriminating malignant from benign intraductal lesions. Most of the studies on pancreatoscopy have been conducted in patients with intraductal papillary mucinous neoplasms (IPMNs) [36–39]. Diagnostic yield of POPS with or without POPS-guided biopsy for malignancy in IPMN are reported, and range from 50 to 68% sensitivity and from 87 to 100% specificity. Diagnostic accuracy is better in main duct IPMN than in side branch IPMN. The pancreatoscopic findings of IPMN include papillary tumor with "fish-egg"-like appearance, granular mucosa, or mucin. Pancreatoscopy also helps in differentiating filling defects seen on a pancreatogram suggestive of a pancreatic stone or a main duct IPMN in these patients, and allows biopsy for histological examination. POPS also helps in accurately identifying the extent of IPMN and identifying surgical margin.

Detection of missed stones

Small stones can be missed during ERCP; these stones can be "drowned" in excessive contrast. In a study, biliary stones were missed in 22% patients on ERCP, which were detected by subsequent cholangioscopy [40]. Cholangioscopy is especially useful in patients where mechanical or electro-hydrolic lithotripsy is performed and a large pneumobilia exists in the bile duct [41].

Therapeutic applications

The main therapeutic indication of cholangioscopy is the management of difficult bile duct stones via intracorporeal lithotripsy. Additional indications for POCPS include selective guide wire placement [42], unexplained hemobilia [43], assessing intraductal biliary ablation therapy [44], management of postliver transplant stricture [45], and extraction of migrated stents [46].

Intracorporeal lithotripsy for biliary calculi

Up to 5–10% of bile duct stones cannot be removed by conventional methods including ERCP and mechanical lithotripsy [47, 48]. Impacted stones, very large stones (≥ 25 mm), and stones above biliary strictures are less likely to be successfully removed by conventional methods. When these measures fail, alternative lithotripsy techniques such as electrohydraulic or laser lithotripsy and surgery may need to be considered.

One of the key advantages of cholangioscopy is the ability to directly visualize and treat large intraductal stones. Cholangioscopy has proven to be valuable in complicated choledocholithiasis, especially in guiding the positioning of an EHL probe or laser fiber on the surface of stone. The direct visualization helps in preventing injury from an EHL probe compared to positioning the EHL probe under fluoroscopy. Success rate of cholangioscopically directed CBD stone removal by these method ranges from 71 to 100% [49, 50].

Electrohydraulic lithotripsy

In this procedure a bipolar lithotripsy probe is used that creates an electric high-voltage spark between two electrodes on the tip of this probe in an aqueous medium. This spark causes expansion of the water and generates hydraulic pressure waves. The energy of these waves is absorbed by the stones and thus the stones are fragmented. An electrohydraulic shock wave generator (Lithotron EL-27; Olympus Medical Systems Co., Tokyo, Japan) set at an output of 2000 V can be used to generate shock waves of increasing frequency (intensity up to 500 mJ). The probe (4.5 F) can be passed through the channel of a mother baby cholangioscope and is usually used in conjunction with a nasobiliary catheter for saline irrigation. The EHL probe can also be passed through the instrument channel

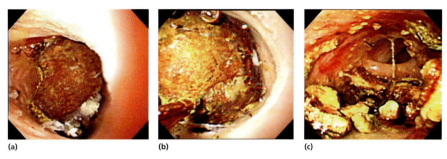

(a)   (b)   (c)

Figure 9.3 Direct cholangioscopy-guided EHL lithotripsy. (a) A large CBD stone. (b) CBD stone being fragmented with EHL probe. (c) Completely fragmented stone.

of the SpyScope, which simultaneously serves for irrigation and aspiration of bile duct fluid and fine pulverized stone debris.

EHL is performed under cholangioscopic guidance (Figure 9.3) to accurately aim the stone and avoid ductal trauma and perforation. The probe is positioned more than 5 mm away from the distal end of a cholangioscope and 1–2 mm from the target calculus. A balloon catheter can be alternatively used if cholangioscopy is not available. The EHL probe is passed through the lumen of a modified balloon catheter and under fluoroscopic guidance the balloon catheter is positioned below the stone. Shock waves are delivered to fragment the stone. Since balloon catheter EHL carries a high risk of complications, it should only be used in cases where conventional cholangioscopic method is not possible. In a study evaluating the role of cholangioscopy, guided EHL reported a stone fragmentation rate of 96% and a final stone clearance rate of 90% [51].

Laser lithotripsy

The holmium:YAG laser and frequency-doubled, double-pulse neodymium:YAG (FREDDY) laser are the two commonly used lasers to crush biliary stones [49, 50, 52]. In holmium laser technology (Medilas H20; Dornier Medtech, Munich, Germany) the energy is delivered via a 365-μm-diameter fiber, with energy levels set at 800–1500 mJ at a frequency of 8–15 Hz. A green aiming beam is used to target the stone, and direct apposition is confirmed via cholangioscopic/flouroscopic view. Laser bursts of less than 5 s are delivered under continuous saline solution irrigation.

Holmium laser energy is rapidly absorbed by water, creating a vaporization bubble that has minimal effects on adjacent tissue. These qualities result in minimal adjacent tissue trauma. However, direct contact with tissue should be avoided and sufficient saline irrigation should be used to prevent adjacent thermal soft tissue effects. The distance between the laser fiber tip and stone is of paramount importance to achieve maximum stone fragmentation [52]. This distance should be 1 to 2 mm to achieve maximum stone fragmentation (Figure 9.4).

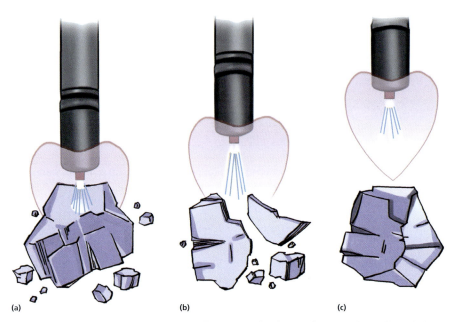

(a) (b) (c)

Figure 9.4 Graphical representation of laser lithotripsy. The distance between the probe and the stone is important to achieve fragmentation of stone. (a) If the distance is less than 1 mm there is a drilling effect without fragmentation. (b) Optimal distance is 1–2 mm to achieve maximum stone fragmentation. (c) Beyond 2 mm the fragmentation effect is lost.

The FREDDY laser system uses wave lengths of 532 nm (20%) and 1064 nm (80%). The green light ignites a plasma at the stone surface, while the infrared laser energy boosts this plasma to form a rapidly collapsing bubble, which produces a strong shock wave that fragments the stones. The FREDDY laser causes minimal or no ductal injury and has been used through the guide wire port of a stone extraction balloon.

Intracorporeal lithotripsy for difficult pancreatic calculi

In difficult pancreatic ductal stones, POPS-guided lithotripsy may be useful in fragmentation and extraction of stones. Pancreatoscopy-guided EHL/LL has been reported with successful pancreatic stone clearance in 69% with clinical success of 74% [53]. In a study [54], laser lithotripsy by POPS has been described with successful pancreatic stone clearance in 100% of cases. The impacted stones or stones that are located above a distal PD stricture are difficult to remove. Dilation of the stricture and pancreatic sphincterotomy are usually required in pancreatoscopy-guided EHL.

Photodynamic therapy for malignant biliary strictures

PDT is a promising novel treatment that has been shown to improve the survival of patients with cholangiocarcinoma.

In this procedure initially a photosensitizer, which is a light-absorbing agent, is administered intravenously. This photosensitizer is selectively taken up by neoplastic tissue. Forty-eight hours later the tumor is irradiated with laser light, which leads to activation of the photosensitizer. Free radical intermediates are formed, which in turn react with oxygen to generate various reactive oxygen species resulting in tumor necrosis. PDT also damages tumor vessels and stimulates an immune response against neoplastic cells.

PDT can be performed during ERCP or using a percutaneous approach. After initial decompression with biliary stents and tissue diagnosis the cancer patient is given a IV photosensitizer. At 48 h after photosensitization repeat ERCP is performed and the stents are removed. Intraductal photoactivation is performed using a laser quartz fiber. The tumor is irradiated for 10–12 min with laser light of wavelength 630 nm with a light dose of 180 J/cm². Oxygen is administered to all patients to optimize the effectiveness of PDT.

A multicenter randomized control trial [55] of repeated PDT with stenting (mean 2.4 sessions) versus stenting alone for irresectable cholangiocarcinoma showed a significant survival advantage in the PDT group as compared to the stent-alone group (493 days compared with 93 days, $P<0.0001$). The monitoring committee discontinued the trial prematurely because of obvious survival advantage in the PDT group. Thirty-one patients with advanced disease who were not randomized initially were later treated with PDT with stenting and showed a median survival of 426 days.

Radiofrequency ablation for malignant biliary strictures and benign hyperplasia

Disadvantages of PDT are the high cost and potential phototoxicity on exposure to sun. RFA has been used for ablation of the tumors in the liver, rectum, and esophagus. Heat energy is utilized to achieve contact coagulative necrosis of surrounding tissue. Endobiliary RFA (Figure 9.5) has recently been used to decrease tumor ingrowth and benign epithelial hyperplasia. This is achieved by using a novel catheter, the HabibEndoHPB (EMcision, London, United Kingdom) catheter, that is a bipolar probe and is 8F in diameter. It is 1.8 m long; compatible with standard duodenoscopes (3.2-mm working channel), and passes over 0.035-in. guidewires [56]. There are two ring electrodes at the distal end of the catheter that provide local coagulative necrosis over a 2.5-cm length. The procedure is performed under general anesthesia using a standard duodenoscope that is advanced up to the papilla. After sphincterotomy and assessment of the stricture length, the ring electrodes are placed exactly at the site of stricture, and energy is delivered using an RFA generator (1500 RF generator; RITA Medical Systems Inc, Fremont, CA). The current setting of the RFA generator is kept at 400 kHz at 7–10 W for 2 min, with a rest period of 1 min before moving the catheter. If the length of the stricture is long, RFA can be applied sequentially without significant overlap of the ablated areas.

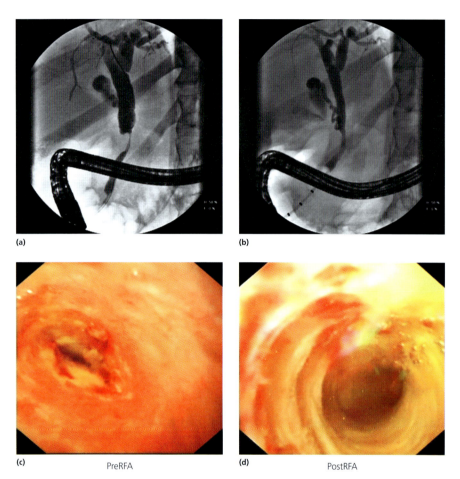

(a)

(b)

(c) PreRFA

(d) PostRFA

Figure 9.5 Endoscopic radiofrequency ablation (RFA) of cholangiocarcinoma. (a and c) Cholangiographic and cholangioscopic images before the RFA. (b) Cholangiographic picture after RFA showing opening of the stricture. (d) Cholangioscopic picture after RFA showing ablated area.

In a recently published study [57] a total of 58 patients underwent 84 RFA procedures. The predominant underlying condition was hilar cholangiocarcinoma (77%). The technical success rate was 100%. Median stent patency after last electively performed RFA was 170 days and median survival was 10.6 months from the time of the first RFA treatment session and 17.9 months from the time of initial diagnosis. Adverse events (AE) including cholangitis, hemobilia, and cholangiosepsis were seen in few patients.

There is scarcity of literature on endobiliary RFA; however, endobiliary RFA seems to be technically feasible and a safe therapeutic option for the palliative treatment of malignant biliary obstruction. Prospective randomized control trial to further quantify the efficacy of this promising new technique is warranted.

Brachytherapy for malignant biliary strictures

Local radiotherapy can be administered in the form of brachytherapy [58, 59], which involves intrabiliary placement of a radioactive source. Intrabiliary brachytherapy can be delivered either by the endoscopic method using a nasobiliary catheter or by the transhepatic route. Six French brachytherapy catheters (Lumencath®, Nucletron, an Elekta company, Elekta AB, Stockholm, Sweden) can be placed through percutaneous transhepatic biliary drainage or nasobiliary catheters under fluoroscopic guidance.

Iridium-192 has been evaluated in patients with biliary cancer to improve stent patency and survival. Radiation therapy is applied to the strictured segment in a calculated dose. Low-dose brachytherapy protocol includes 30–45 Gy (3000–4500 rad) over 24–60 h. Radiosensitizing chemotherapeutic agents such as 5-fluorouracil (5-FU) can be used simultaneously in some cases. Post radiotherapy it is important to ensure adequate biliary drainage by placing biliary stents. The AE associated with this procedure include cholangitis, duodenal ulcers, bilioenteric fistula, and hemobilia.

Complications of cholangioscopy

POCP is usually safe; however, the AE of ERCP such as bleeding and perforation can occur during a sphincterotomy. Pancreatitis is a rare AE but has been reported when a large-diameter cholangioscope is used without a adequate sphincterotomy. Cholangitis is a major concern, especially when dealing with a patient with PSC or complex strictures or stones. In a retrospective analysis [60], AEs from POCP were found to be more than double of those of ERCP alone. POCP was associated with a significantly higher rate of cholangitis, possibly because of constant irrigation of saline that is required during the procedure. Hemobilia has been reported in patients undergoing intracorporal lithotripsy. Fatal air embolism has been reported, and the careful use of CO_2 for insufflation has been recommended.

Conclusion

POCPS is an important additional modality during ERCP. POCPS aids in direct visualization, tissue acquisition, and treatment of the biliary and pancreatic ductal pathology. This technology is, unfortunately, limited to tertiary centers because of the cost involved in acquisition and maintenance. However, recent advancements in electronic video chip technology, introduction of catheter-based cholangiopancreatoscopy, and the development of ultrathin gastroscope has renewed interest among endoscopists to perform POCPS more routinely. Currently, the most common indications for POCPS are stone therapy, evaluation of indeterminate biliary strictures, and IPMN. More refinement in the scope with four-way steering, irrigation, and better image quality are desirable. Newer intraductal therapies including PDT and RFA are emerging. Large multicentric randomized trials are required before they can be routinely recommended.

References

1 Devereaux CE, Binmoeller KF. Endoscopic retrograde cholangiopancreatography in the next millennium. Gastrointest Endosc Clin North Am 2000 Jan;10(1):117–33.

2 MacEneaney P, Mitchell MT, McDermott R. Update on magnetic resonance cholangiopancreatography. Gastroenterol Clin North Am 2002;31:731–46.

3 Tripathi RP, Batra A, Kaushik S. Magnetic resonance cholangiopancreatography: evaluation in 150 patients. Indian J Gastroenterol 2002;21:105–9.

4 Rosch T, Hofrichter K, Frimberger E, *et al*. ERCP or EUS for tissue diagnosis of biliary strictures? A prospective comparative study. Gastrointest Endosc 2004;60:390–6.

5 Nguyen NQ, Binmoeller KF, Shah JN. Cholangioscopy and pancreatoscopy (with videos). Gastrointest Endosc 2009 Dec;70(6):1200–10.

6 Takada T, Suzuki S, Nakamura K, *et al*. Percutaneous transhepatic cholangioscopy as a new approach to the diagnosis of biliary disease. Gastroenterol Endosc 1974;16:106–11.

7 Nakajima M, Akasaka Y, Fukumoto K, Mitsuyoshi Y, Kawai K. Peroral cholangiopancreatosocopy (PCPS) under duodenoscopic guidance. Am J Gastroenterol 1976 Sep;66(3):241–7.

8 Rosch W, Koch H, Demling L. Peroral cholangioscopy. Endoscopy 1976;8:172–5.

9 Nakajima M, Mukai H, Kawai K. Peroral cholangioscopy and pancreatoscopy. In: Sivak MV, editor. Gastrointestinal Endoscopy. 2nd ed. Philadelphia: WB Saunders, 2000: 1055–68.

10 Kodama T, Imamura Y, Sato H, *et al*. Feasibility study using a new small electronic pancreatoscope: description of findings in chronic pancreatitis. Endoscopy 2003;35(4):305–10.

11 Kodama T, Koshitani T, Sato H, *et al*. Electronic pancreatoscopy for the diagnosis of pancreatic diseases. Am J Gastroenterol 2002;97(3):617–22.

12 Kodama T, Tatsumi Y, Sato H, *et al*. Initial experience with a new peroral electronic pancreatoscope with an accessory channel. Gastrointest Endosc 2004;59(7):895–900.

13 Itoi T, Neuhaus H, Chen YK. Diagnostic value of image-enhanced video cholangiopancreatoscopy. Gastrointest Endosc Clin North Am 2009 Oct;19(4):557–66.

14 Itoi T, Sofuni A, Itokawa F, *et al*. Peroral cholangioscopic diagnosis of biliary-tract diseases by using narrow-band imaging (with videos). Gastrointest Endosc 2007 Oct;66(4):730–6.

15 Chen YK. Preclinical characterization of the Spyglass peroral cholangiopancreatoscopy system for direct access, visualization, and biopsy. Gastrointest Endosc 2007 Feb;65(2): 303–11.

16 Chen YK, Pleskow DK. SpyGlass single-operator peroral cholangiopancreatoscopy system for the diagnosis and therapy of bile-duct disorders: a clinical feasibility study (with video). Gastrointest Endosc 2007 May;65(6):832–41.

17 Hoffman A, Kiesslich R, Bittinger F, Galle PR, Neurath MF. Methylene blue-aided cholangioscopy in patients with biliary strictures: feasibility and outcome analysis. Endoscopy. 2008 Jul;40(7):563–71.

18 Hoffman A, Kiesslich R, Moench C, *et al*. Methylene blue-aided cholangioscopy unravels the endoscopic features of ischemic-type biliary lesions after liver transplantation. Gastrointest Endosc 2007 Nov;66(5):1052–8.

19 Larghi A, Waxman I. Endoscopic direct cholangioscopy by using an ultra-slim upper endoscope: a feasibility study. Gastrointest Endosc 2006;63:853–7.

20 Waxman I, Chennat J, Konda V. Peroral direct cholangioscopic-guided selective intrahepatic duct stent placement with an ultraslim endoscope. Gastrointest Endosc 2010;71(4):875–8.

21 Moon JH, Ko BM, Choi HJ, *et al.* Intraductal balloon-guided direct peroral cholangioscopy with an ultraslim upper endoscope (with videos). Gastrointest Endosc 2009;70(2): 297–302.

22 Choi HJ, Moon JH, Ko BM, *et al.* Overtube-balloon-assisted direct peroral cholangioscopy by using an ultra-slim upper endoscope (with videos). Gastrointest Endosc 2009;69(4): 935–40.

23 Tsou YK, Lin CH, Tang JH, Liu NJ, Cheng CL. Direct peroral cholangioscopy using an ultraslim endoscope and overtube balloon-assisted technique: a case series. Endoscopy 2010;42:681–3.

24 Tajiri, H, Kobayashi, M, Niwa, H, Furui S. Clinical application of an ultra-thin pancreato-scope using a sequential video converter. *Gastrointest Endosc* 1993;**39**:371–74.

25 Meining A, Frimberger E, Becker V, *et al.* Detection of cholangiocarcinoma in vivo using miniprobe-based confocal fluorescence microscopy. Clin Gastroenterol Hepatol 2008 Sep;6(9):1057–60.

26 Meining A, Shah RJ, Slivka A, *et al.* Classification of probe-based confocal laser endomicros-copy findings in pancreaticobiliary strictures. Endoscopy 2012 Mar;44(3):251–7.

27 Glasbrenner B, Ardan M, Boeck W, *et al.* Prospective evaluation of brush cytology of biliary strictures during endoscopic retrograde cholangiopancreatography. Endoscopy 1999 Nov;31(9):712–7.

28 Fogel EL, deBellis M, McHenry L, *et al.* Effectiveness of a new long cytology brush in the evaluation of malignant biliary obstruction: a prospective study. Gastrointest Endosc 2006 Jan;63(1):71–7.

29 Ornellas LC, Santos Gda C, Nakao FS, Ferrari AP. Comparison between endoscopic brush cytology performed before and after biliary stricture dilation for cancer detection. Arq Gastroenterol 2006 Jan–Mar;43(1):20–3.

30 Parsi MA, Li A, Li CP, Goggins M. DNA methylation alterations in endoscopic retrograde chol-angiopancreatography brush samples of patients with suspected pancreaticobiliary disease. Clin Gastroenterol Hepatol 2008 Nov;6(11):1270–8.

31 Seo DW, Lee SK, Yoo KS, Kang GH, Kim MH. Cholangioscopic findings in bile duct tumors. Gastrointest Endosc 2000 Nov;52(5):630–4.

32 Kim HJ, Kim MH, Lee SK, *et al.* Tumor vessel: a valuable cholangioscopic clue of malignant biliary stricture. Gastrointest Endosc 2000 Nov;52(5):635–8.

33 Fukuda Y, Tsuyuguchi T, Sakai Y, Tsuchiya S, Saisyo H. Diagnostic utility of peroral cholan-gioscopy for various bile-duct lesions. Gastrointest Endosc 2005 Sep;62(3):374–82.

34 Chen YK, Parsi MA, Binmoeller KF, *et al.* Peroral cholangioscopy (POC) using a disposable steerable single operator catheter for biliary stone therapy and assessment of indeterminate strictures—A multicenter experience using SpyGlass. Gastrointest Endosc 2009;AB264–5.

35 Ramchandani M, Reddy DN, Gupta R, *et al.* Role of single-operator peroral cholangioscopy in the diagnosis of indeterminate biliary lesions: a single-center, prospective study. Gastrointest Endosc 2011 Sep;74(3):511–9.

36 Yelamali A, Mansard MJ, Dama R, *et al.* Intraoperative pancreatoscopy with narrow band imaging: a novel method for assessment of resection margins in case of intraductal papillary mucinous neoplasm. Surg Endosc 2012 Dec;26(12):3682–5.

37 Miura T, Igarashi Y, Okano N, Miki K, Okubo Y. Endoscopic diagnosis of intraductal papil-lary-mucinous neoplasm of the pancreas by means of peroral pancreatoscopy using a small-diameter videoscope and narrow-band imaging. Dig Endosc 2010 Apr;22(2):119–23.

38 Itoi T, Sofuni A, Itokawa F, *et al.* Initial experience of peroral pancreatoscopy combined with narrow-band imaging in the diagnosis of intraductal papillary mucinous neoplasms of the pancreas (with videos). Gastrointest Endosc 2007 Oct;66(4):793–7.

39 Yamaguchi T, Shirai Y, Ishihara T, *et al*. Pancreatic juice cytology in the diagnosis of intra-ductal papillary mucinous neoplasm of the pancreas: significance of sampling by peroral pancreatoscopy. Cancer 2005 Dec 15;104(12):2830–6.

40 Huang SW, Lin CH, Lee MS, Tsou YK, Sung KF. Residual common bile duct stones on direct peroral cholangioscopy using ultraslim endoscope. World J Gastroenterol 2013 Aug 14;19(30):4966–72.

41 Itoi T, Sofuni A, Itokawa F, *et al*. Evaluation of residual bile duct stones by peroral cholan-gioscopy in comparison with balloon-cholangiography. Dig Endosc 2010 Jul;22 Suppl 1:S85–9.

42 Parsi MA. Peroral cholangioscopy-assisted guidewire placement for removal of impacted stones in the cystic duct remnant. World J Gastrointest Surg 2009;1:59–61.

43 Hayashi S, Baba Y, Ueno K, Nakajo M. Small arteriovenous malformation of the common bile duct causing hemobilia in a patient with hereditary hemorrhagic telangiectasia. Cardiovasc Intervent Radiol 2008 Jul;31 Suppl 2:S131–4.

44 Monga A, Gupta R, Ramchandani M, *et al*. Endoscopic radiofrequency ablation of cholan-giocarcinoma: new palliative treatment modality (with videos). Gastrointest Endosc 2011 Oct;74(4):935–7.

45 Parsi MA, Guardino J, Vargo JJ. Peroral cholangioscopy-guided stricture therapy in living donor liver transplantation. Liver Transpl 2009;15:263–5.

46 Maydeo A, Kwek A, Bhandari S, Bapat M, Mathew P. SpyGlass pancreatoscopy-guided cannulation and retrieval of a deeply migrated pancreatic duct stent. Endoscopy 2011;43 Suppl 2 UCTN:E137–8.

47 Van Dam J, Sivak MV Jr. Mechanical lithotripsy of large common bile duct stones. Cleve Clin J Med 1993;60(1):38–42.

48 Tandan M, Reddy DN, Santosh D, *et al*. Extracorporeal shock wave lithotripsy of large diffi-cult common bile duct stones: efficacy and analysis of factors that favor stone fragmentation. J Gastroenterol Hepatol 2009 Aug;24(8):1370–4.

49 Neuhaus H, Hoffmann W, Zillinger C, Classen M. Laser lithotripsy of difficult bile duct stones under direct visual control. Gut 1993 Mar;34(3):415–21.

50 Jakobs R, Pereira-Lima JC, Schuch AW, *et al*. Endoscopic laser lithotripsy for complicated bile duct stones: is cholangioscopic guidance necessary? Arq Gastroenterol 2007 Apr–Jun;44(2): 137–40.

51 Arya N, Nelles SE, Haber GB, Kim YI, Kortan PK. Electrohydraulic lithotripsy in 111 patients: a safe and effective therapy for difficult bile duct stones. Am J Gastroenterol 2004 Dec;99(12):2330–4.

52 Patel SN, Rosenkranz L, Hooks B, *et al*. Holmium-yttrium aluminum garnet laser lithotripsy in the treatment of biliary calculi using single-operator cholangioscopy: a multicenter experience(with video). Gastrointest Endosc 2014 Feb;79(2):344–8.

53 Alatawi A, Leblanc S, Vienne A, *et al*. Pancreatoscopy-guided intracorporeal laser lithotripsy for difficult pancreatic duct stones: a case series with prospective follow-up (with video). Gastrointest Endosc 2013 Jul;78(1):179–83.

54 Maydeo A, Kwek BE, Bhandari S, Bapat M, Dhir V. Single-operator cholangioscopy-guided laser lithotripsy in patients with difficult biliary and pancreatic ductal stones (with videos). Gastrointest Endosc 2011 Dec;74(6):1308–14.

55 Ortner ME, Caca K, Berr F, *et al*. Successful photodynamic therapy for nonresectable chol-angiocarcinoma: a randomized prospective study. Gastroenterology 2003 Nov;125(5): 1355–63.

56 Steel AW, Postgate AJ, Khorsandi S, *et al*. Endoscopically applied radiofrequency ablation appears to be safe in the treatment of malignant biliary obstruction. Gastrointest Endosc. 2011 Jan;73(1):149–53.

57 Dolak W, Schreiber F, Schwaighofer H, *et al.* Endoscopic radiofrequency ablation for malignant biliary obstruction: a nationwide retrospective study of 84 consecutive applications. Surg Endosc 2014 Mar;28(3):854–60.

58 Deodato F, Clemente G, Mattiucci GC, *et al.* Chemoradiation and brachytherapy in biliary tract carcinoma: long-term results. Int J Radiat Oncol Biol Phys 2006;64:483–488.

59 Shin HS, Seong J, Kim WC, *et al.* Combination of external beam irradiation and high-dose-rate intraluminal brachytherapy for inoperable carcinoma of the extrahepatic bile ducts. Int J Radiat Oncol Biol Phys 2003;57:105–112.

60 Sethi A, Chen YK, Austin GL, *et al.* ERCP with cholangiopancreatoscopy may be associated with higher rates of complications than ERCP alone: a single-center experience. Gastrointest Endosc 2011 Feb;73(2):251–6.

CHAPTER 10

Sphincter of Oddi Manometry

Evan L. Fogel & Stuart Sherman

Digestive and Liver Disorders, Indiana University Health, University Hospital, Indianapolis, USA

KEY POINTS

- Sphincter of Oddi manometry (SOM) may be considered in the evaluation of patients with *disabling* abdominal pain suspected to be of pancreatobiliary origin, or idiopathic pancreatitis.

- Basic endoscopic retrograde cholangiopancreatography (ERCP) skills are essential for performance of SOM, as this cannot be accomplished without selective cannulation of the pancreatic duct and bile duct.

- Medications that may relax or stimulate the sphincter should be avoided for at least 8–12 h prior to performance of SOM and during the manometric session.

- Appropriate training in technical performance of SOM and interpretation of manometry tracings is required for both the endoscopist and the manometrist.

The sphincter of Oddi (SO) is a complex smooth muscle structure surrounding the terminal common bile duct, main pancreatic duct, and the common channel, when present (Figure 10.1). The high-pressure zone generated by the sphincter varies from 4 to 10 mm in length. The SO regulates the flow of bile and pancreatic exocrine juice, and prevents duodenum-to-duct reflux (i.e., maintains a sterile intraductal environment). The SO possesses a basal pressure and phasic contractile activities; the former appears to be the predominant mechanism regulating flow of pancreatobiliary secretions. Although phasic SO contractions may aid in regulating bile and pancreatic juice flow, their primary role appears to be maintaining a sterile intraductal milieu.

Sphincter of Oddi dysfunction (SOD) refers to an abnormality of SO contractility. It is a benign noncalculous obstruction to the flow of bile or pancreatic juice through the pancreatobiliary junction (i.e., the SO). This may cause pancreaticobiliary-type pain, cholestasis, and/or recurrent pancreatitis. The most definitive development in our understanding of the pressure dynamics of the SO came with the advent of SOM. SOM is the only available method to measure

---

ERCP: The Fundamentals, Second Edition. Edited by Peter B. Cotton and Joseph Leung.
Companion Website: www.wiley.com\go\cotton\ercp

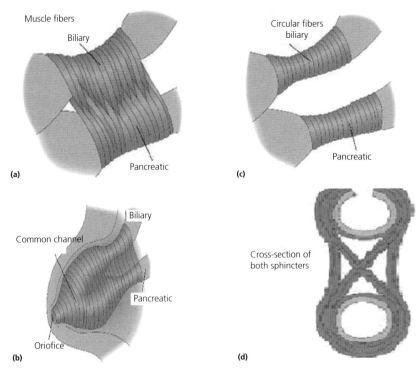

Figure 10.1 (a–d) Schematic representation of the sphincter of Oddi, demonstrating the circular smooth muscle that surrounds the common channel, distal common bile duct, and pancreatic duct. Source: Fogel EL, Sherman S, Lehman GA. Sphincter of Oddi Manometry. In: Cohen, J (ed). Successful Training in Gastrointestinal Endoscopy. Oxford: John Wiley and Sons 2011:324-331. Reproduced with permission of Wiley & Sons.

SO motor activity directly [2, 3]. SOM is considered by most authorities to be the most accurate means to evaluate patients for sphincter dysfunction [4, 5]. Although SOM can be performed intraoperatively [6–8] and percutaneously [9], it is most commonly done in the ERCP setting. The use of manometry to detect motility disorders of the SO is similar to its use in other parts of the gastrointestinal (GI) tract. However, performance of SOM is more technically demanding and hazardous, with complication rates (in particular, pancreatitis) approaching 20% in several series. Its use, therefore, should be reserved for patients with clinically significant or disabling symptoms. One needs to appreciate, however, that SOM is not likely an independent risk factor for post-ERCP pancreatitis when the aspirating manometry catheter is used (see discussion later). Questions remain as to whether the short-term observations (2–10 min recordings per pull-through) reflect the "24-h pathophysiology" of the sphincter [10–14]. Despite these problems, SOM has slowly gained more widespread application after three decades of evaluation, although lingering doubts as to its clinical utility do remain [15]. In this review, we will discuss the technique of SOM, with an emphasis on the technical and cognitive skill sets required. Specific indications for SOM are discussed elsewhere in this book (Section 17.3).

Method of SOM

Sedation

SOM is usually performed at the time of ERCP. The initial step in performing SOM, therefore, is to administer adequate sedation that will result in a comfortable, cooperative, motionless patient. All drugs that relax (anticholinergics, nitrates, calcium channel blockers, glucagon) or stimulate (narcotics, cholinergic agents) the sphincter should be avoided for at least 8–12 h prior to manometry and during the manometric session. Early studies with midazolam and diazepam suggested that these benzodiazepines do not interfere with SO manometric parameters and therefore are acceptable sedatives for SOM [16–20]. While one study did demonstrate a decrease in mean basal sphincter pressure in 4 of 18 patients (22%) receiving midazolam [21], these results have not been duplicated to date. Opioids had traditionally been avoided during SOM because of indirect evidence suggesting that these agents caused SO spasm [22–28]. However, two prospective studies [29, 30] have demonstrated that meperidine, at a dose of ≤ 1 mg/kg, does not affect the basal sphincter pressure but does alter phasic wave characteristics. Since the basal sphincter pressure generally is the only manometric criterion used to diagnose SOD and determine therapy, meperidine may be used to facilitate moderate sedation for manometry. Recent preliminary data also suggests that a low dose of fentanyl, administered topically, does not affect the basal sphincter pressure [31]. Confirmatory data are awaited. Patients referred for SOM may take large doses of narcotics on a daily basis and frequently prove difficult to sedate at ERCP. Adjunctive agents for moderate sedation, therefore, have been sought. Our group demonstrated that droperidol did not significantly alter SOM results; concordance (normal vs. abnormal basal sphincter pressure) was seen in 30 of 31 patients [32]. Wilcox and colleagues [33], on the other hand, suggested that droperidol did in fact influence SOM parameters. However, in their series of 41 patients, ERCP and SOM were carried out under general anesthesia in all but 7 patients. Indeed, an increasing recent trend has been to perform ERCP under general anesthesia or monitored anesthesia care (MAC). While it has been suggested that SO motor function is not influenced by general anesthesia [2], the effects of newer anesthetic agents are unknown, making interpretation of their results problematic. In one study, ketamine did not significantly alter SOM parameters, with concordance noted in 28 of 30 (93%) patients [34]. Limited experience with propofol suggests that this drug also does not affect the basal sphincter pressure [35, 36], but further study is required before routine use of ketamine or propofol for SOM is recommended. If glucagon must be used to achieve cannulation, a 15-min waiting period is required to restore the sphincter to its basal condition.

Equipment

Virtually all standards have been established with 5 French (Fr) catheters; therefore, these should be used. Triple-lumen catheters are state of the art and are available from several manufacturers. These are available in both long-nose and short-nose configurations (Figure 10.2). Catheters with a long intraductal tip may help secure the catheter within the bile duct, but such a long nose is commonly a hindrance if pancreatic manometry is desired. A sleeve catheter is a perfused channel system that records pressure along its length, potentially limiting motion artifacts during performance of SOM [38]. Limited data from Australia suggests that this sleeve method is comparable to standard SOM with triple-lumen catheters, possibly with lower pancreatitis rates [39], but more data are needed. Over-the-wire (monorail) catheters can be passed after first securing one's position within the duct with a guide wire. Whether this guide wire influences basal sphincter pressure has not been definitively elucidated (see discussion later). Some triple-lumen catheters will accommodate a 0.018- or 0.021-in. diameter guide wire passed through the entire length of the catheter and can be used to facilitate cannulation or maintain position in the duct. Guide wire–tipped catheters are also being evaluated. Early experience with performance of SOM using perfusion systems demonstrated unacceptably high postprocedure pancreatitis rates [40–43]. Presumably, overdistension of small-caliber pancreatic ducts may lead to this complication. Aspiration catheters (Figure 10.3) in which one recording port is sacrificed to permit both end- and side-hole aspiration of intraductal juice and the perfusing fluid are therefore highly recommended for pancreatic manometry. These catheters have been shown to reduce the frequency of post-SOM pancreatitis while accurately recording sphincter pressures [42]. Most centers prefer to perfuse the catheters at 0.25 ml/channel/min using a low-compliance pump (Figure 10.4). Lower perfusion rates will give accurate basal sphincter pressure measurements, but will not give accurate

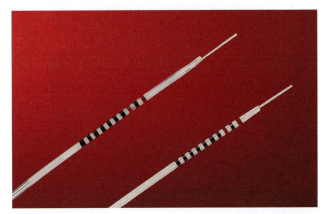

Figure 10.2 Long- and short-nose manometry catheters. Source: Fogel EL. Sphincter of Oddi Manometry. In: Baron TH, Kozarek RA, Carr-Locke DL (eds.): ERCP 2nd Edition. Philadelphia: Elsevier (Saunders) 2013: 124–137. Reproduced with permission of Elsevier.

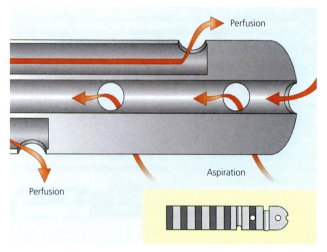

Figure 10.3 Schematic representation of a modified triple-lumen aspirating catheter. Source: Fogel EL, Sherman S, Lehman GA. Sphincter of Oddi Manometry. In: Cohen, J (ed). Successful Training in Gastrointestinal Endoscopy. Oxford: John Wiley and Sons 2011: 324–331. Reproduced with permission of Wiley & Sons.

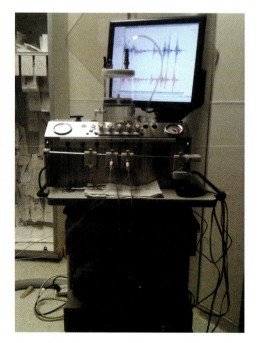

Figure 10.4 Photograph of a perfusion pump and accompanying monitor. Source: Fogel EL. Sphincter of Oddi Manometry. In: Baron TH, Kozarek RA, Carr-Locke DL (eds.): ERCP 2nd Edition. Philadelphia: Elsevier (Saunders) 2013: 124–137. Reproduced with permission of Elsevier.

phasic wave information. The perfusate is generally distilled water, although physiological saline needs further evaluation. The latter may crystallize in the capillary tubing of perfusion pumps and must be flushed out frequently. Solid-state catheters [43, 44] and microtransducer manometry systems [45] are also available and have been used by some investigators in an attempt to avoid volume loading of the biliopancreatic system during perfusion manometry [44, 46]. Preliminary data from a few centers demonstrate comparable SOM results to those achieved with perfusing catheters [43, 45]. More recently, Draganov and colleagues [47] performed SOM using both the aspirating triple-lumen water-perfused catheter and solid-state catheter in 30 patients. There was complete agreement on the final results of SOM (normal/abnormal) between the two groups (accuracy 100%).

Technical performance of SOM (see accompanying video)

SOM requires selective cannulation of the bile duct and/or pancreatic duct. Maximal efficiency is achieved by combining ERCP and SOM in a single session. It is preferable to perform cholangiography and/or pancreatography prior to performance of SOM, as certain findings (e.g., common bile duct stone) may obviate the need for SOM. This can simply be done by injecting contrast media through one of the perfusion ports. Alternatively, the duct entered can be identified by gently aspirating on any port (Figure 10.5). The appearance of yellow-colored fluid in the endoscopic view indicates entry into the bile duct. Clear aspirate indicates that the pancreatic duct has been entered. This technique may prove useful when attempting to access the bile duct following pancreatic SOM, as repeated pancreatic duct injections may increase post-ERCP pancreatitis rates [48]. If clear fluid is seen in the catheter, suggesting

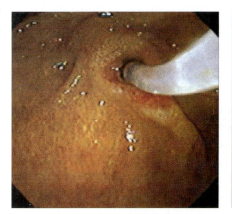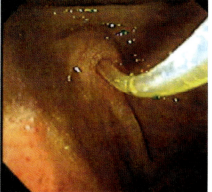

Figure 10.5 The duct entered during sphincter of Oddi manometry can be identified by aspirating the catheter. Clear fluid indicates pancreatic duct entry, whereas yellow fluid signifies entry into the bile duct. Source: Fogel EL, Sherman S, Lehman GA. Sphincter of Oddi Manometry. In: Cohen, J (ed). Successful Training in Gastrointestinal Endoscopy. Oxford: John Wiley and Sons 2011:324-331. Reproduced with permission of Wiley & Sons.

pancreatic duct entry, the catheter position is altered to achieve a more favorable angle for biliary cannulation. Blaut and colleagues [49] have shown that injection of contrast into the biliary tree prior to SOM does not significantly affect sphincter pressure characteristics. Similar evaluation of the pancreatic sphincter after contrast injection has not been reported. One must be certain that the catheter is not impacted against the wall of the duct in order to ensure accurate pressure measurements. On occasion, selective deep cannulation of the desired duct may only be achieved with a guide wire. However, stiffer shafted nitinol core guide wires used for this purpose commonly increase basal biliary sphincter pressure measured at ERCP by 50–100% [50]. Therefore, when wire-guided cannulation is performed, we recommend withdrawing the wire back into the catheter, outside of the duct and not traversing the sphincter, during performance of SOM. Alternatively, stiff guide wires need to be avoided or very soft-core guide wires must be used. Once deep cannulation is achieved and the patient acceptably sedated, the catheter is withdrawn across the sphincter at 1–2 mm intervals by standard station pull-through technique. Ideally, both the pancreatic and bile ducts should be studied. Current data indicate that an abnormal basal sphincter pressure may be confined to one side of the sphincter in 35–65% of patients with abnormal manometry [51–56], and thus one sphincter segment may be dysfunctional and the other normal. Raddawi and colleagues [53] reported that an abnormal basal sphincter pressure was more likely to be confined to the pancreatic duct segment in patients with pancreatitis and to the bile duct segment in patients with biliary-type pain and elevated liver function tests.

Abnormalities of the basal sphincter pressure should ideally be observed for at least 30 s in each lead and be seen on two or more separate pull-throughs. From a practical clinical standpoint, we settle for one pull-through from each duct if the readings are clearly normal or abnormal. It is important that there be no kinking or impaction of the catheter to cause spurious pressure rises or artifacts that might impair interpretation of the manometry tracing. During the pull-through, it is necessary to establish good communication between the endoscopist and the manometrist who is reading the tracing as it rolls off the recorder or appears on the computer screen. This permits optimal positioning of the catheter in order to achieve interpretable tracings. Alternatively, electronic manometry systems with a television screen can be mounted near the endoscopic image screen to allow the endoscopist to view the manometry tracing during endoscopy. This can be particularly helpful when vigorous duodenal motility is present, necessitating constant attention be paid to catheter position in the duodenal lumen. Once the baseline study is completed, agents to relax or stimulate (e.g., cholecystokinin) the SO can be given and manometric and pain response monitored. The value of these provocative maneuvers for routine use needs further study before widespread application is recommended.

Interpretation criteria

Criteria for interpretation of a manometry tracing are relatively standard; how-ever, they may vary somewhat from center to center. Some areas where there may be disagreement in interpretation include the required duration of basal sphincter pressure elevation, the number of leads in which basal pressure eleva-tion is required, and the role of averaging pressures from the three (or two in an aspirating catheter) recording ports. Our recommended method for reading the manometry tracings is first to define the "zero" duodenal baseline before and after the pull-through. Alternatively, intraduodenal pressure can be continuously recorded from a separate intraduodenal catheter attached to the endoscope. The highest basal pressure (defined as the pressure above the zero duodenal baseline; Figure 10.6) that is sustained for at least 30s is then identified. From the four lowest amplitude points in this zone, the mean of these readings is taken as the

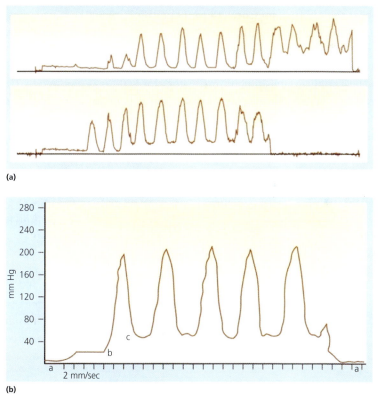

(a)

(b)

Figure 10.6 (A) An abnormal station pull-through at sphincter of Oddi manometry. The study has been abbreviated to fit onto one page. (B) Schematic representation of one lead of this tracing. (*a*) baseline duodenal 0 reference. (*b*) intraductal (pancreatic) pressure of 20 mmHg (abnormal). (*c*) basal pancreatic sphincter pressure of 45 mmHg (abnormal). Phasic waves are 155–175 mmHg in amplitude and 6 s in duration (normal). Source: Fogel EL. Clinical Perspectives in Gastroenterology 2001;165-173. Reproduced with permission of Elsevier.

basal sphincter pressure for that lead for that pull-through. The basal sphincter pressure for all interpretable observations is then averaged; this is the final basal sphincter pressure. The amplitude of phasic wave contractions is measured from the beginning of the slope of the pressure increase from the basal pressure to the peak of the contraction wave. Four representative waves are taken for each lead and the mean pressure determined. The number of phasic waves per minute and the duration of phasic waves can also be determined. Most authorities use only the basal sphincter pressure as an indicator of pathology of the SO. However, data from Johns Hopkins University [58] suggest that intrabiliary pressure, which is easier to measure than SO pressure, correlates with basal sphincter pressure. In this study, intrabiliary pressure was significantly higher in patients with SOD than those with normal basal biliary sphincter pressure (20 vs. 10 mmHg; $P<0.01$). In a similar study, the Milwaukee group [59] found that increased pancreatic duct pressure correlated with increased pancreatic basal sphincter pressure ($P<0.001$). Pancreatic duct pressure was significantly higher in SOD patients as compared with those with normal pressure (18 vs. 11 mmHg; $P<0.0001$). A pancreatic duct pressure greater than 20 mmHg was 90% specific and 30% sensitive for the diagnosis of SOD. These studies await confirmation but support the theory that increased intrabiliary and/or intrapancreatic pressure is a cause of pain in SOD.

The best study establishing normal values for SOM was reported by Guelrud and associates [12]. Fifty asymptomatic control patients were evaluated and repeated on 2 occasions in 10 subjects. This study established normal values for intraductal pressure, basal sphincter pressure, and phasic wave parameters (see Table 10.1). Moreover, the reproducibility of SOM was confirmed (see later). A potential limitation of this study, however, was the exclusion of patients with difficult cannulation or failed deep cannulation. Potentially, patients with small-caliber ducts might prove difficult to cannulate with a 5 Fr catheter, leading to a high-pressure zone on a purely structural basis, unrelated to muscle con-

Table 10.1 Suggested standard for abnormal values for endoscopic sphincter of Oddi manometry obtained from 50 volunteers without abdominal symptoms (Guelrud et al, 1990 [11] Reproduced with permission of Springer Science and Business Media).

Basal sphincter pressure*	>35 mmHg
Basal ductal pressure	>13 mmHg
Phasic contractions	
Amplitude	>220 mmHg
Duration	>8 s
Frequency	>10/min

Values were obtained by adding three standard deviations to the mean (mean obtained by averaging the results on two to three station pull-throughs). Data combine pancreatic and biliary studies.

*Basal pressures determined by (i) reading the peak basal pressure (i.e., highest single lead as obtained using a triple-lumen catheter); (ii) obtaining the mean of these peak pressures from multiple-station pull-throughs.

traction or spasm [15]. Despite this criticism, most authorities interchangeably use 35 or 40 mmHg as the upper limits of normal for mean basal SO pressure. Such upper limits of normal values are mean values plus 3 standard deviations. More studies are needed to determine if 2 or 2.5 standard deviations above the mean would be more appropriate.

Interobserver variability for reading SOM is minimal when the observers are experienced in reading these tracings [60].

Reproducibility of SOM

It has been questioned whether the short-term pressure recording obtained during SOM reflects the "24-h pathophysiology" of the sphincter, as patients with SOD may have intermittent, episodic symptoms [14]. If the basal sphincter pressure does vary over time, performance of SOM on two separate occasions may lead to different results and affect therapy. Three studies have demonstrated reproducibility of biliary SOM in 34 of 36 symptomatic patients overall [11, 13], and 10 of 10 healthy volunteers [12]. However, reproducibility of pancreatic SOM was found in only 58% (7/12) and 40% (12/30) of persistently symptomatic patients with previously normal SOM at two large referral centers [10, 14]. Other studies have also shown that SO basal pressures are not constant [61–63], perhaps due to the inherent physiological fluctuation of SO motor activity. Newer devices capable of portable, ambulatory, prolonged SOM would be of interest.

Complications of SOM

Several studies have indicated that pancreatitis is the most common major complication after SOM. Historically, using standard perfused catheters, pancreatitis rates over 20% have been reported, especially following manometric evaluation of the pancreatic duct. Such high complication rates have limited more widespread use of SOM. Placement of a small-diameter, protective, temporary pancreatic stent is now considered to be the standard of care in these high-risk patients [64, 65]. In addition, a recently completed multicenter randomized controlled trial demonstrated that rectal indomethacin (100 mg) decreased pancreatitis rates post-ERCP by 46% in high-risk patients (16.9% placebo group to 9.2% indomethacin group, $P = 0.005$), the majority of which were suspected/documented SOD [66]. Further studies to determine the optimal dose of indomethacin, as well as a direct comparison of pancreatic duct stent placement versus indomethacin alone, are planned or under way. A variety of other methods to decrease the incidence of postmanometry pancreatitis have been proposed. These include (i) the use of an aspiration catheter; (ii) gravity drainage of the pancreatic duct after manometry; (iii) decrease in the perfusion rate to 0.05–0.10 ml/lumen/min; (iv) limiting pancreatic duct manometry time to less than 2 min (or avoiding pancreatic manometry); (v) using the microtransducer or solid-state (nonperfused) systems. In a prospective randomized study, Sherman and colleagues [42] found that the aspirating catheter (this catheter allows for aspiration of the perfused fluid from end and side holes while accurately recording pressure from the two remaining sideports) reduced the frequency of pancreatic duct manometry-induced pancreatitis from 31 to 4% ($P=0.01$). The reduction in pancreatitis with use of this catheter in the pancreatic duct and the very low incidence of pancreatitis after bile duct manometry lend support to the notion that increased pancreatic duct hydrostatic pressure is a major cause of this complication. Thus, we routinely aspirate pancreatic juice and perfusate when we study the pancreatic duct by SOM.

In summary, mastery of the fundamentals of ERCP and appropriate training is necessary for the physician who evaluates patients with SOM. At a minimum, the endoscopist must be skilled in diagnostic ERCP, since performance of SOM cannot be accomplished without selective cannulation of the pancreatic duct and bile duct. The physician must be aware of the limitations on sedation imposed by manometry, and be familiar with the equipment needed to perform the procedure. Technical skills in manometric pressure recording techniques must be acquired, limiting the maneuvers that may lead to recording artifacts. Appropriate training in interpretation of manometry tracings is essential for both the endoscopist and the manometrist. An expert panel has stated in their position paper that training should be obtained at a pancreatobiliary center that routinely performs SOM [3]. While there are no society guidelines recommending specific numbers of procedures that need to be performed during training, a minimum of 100 SOM studies performed during the course of a 3-year clinical GI fellowship or an advanced 4th-year fellowship seems reasonable. There is no substitute for practice and experience.

TIPS AND TRICKS

1 When guide wire cannulation is needed to achieve deep cannulation, pull the wire back into the catheter during SOM, as having the wire across the sphincter may influence manometry results.

2 Ensure that there is no kinking or impaction of the catheter during SOM to cause spurious pressure rises or artifacts that might impair interpretation of the manometry tracing.

3 Following cannulation, aspiration of fluid via the manometry catheter allows for identification of the duct entered (yellow bile; clear, pancreatic), thus limiting pancreatic duct injections and potentially lowering post-ERCP pancreatitis rates.

References

1 Fogel EL, Sherman S, Lehman GA. Sphincter of Oddi manometry. In: Cohen, J (ed). *Successful Training in Gastrointestinal Endoscopy*. Oxford: John Wiley and Sons, 2011:324–31.
2 Gandolfi L, Corazziari E. The international workshop on sphincter of Oddi manometry. *Gastrointest Endosc* 1986;32:46–9.

3 Hogan WJ, Sherman S, Pasricha P, Carr-Locke D. Sphincter of Oddi manometry (position paper). *Gastrointest Endosc* 1997;45:342–8.

4 Lehman GA. Endoscopic sphincter of Oddi manometry: a clinical practice and research tool. *Gastrointest Endosc* 1991;37:490–2.

5 Lans JL, Parikh NP, Geenen JE. Application of sphincter of Oddi manometry in routine clinical investigations. *Endoscopy* 1991;23:139–43.

6 Sherman S, Hawes RH, Madura JA, Lehman GA. Comparison of intraoperative and endoscopic manometry of the sphincter of Oddi. *Surg Gynecol Obstet* 1992;175:410–8.

7 Funch-Jensen P, Diederich P, Kragland K. Intraoperative sphincter of Oddi manometry in patients with gallstones. *Scand J Gastroenterol* 1984;19:931–6.

8 Oster MJ, Csendes A, Funch-Jensen P, Skjoldborg H. Intraoperative pressure measurements of the choledochoduodenal junction, common bile duct, cysticocholedochal junction and gallbladder in humans. *Surg Gynecol Obstet* 1980;150:385–9.

9 Hong SJ, Lee MS, Joo JH, et al. Long-term percutaneous transhepatic manometry of sphincter of Oddi during fasting and after feeding. *Korean J Gastroenterol* 1995;27:423–32.

10 Varadarajulu S, Hawes RH, Cotton PB. Determination of sphincter of Oddi dysfunction in patients with prior normal manometry. *Gastrointest Endosc* 2003;58:341–4.

11 Thune A, Scicchitano J, Roberts-Thomson I, Toouli J. Reproducibility of endoscopic sphincter of Oddi manometry. *Dig Dis Sci* 1991;36:1401–5.

12 Guelrud M, Mendoza S, Rossiter G, Villegas MI. Sphincter of Oddi manometry in healthy volunteers. *Dig Dis Sci* 1990;35:38–46.

13 Geenen JE, Hogan WJ, Dodds WJ, et al. The efficacy of endoscopic sphincterotomy after cholecystectomy in patients with suspected sphincter of Oddi dysfunction. *N Engl J Med* 1989;320:82–7.

14 Khashab MA, Fogel EL, Sherman S, et al. Frequency of sphincter of Oddi dysfunction in patients with previously normal sphincter of Oddi manometry studies. *Gastrointest Endosc* 2008;67:108.

15 Haber GB, Sphincter of Oddi manometry: still a valid gold standard? *Endoscopy* 2010;42: 413–5.

16 Nebel OT. Manometric evaluation of the papilla of Vater. *Gastrointest Endosc* 1975;21:126–8.

17 Staritz M, Meyer Zum Buschenfelde KH. Investigation of the effect of diazepam and other drugs on the sphincter of Oddi motility. *Ital J Gastroenterol* 1986;18:41–3.

18 Cuer JC, Dapoigny M, Bommelaer G. The effect of midazolam on motility of the sphincter of Oddi in human subjects. *Endoscopy* 1993;25:384–6.

19 Rolny P, Arleback A. Effect of midazolam on sphincter of Oddi motility. *Endoscopy* 1993;25:381–3.

20 Ponce Garcia J, Garrigues V, Sala T, et al. Diazepam does not modify the motility of the sphincter of Oddi [letter]. *Endoscopy* 1988;20:87.

21 Fazel A, Burton FR. A controlled study of the effect of midazolam on abnormal sphincter of Oddi motility. *Gastrointest Endosc* 2002;55:637–40.

22 Economou G, Ward-McQuaid JN. A cross-over comparison of the effect of morphine, pethidine, pentazocine, and phenazocine on biliary pressure. *Gut* 1971;12:218–21.

23 Greenstein AJ, Kaynan A, Singer A, Dreiling DA. A comparative study of pentazocine and meperidine on the biliary passage pressure. *Am J Gastroenterol* 1972;58:417–27.

24 Radnay PA, Brodman E, Mankikar D, Duncalf D. The effect of equianalgesic doses of fentanyl, morphine, meperidine and pentazocine on common bile duct pressure. *Anaesthesist* 1980;29:26–9.

25 McCammon RL, Stoelting R, Madura JA. Reversal of fentanyl-induced spasm of the sphincter of Oddi. *Surg Gynecol Obstet* 1983;156:329–34.

26 Joehl RJ, Koch KL, Nahrwold DL. Opioid drugs cause bile duct obstruction during hepatobiliary scans. *Am J Surg* 1984;147:134–8.

27 Helm JF, Venu RP, Geenen JE, et al. Effects of morphine on the human sphincter of Oddi. *Gut* 1988;29:1402–7.

28 Thune A, Baker RA, Saccone GTP, et al. Differing effects of pethidine and morphine on human sphincter of Oddi motility. *Br J Surg* 1990;77:992–5.

29 Sherman S, Gottlieb K, Uzer MF, et al. Effects of meperidine on the pancreatic and biliary sphincter. *Gastrointest Endosc* 1996;44:239–42.

30 Elta GH, Barnett JL. Meperidine need not be proscribed during sphincter of Oddi manometry. *Gastrointest Endosc* 1994;40:7–9.

31 Koo HC, Moon JH, Choi HJ, et al. Effect of transdermal fentanyl patch on sphincter of Oddi—for application of pain management in pancreatitis. *Gastrointest Endosc* 2009;69:270.

32 Fogel EL, Sherman S, Bucksot L, et al. Effects of droperidol on the pancreatic and biliary sphincters. *Gastrointest Endosc* 2003;58:488–92.

33 Wilcox CM, Linder J. Prospective evaluation of droperidol on sphincter of Oddi motility. *Gastrointest Endosc* 2003;58:483–7.

34 Varadarajulu S, Tamhane A, Wilcox CM. Prospective evaluation of adjunctive ketamine on sphincter of Oddi motility in humans. *J Gastro Hepatol* 2008;23:e405–9.

35 Goff JS. Effect of propofol on human sphincter of Oddi. *Dig Dis Sci* 1995;40:2364–7.

36 Schmitt T, Seifert H, Dietrich CF, et al. Sedation with propofol during endoscopic sphincter of Oddi manometry. *Z Gastroenterol* 1999;37:219–27.

37 Fogel EL. Sphincter of Oddi manometry. In: Baron TH, Kozarek RA, Carr-Locke DL (eds.), ERCP 2nd Edition. Philadelphia: Elsevier (Saunders), 2013:124–37.

38 Craig AG, Omari T, Lingenfelser T, et al. Development of a sleeve sensor for measurement of sphincter of Oddi motility. *Endoscopy* 2001;33:651–657.

39 Kawamoto M, Geenen J, Omari T, et al. Sleeve sphincter of Oddi (SO) manometry: a new method for characterizing the motility of the sphincter of Oddi. *J Hepatobiliary Pancreat* Surg 2008;15:391–396.

40 Maldonado ME, Brady PG, Mamel JJ, Robinson B. Incidence of pancreatitis in patients undergoing sphincter of Oddi manometry. *Am J Gastroenterol* 1999;94:387–90.

41 Meshkinpour H, Kay L, Mollot M. The role of the flow-rate of the pneumohydraulic system on post-sphincter of Oddi manometry. *J Clin Gastroenterol* 1992;14:236–9.

42 Sherman S, Troiano FP, Hawes RH, Lehman GA. Sphincter of Oddi manometry: decreased risk of clinical pancreatitis with use of a modified aspirating catheter. *Gastrointest Endosc* 1990:36:462–6.

43 Tanaka M, Ikeda S. Sphincter of Oddi manometry: comparison of microtransducer and perfusion methods. *Endoscopy* 1988;20:184–8.

44 Tanaka M, Ikeda S, Nakayama F. Nonoperative measurement of pancreatic and common bile duct pressures with a microtransducer catheter and effects of duodenoscopic sphincterotomy. *Dig Dis Sci* 1981;26:545–53.

45 Wehrmann T, Stergiou N, Schmitt T, et al. Reduced risk for pancreatitis after endoscopic microtransducer manometry of the sphincter of Oddi: a randomized comparison with the perfusion manometry technique. *Endoscopy* 2003;35:472–7.

46 Frenz MB, Wehrmann T. Solid state manometry catheter: impact on diagnosis post-study pancreatitis. *Curr Gastroenterol Rep* 2007;9:171–4.

47 Draganov PV, Kowalczyk L, Forsmark CE. Prospective trial comparing solid-state catheter and water-perfusion triple-lumen catheter for sphincter of Oddi manometry done at the time of ERCP. *Gastrointest Endosc* 2009;70:92–5.

48 Freeman ML, DiSario JA, Nelson DB, et al. Risk factors for post-ERCP pancreatitis: a prospective, multicenter study. *Gastrointest Endosc* 2001;54:425–34.

49 Blaut U, Sherman S, Fogel E, Lehman GA. Influence of cholangiography on biliary sphincter of Oddi manometric parameters. *Gastrointest Endosc* 2000;52:624–9.

50 Blaut U, Sherman S, Fogel EL, et al. The influence of variable stiffness guidewires on basal biliary sphincter pressure measured at ERCP. *Gastrointest Endosc* 2002:55:83.

51 Eversman D, Fogel EL, Rusche M, et al. Frequency of abnormal pancreatic and biliary sphincter manometry compared with clinical suspicion of sphincter of Oddi dysfunction. *Gastrointest Endosc* 1999;50:637–41.

52 Aymerich RR, Prakash C. Aliperti G. Sphincter of Oddi manometry: is it necessary to measure both biliary and pancreatic sphincter pressure? *Gastrointest Endosc* 2000;52:183–6.

53 Raddawi HM, Geenen JE, Hogan WJ, et al. Pressure measurements from biliary and pancreatic segments of sphincter of Oddi. Comparison between patients with functional abdominal pain, biliary or pancreatic disease. *Dig Dis Sci* 1991;36:71–4.

54 Rolny P, Arleback A, Funch-Jensen P, et al. Clinical significance of manometric assessment of both pancreatic duct and bile duct sphincter in the same patient. *Scand J Gastroenterol* 1989;24:751–4.

55 Silverman WB, Ruffalo TA, Sherman S, et al. Correlation of basal sphincter pressures measured from both the bile duct and pancreatic duct in patients with suspected sphincter of Oddi dysfunction. *Gastrointest Endosc* 1992;38:440–3.

56 Chan YK, Evans PR, Dowsett JF, et al. Discordance of pressure recordings from biliary and pancreatic duct segments in patients with suspected sphincter of Oddi dysfunction. *Dig Dis Sci* 1997;42:1501–6.

57 Fogel EL, Sherman S. Performance of sphincter of Oddi manometry. *Clin Perspect Gastroenterol* 2001;May/June:165–73.

58 Kalloo AN, Tietjen TG, Pasricha PJ. Does intrabiliary pressure predict basal sphincter of Oddi pressure? A study in patients with and without gallbladders. Gastrointest Endosc 1996;44:696–9.

59 Fazel A, Catalano M, Quadri A, Geenen J. Pancreatic ductal pressures: a potential surrogate marker for pancreatic sphincter of Oddi dysfunction. *Gastrointest Endosc* 2002;55:92.

60 Smithline A, Hawes R, Lehman G. Sphincter of Oddi manometry: interobserver variability. Gastrointest Endosc 1993;39:486–91.

61 Guelrud M, Rossiter A, Souney PF, et al. The effect of transcutaneous nerve stimulation on sphincter of Oddi pressure in patients with biliary dyskinesia. *Am J Gastroenterol* 1991;86:581–5.

62 Lee SK, Kim MH, Kim HJ, et al. Electroacupuncture may relax the sphincter of Oddi in humans. *Gastrointest Endosc* 2001; 53:211–6.

63 Torsoli A, Corazziari E, Habib FI, et al. Frequencies and cyclical pattern of the human sphincter of Oddi phasic activity. *Gut* 1986;27:363–9.

64 Singh P, Das A, Isenberg G, et al. Does prophylactic pancreatic stent placement reduce the risk of post-ERCP acute pancreatitis? A meta-analysis of controlled trials. *Gastrointest Endosc* 2004;60:544–50.

65 Saad AM, Fogel EL, McHenry L, et al. Pancreatic duct stent placement prevents post-ERCP pancreatitis in patients with suspected sphincter of Oddi dysfunction but normal manometry results. *Gastrointest Endosc* 2008;67:255–61.

66 Elmunzer BJ, Scheiman JM, Lehman GA, et al. A randomized trial of rectal indomethacin to prevent post-ERCP pancreatitis. *N Eng J Med* 2012;366:1414–22.

CHAPTER 11

Endoscopic ampullectomy

Michael Bourke

University of Sydney, Sydney, Australia
Westmead Hospital, Westmead, Australia

KEY POINTS

- Ampullectomy is a safe and effective technique for the treatment of neoplastic papillary lesions.
- Significant complications may occur and thus significant endoscopist and team expertise are necessary.
- Appropriate tertiary-level surgical and interventional radiology support is mandatory.
- Patient comorbidities must be carefully considered and factored into the therapeutic approach.
- Careful multimodality radiological and endoscopic staging is required before proceeding, particularly for large lesions.
- Endoscopic biopsies may not be representative of underlying pathology.
- Pancreatic stents should be placed to minimize the risk of pancreatitis. This should be done promptly as bleeding may ensue and make this difficult.
- Delayed bleeding is the most frequent complication. It may be severe and life-threatening, particularly in those with significant comorbid illness. Both patients and clinicians must be prepared to deal with this.

Introduction

Endoscopic ampullectomy offers a minimally invasive method for effectively treating mucosal and some superficial submucosal lesions of the ampulla of Vater and surrounding periampullary region, with high success and relative safety [1]. These lesions would otherwise require surgical intervention, including pancreaticoduodenectomy (Whipple's procedure). Here I provide a practical guide to undertaking safe endoscopic ampullectomy, highlight some of the common difficulties with this therapy, and strategies to deal with these challenges.

ERCP: The Fundamentals, Second Edition. Edited by Peter B. Cotton and Joseph Leung.
© 2015 John Wiley & Sons, Ltd. Published 2015 by John Wiley & Sons, Ltd.
Companion Website: www.wiley.com\go\cotton\ercp

Lesion assessment and staging

At the initial endoscopy the lesion should be assessed by careful observation and biopsy. This should avoid the pancreatic orifice, generally located in the 5 o'clock position. Assuming the neoplasm involves most of the ampulla, as is usually the case, maximize safety by taking samples from the superior left-hand quadrant of the papilla between 9 o'clock and 1 o'clock, unless an obvious area of invasive disease exists. In this case it should be directly targeted. A careful tissue sampling approach is especially important for small lesions without pancreatic duct (PD) dilatation, where the risk of postbiopsy pancreatitis is greatest, for example, in familial adenomatous polyposis (FAP). If there is discordance between the anticipated pathology based on endoscopic appearances and the biopsy results, then the situation needs to be carefully reviewed, including multimodality staging and further endoscopic assessment and biopsy to ensure correct histology.

Most lesions are tubulovillous adenomas, but occasionally other submucosal lesions are encountered including carcinoid tumors and gangliocytic paragangliomas. Benign adenomatous lesions are soft, freely mobile, and devoid of ulceration. If the papilla is firm to probing with a sphincterotome, relatively fixed or ulcerated, then malignancy should be considered and if endoscopic treatment is being contemplated then complete staging is necessary irrespective of the biopsy results, which may not be representative.

Complete assessment and staging may include endoscopic ultrasound (EUS), magnetic resonance cholangiopancreatography (MRCP), contrast-enhanced multidetector computed tomography (CT), and careful cholangiopancreatography, usually at the time of ampullectomy. These modalities are used to define the nature and extent of the lesion, in particular assessing for evidence of submucosal invasion or lymph node metastasis and the presence and extent of any intraductal extension (IDE) [2, 3]. When concern for any of these features exists, staging should always be multimodal and comprehensive. No one test has proven to be definitive and they are often complementary.

EUS can detect IDE, assess depth of invasion, and identify pathological lymphadenopathy. It can be used for tissue sampling in cases where the diagnosis remains unclear, for example, in submucosal lesions. Its accuracy at T staging has been reported at between 60 and 75%, improving at higher T stages [3, 4]. MRCP provides noninvasive assessment of the distal common bile duct (CBD) and PD to detect for ductal dilatation, IDE, and anatomical variants such as pancreas divisum. Its accuracy in predicting IDE is uncertain, but it is certainly useful to exclude major extensions beyond the duodenal wall (Figure 11.1). Despite multimodality staging as outlined earlier, on occasion IDE may only be identified at endoscopic cholangiography at the time of resection. If IDE is limited to the papilla (and not beyond the duodenal wall) then en bloc excision can still be achieved. Endoscopic image enhancement, such as narrow band imaging, may be useful in defining the margins of the lesion [5], although this is generally not difficult.

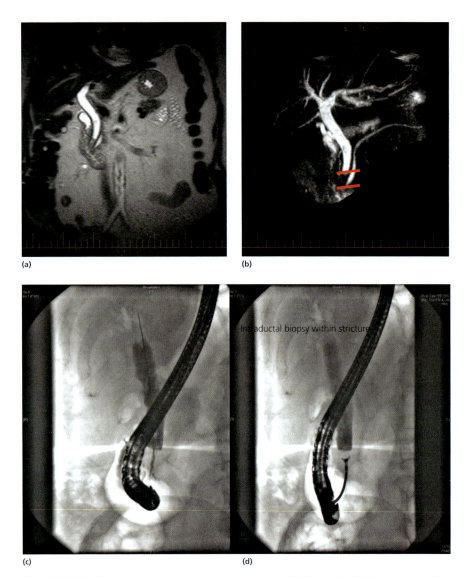

(a)

(b)

(c)

(d)

Figure 11.1 Significant intraductal extension suggested by MRCP (a, b), ERCP at the time of anticipated ampullectomy shows a shouldered stricture (c) that is probably malignant. An intraductal biopsy is taken (d).

For small (<15 mm) obviously benign lesions comprehensive staging is not necessary and careful cholangiopancreatography at the time of ampullectomy will often suffice. It is, however, helpful to have a prior MRCP, as in keeping with the general population, approximately 7% of patients scheduled for ampullectomy have pancreas divisum, and knowledge of this prior to the procedure averts the frustrating and potentially anxiety-provoking scenario of prolonged and ultimately failed PD cannulation.

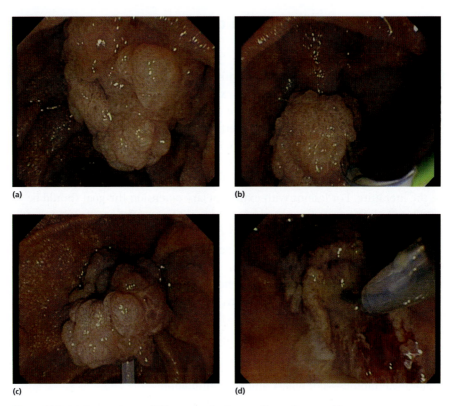

Figure 11.2 (a) A granular or villiform exophytic ampullary adenoma. These are most common and are usually benign. (b) The sphincterotome is used to move the neoplasm around so its margins can be evaluated and the length and size of the intramural segment of bile duct assessed. (c) The snare is closed tightly around the lesion. (d) The papilla and neoplasm have been removed and the pancreatic duct is cannulated with a guide wire.

There is no widely accepted endoscopic classification system for ampullary adenomas. My view is that they may be broadly grouped into three types [6]:

1 *Granular or villiform exophytic lesions* are most commonly encountered (>85%) and are usually benign. They may also have a laterally spreading component (termed laterally spreading tumor of the papilla or LST-P), extending onto the duodenal wall beyond the papilla (Figure 11.2a) [7].

2 *Smooth elevated lesions* are less frequent (10%) but probably have a greater risk for invasive disease.

3 *Umbilicated lesions* are uncommon. They are characterized by neoplastic tissue at the biliary orifice that may be exophytic, with a swollen otherwise feature-less mucosa overlying the papilla. This appearance is due to IDE of the neoplasm within the intrapapillary portion of the CBD and possibly beyond the duodenal wall. An unknown proportion of these lesions are primary distal biliary epithelial neoplasms. They also have a significant risk of invasive disease.

Endoscopic resection technique

General principles

For conventional papillary adenomas without extrapapillary extension, complete papillectomy with concomitant en bloc excision of the entire neoplasm should be the goal. To achieve this I favor complete single stage excision of the papilla to the plane of the duodenal wall. This method minimizes recurrence due to subtle IDE within the papilla [6, 7]. This type of recurrence is difficult to both detect and treat as the area tends to concert in upon itself after the initial intervention, limiting subsequent access. It accounts for the majority of the recurrences reported in the literature. For lesions with extrapapillary extension the goal should be to remove the lesion in as few pieces as safely possible, and the papilla itself should be excised as one. En bloc resection has many advantages including more accurate histological assessment and negligible recurrence. Endoscopic ampullectomy is an advanced therapeutic intervention that requires significant prior training, expertise and judgment to safely and effectively perform the procedure. Repeat intervention for partially resected lesions is difficult and entails an increased risk of complications due to the disruption of the underlying anatomy and submucosal fibrosis.

Equipment

- Sphincterotomes—For biliary and PD cannulation.
- Hydrophylic guide wires—For stent placement and duct access.
- Injection catheters including spring loaded (e.g., Carr-Lock needle, US Endoscopy, Cleveland, OH, USA)—In case of extrapapillary extension requiring submucosal injection and application of endoscopic mucosal resection (EMR) principles, and occasionally for injection therapy for bleeding.
- A range of stiff thin wire snares—No single snare meets all needs. I choose snares of suitable shape and size with reference to the morphology of the neoplasm.
- Coagulation forceps (Coag grasper Olympus Medical Corporation, Tokyo, Japan)—Brisk bleeding is not uncommon and the endoscopist must be prepared for it.
- Endoscopic clips—May be required for bleeding, deep tissue injury, or perforation.
- Biliary stents—Plastic 10 Fr, and metal fully covered removable, 8- and 10-mm diameter.
- Pancreatic stents—5 Fr plastic, proximal flange, and single distal pigtail.
- Retrieval nets.
- Microprocessor-controlled electrosurgical generator.

I recommend the use of stiff thin wire snare, with wires of approximately 0.3-mm diameter. The thin wire maximizes current density for swift transection of the papillary mechanism, minimizing the risk of "stalling" and limiting dispersion of the energy, which may cause unnecessary injury to the pancreatic orifice, increasing the risk of a late stenosis. Snare size should be closely adapted to the size of the target. Oval or hexagonal snares of approximately 10–20 mm are ideal for most conventional adenomas. The close approximation of lesion and snare size affords precision in tissue capture, ensuring an R0 excision where this is technically feasible. If the snare is too large, particularly if it is too long, it will buckle above the papilla, losing contact with the duodenal wall and risking an oblique transection of the papilla compromising the possibility of an R0 excision.

Microprocessor-controlled electrosurgical generators capable of delivering alternating cycles of high-frequency short-pulse cutting with more prolonged coagulation current are required (ERBE VIO 300 Tübingen, Germany; Olympus ESG-100, Tokyo, Japan). These generators sense tissue impedance via signals from the return electrode and adjust power output accordingly. As the tissue to be transected usually includes the muscle of the papillary mechanism, which may be resistant to division, these generators minimize the likelihood of "stalling." For endoscopic ampullectomy I use ERBE electrosurgical generators with the setting of Endocut Q, effect 3.

Resection technique

Endoscopic cholangiopancreatography is important for staging and should be undertaken prior to endoscopic ampullectomy. This is the most sensitive means of detecting subtle IDE. The clues are both tactile and visual. Fixed resistance to the passage of the sphincterotome across the papilla or a shouldered stenosis in the distal CBD or PD suggests the possibility of a malignant process and endoscopic treatment may need to be reconsidered. Prior cannulation also facilitates access to the PD after ampullectomy. If difficulty is encountered subsequently, photodocumentation of the orientation of the sphincterotome and position on the papilla at the time of PD cannulation may assist with localization of the orifice. Contrast escaping from the orifice may also help. Although methylene blue within the contrast is reported as a cannulation aid, in practice I don't find it useful. On occasion deep cannulation may be difficult. In this case it may be best to perform cholangio-pancreatography post resection. Exhaustive attempts at cannulation may not be helpful and may unnecessarily prolong the procedure and increase the risks of pancreatitis. Here again, a prior high-quality MRCP is invaluable.

After careful lesion assessment, an endoscopic resection plan is formulated. In most cases this is a direct en bloc papillectomy, aiming for an R0 resection with lateral and deep margins free of neoplasia (Figures 11.2–11.5). This minimizes the risk of recurrence.

- Orientate the lesion so that an en-face view is obtained with a stable duodenoscope position.
- For small lesions (<20 mm), complete, en bloc resection of the entire papilla without submucosal injection should be performed. This is also feasible for

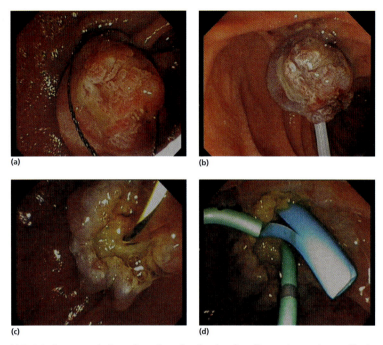

Figure 11.3 (a) The snare tip is anchored on the duodenal wall superior to the papilla, just a few millimeters above the point of reflection of the papillary mound onto the duodenal wall and usually slightly to the right, approximating 1 o'clock, closed tightly around the lesion. It is then opened parallel to the long axis of the papilla. (b) The snare is closed tight. (c) The papilla has been removed and the pancreatic duct cannulated, and bile is flowing from the bile duct. (d) Stents have been placed into both ducts.

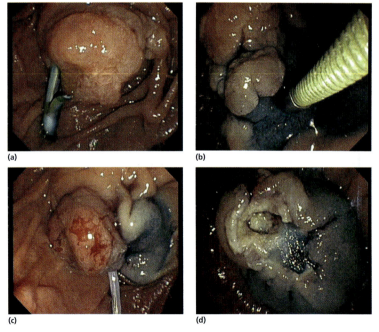

Figure 11.4 (a) A bulky lesion. (b) A submucosal injection is made beneath a small vertical extension. (c) The lesion is captured with the snare, which is closed maximally and the elevator then opened fully. (d) The lesion has been excised in a single piece.

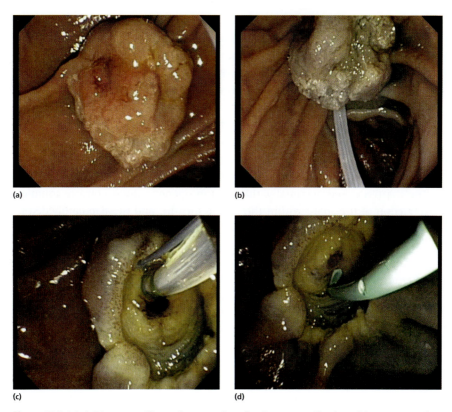

(a)

(b)

(c)

(d)

Figure 11.5 (a) A 20-mm papillary adenoma; there has been a small prior sphincterotomy that creates the appearance of an apparent depression in the middle of the lesion. Sphincterotomy may compromise complete resection and is best avoided prior to ampullectomy. (b) The lesion is completely enclosed within the snare. (c) The bile duct is cannulated and lifted vertically to expose the pancreatic duct orifice. (d) A pancreatic duct stent is being placed.

larger (>30 mm) lesions where the point of attachment does not exceed the boundaries of the papillary mound. In this case move the lesion up, down, and sideways with the sphincterotome or snare prior to resection to assess the lesions boundaries and evaluate the length and size of the intramural segment of bile duct beyond the margins of the neoplasm (Figure 11.2b).

- To resect the papilla the snare should be opened in a line approximating the long axis of the mound. This is done as follows. With the snare only partially opened, the snare tip is anchored on the duodenal wall superior to the papilla, just a few millimeters above the point of reflection of the papillary mound onto the duodenal wall and usually slightly to the right, approximating the 1 o'clock assuming that the true long axis of the papilla is at 12 o'clock (Figure 11.3a). In practice this slight right-sided positioning avoids the snare disimpacting and sliding off to the left. The snare is then slowly opened and positioned over the papilla, by gently pushing the duodenoscope distally whilst slowly opening the elevator and the snare simultaneously with gentle force keeping the snare tip impacted in the duodenal wall above. This has been termed the fulcrum technique. Once the snare has been placed over the papilla in this manner, it is closed maximally, as tight as possible without losing contact with the point of impaction above. The entrapped papilla should be independently mobile relative to the duodenal wall behind. This is assessed by opening the elevator completely and moving the snare back and forth; the entrapped tissue should slide freely for a short distance over the duodenal wall. If it is comparatively fixed this implies entrapment of deeper structures or invasive disease. You may elect to release (even momentarily) and recapture.

- The snare is closed maximally, the elevator opened fully (to ensure complete retraction of the snare within the plastic sheath), and the papilla divided by continuous application of current (as described earlier). This takes approximately two to three times (sometimes disconcertingly) as long as a polyp stalk of comparable size, usually 3–4 s.

- After resection the snare catheter should be used to lift the specimen above the papilla. If the patient is in the prone endoscopic retrograde cholangiopancreatography (ERCP) position it will then drop into the duodenal cap. Antiperistaltic agents such as hyoscine butylbromide, 10 mg, or glucagon, 1 mg, should be given just prior to ampullectomy to prevent distal migration of the specimen.

- Lesions with predominant vertical extrapapillary extension (usually Paris 0 – Is + IIa) [8] should be treated by initial maximal papillectomy in the vertical plane and beyond the inferior aspect of the true papilla. Submucosal injection should be used if it is possible to perform an en bloc excision of the entire lesion (extent <30 mm), in which case only the extrapapillary component should be elevated (Figure 11.4).

- Submucosal injection should not be placed directly into the papillary region; the papilla is relatively fixed to the duodenal wall and cannot be meaningfully elevated but rather the fluid may disperse laterally causing a sunken papilla and interfere with resection.

- Lesions with predominant lateral extrapapillary extension (LST-P, usually Paris 0 – IIa + Is) should be treated with submucosal injection and EMR at one edge, working sequentially from the distal aspect on one side and then the other to isolate the papilla, allowing subsequent en bloc papillectomy (Figure 11.4).

- When injection is required (for extrapapillary extension) most centers use an injection solution based on normal saline. We prefer succinylated gelatin, which is widely available in Australia and Europe. It is an inexpensive and safe colloidal solution that is commonly used for intravenous fluid resuscitation. In a double-blind controlled trial it significantly improved technical outcomes compared to normal saline in colonic EMR [9] although no evidence exists to quantify the magnitude of benefit in the duodenum. A biologically inert blue dye such as indigo carmine in a concentration of 0.04% is used in the injection solution to define the perimeter of the lesion, delineate the extent of the submucosal cushion, and confirm that one is working in the correct tissue plane. Dilute epinephrine in a concentration of 1:100,000 is also added to the injection solution.

- The PD should be accessed and stented as the first priority after the papillectomy. Level one evidence confirms that PD stent placement reduces the risk of pancreatitis [10]. After an initial hiatus, bleeding of varying intensity (mild venous oozing or major arterial bleeding) often ensues. This will often obscure the PD orifice and frustrate attempts at PD cannulation, creating unnecessary stress for the endoscopist. So prompt PD stent placement is advisable and it wise to have this equipment ready. If the PD orifice is not obvious, then if the CBD can be cannulated, lift this vertically to expose the PD orifice (Figure 11.5). The bile duct should then be cannulated. If there is concern of IDE on cholangiogram, sweeping with a stone extraction balloon can be used to try and expose this tissue, though a biliary sphincterotomy is usually required. Further snare resection of this tissue may then be performed, even within the distal bile duct [11].

- Intraprocedural bleeding is common [12] and can hamper visualization, further hindering stent placement. The endoscopist should have available, and be familiar with, a range of hemostatic devices including injectors, hemostatic clips, and coagulating forceps. Major bleeding is often best treated using coagulating forceps, but several therapeutic modalities may be required. For hemostasis with coagulating forceps I use "soft coagulation" 80 W, effect 4, with an ERBE generator. The bleeding point is grasped and gently tented away from the wall, before energy is applied (Figure 11.6). The soft coagulation mode caps the voltage to <200 V and thus limits carbonization and deep tissue injury. Theoretically, once the tissue is desiccated, tissue resistance rises rapidly and current can no longer flow and thus thermal damage ceases. It has recently been shown to be safe and effective in the colon even when using a snare tip [13].

Pancreatic stenting

The first priority after resection of the papilla is to place a pancreatic stent to reduce the risk of pancreatitis [10]. I prefer a short (3–5 cm, so it does not cross the genu) 5 Fr single-pigtail pancreatic stent with an internal flange. A plain X-ray in the fasting patient is obtained at day 14 and this stent can then be removed the same day if it is still in situ. It is important to ensure and document that the stent has passed or been removed, if left in situ beyond a few weeks it may result in PD injury or stricture. See Box 11.1 for tips on achieving pancreatic cannulation.

Biliary stenting and sphincterotomy

In contrast to PD stenting the evidence for routine biliary stent placement after ampullectomy is weak and the decision to proceed with biliary stenting should be individualized. It may be beneficial if there is the potential for major

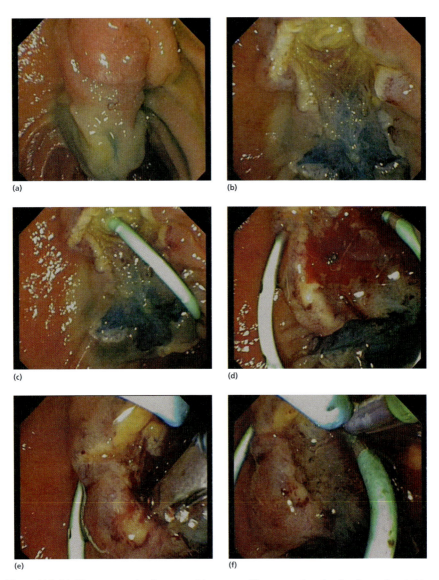

Figure 11.6 (a) 20-mm smooth adenoma with extrapapillary extension that has been elevated by submucosal injection. (b) The lesion has been excised en bloc. (c) A pancreatic stent has been placed. (d) Brisk bleeding ensues from the left-hand edge of the mucosal defect. (e) Coagulating forceps are used to treat the bleeding point. (f) The bleeding point has been effectively coagulated. A biliary stent has also been placed in case of further bleeding. The sphincterotome is being used to lift the stent up to visualize the bleeding point.

bleeding. In this case it may reduce the risk of ascending cholangitis from hemobilia and serve to orientate the endoscopist when a second procedure is required as the bile duct orifice is often obscured by a clot, in which case the stent can be glimpsed or localized fluoroscopically. Stent placement is also

---

Box 11.1 Tips for successful pancreatic duct (PD) cannulation after ampullectomy.

1 If possible, cannulate PD (and CBD) prior to ampullectomy and obtain a pancreatogram to determine the location of the pancreatic orifice and direction of the PD.

2 Remember the anatomical relationship between biliary and pancreatic orifices. If imagined on a clock face, the CBD is at 11 o'clock and the PD usually at 5 o'clock, although aberrant relationships occur in 5% (Figure 11.6).

3 Attempt PD cannulation as the first maneuver after ampullectomy whilst visualization is optimal.

4 If the PD cannot be identified then cannulate the distal aspect of the CBD with a sphincterotome and lift it up to "stretch" the pancreatic orifice and improve visibility (Figure 11.6).

5 Be wary of underlying pancreas divisum. The benefit of stenting the ventral duct is limited and attempts to do so can be frustrating.

---

important if there is concern over retroduodenal perforation; here it will ensure correct bile flow into the duodenum and potentially seal a small defect. In this situation I choose a fully covered self-expanding 8–10-mm-diameter removable metal stent depending on the native bile duct size. Too large a stent and the patient will have significant pain. The extra compressive force minimizes the migration risk and possibly by tamponade reduces the postprocedural bleeding risk. Biliary sphincterotomy may be considered if there is concern for stenosis of the orifice (e.g., a slow transection of the papilla) though evidence to recommend routine sphincterotomy is lacking and I do not recommend it.

Thermal ablation

We do not routinely apply thermal ablation (argon plasma coagulation (APC)) during ampullectomy as complete tissue destruction cannot be ensured. For advanced tissue resection in the colon, the use of APC is an independent predictor of recurrence [14]. Similar high-level data for ampullectomy are lacking, but it is reasonable to assume that the situation is similar. Instead, we prefer to completely resect all neoplastic tissue using a stiff thin wire snare. In the EMR situation with laterally spreading lesions we include a small cuff of normal tissue. If there is a diminutive recurrence or a residual lesion at either duct orifice not amenable to snare excision, I prefer to treat this with snare tip soft coagulation, using settings as described for hemostasis (with coagulating forceps above). Briefly, the snare tip is positioned so that it only just exits the plastic sheath of the snare, it is then gently touched against the residual tissue and current applied in short 1–3 s bursts; this results in precise, predictable tissue destruction without carbonization and scatter, a common problem with APC.

Specimen processing, postprocedural care, and endoscopic follow-up

All specimens should be retrieved for histological assessment. Commercially available 2–3-cm nets are the best option for multiple-specimen retrieval. The papillary resection and specimens larger than 15 mm should be flattened on a cork board and their margins pinned. Pinning of specimens (particularly after en bloc excision) prevents curling of the tissue within the formalin and facilitates more accurate histological assessment, allowing the pathologist to report on lateral and deep margins of excision.

After ampullectomy patients are kept in first-stage recovery for 2 h with abdominal examination before moving to second-stage recovery. They remain fasting for 4 h postprocedure and then commence a clear liquid diet. If the procedure is very straightforward and the patient is young with limited comorbidity then same-day discharge with close follow-up by phone call on day 1 is acceptable. Other patients are admitted to hospital, usually just for one night. Either way, whether the goal is inpatient or outpatient management, ampullectomy procedures are best scheduled in the morning so that, if there is an obvious or suspected complication, appropriate investigations, cross-team consultations, and management decisions can be considered and made in hours when the institutions' full resources are at hand, rather than in the middle of the night.

Endoscopic surveillance should be performed at 4–6 months and continue annually for 3–5 years as there is a small risk of late recurrence, despite a normal early follow-up examination. On each occasion the ampullectomy site is carefully examined, including photodocumentation and biopsy. If there is a residual lesion, this is generally diminutive and easily excised (or ablated if excision is not possible).

Complications and management

The most serious complications are perforation, bleeding, and pancreatitis and all are potentially lethal in their most severe forms [15–17]. Identification of high-risk patients, early recognition of complications, and aggressive management ameliorates their frequency and severity. The incidences of the most concerning complications are summarized in Table 11.1.

Bleeding

This is the most frequent complication as the duodenum is highly vascular and is thus at high risk of both early and delayed bleeding, particularly with resection of extensive and laterally spreading lesions [7–18]. Delayed bleeding is common and should in general be managed as for bleeding after endoscopic sphincterotomy. For patients with melena without hemodynamic

Table 11.1 Incidence of ampullectomy complications.

Complication	Incidence (%)
Bleeding	2–30
Pancreatitis	3–25
Perforation	0–8
Cholangitis	0–5
Papillary stenosis in follow-up	0–8

compromise I generally do not perform endoscopy as many will settle spontaneously. If major bleeding is a significant possibility then temporary biliary stenting is helpful to prevent obstructing hemobilia and localize the ampullectomy bed (and the likely bleeding site) amidst the brisk bleeding at the time of urgent endoscopy. For focal arterial bleeding coagulating forceps using soft coagulation as described earlier (80 W, effect 4–6 on the ERBE generator) is preferred. Clipping may be useful but can be difficult over the elevator of the duodenoscope. Consider removing the outer sheath of the clipping catheter. Care should be taken as it may be possible to tear the relatively fixed retroperitoneal duodenal wall with clips. Angiographic embolization is a useful option for endoscopically uncontrollable or massive hemorrhage.

As bleeding is frequent and may be massive, the patient's comorbidities and medications must always be very carefully considered against their bleeding risk, including their ability to tolerate the substantial physiological insult of major gastrointestinal hemorrhage. Malignant transformation in asymptomatic ampullary adenomas is generally slow and intervention in those with significant comorbidity, particularly the elderly to remove the lesion, may constitute a greater threat to life than the neoplasm itself.

Perforation

A control film at the start of the case with the duodenum inflated is important. The gas pattern can be compared against a similar film (with the patient and X-ray arm in the same position) taken at completion. Evidence for extraluminal gas can be used as an early warning prompting further assessment and/or treatment. Careful inspection of the resection defect must always be undertaken to assess for areas of deep or transmural injury. If there is any doubt consider placing a fully covered removable metal stent, bile duct diameter permitting, to anchor the distal CBD against the surrounding tissues and ensure bile flow into the duodenum. In my view CO_2 insufflation is now mandatory for all advanced endoscopic resection including ampullectomy, since it significantly reduces postprocedural pain. In case of perforation there are also theoretical advantages, due to reduced transmural pressure and enhanced resorption of escaped gas.

Endoscopic features are less reliable at determining deep resection than in other sites and so a high clinical index of suspicion must be maintained during postprocedural clinical assessment. Ongoing pain should prompt radiological assessment and surgical review. The absence of free intraperitoneal or subdiaphragmatic gas on plain X-rays does not exclude perforation, which is usually retroperitoneal. CT (preferably with oral contrast) is more sensitive and is the best test if there is genuine concern. Seeking a plain X-ray simply delays definitive exclusion of perforation. Oral contrast is very helpful to ascertain if there is an ongoing leak, the absence of which may allow conservative management, especially if there is no extramural fluid. Multidisciplinary management between medical and surgical teams is necessary to achieve the best possible clinical outcome. Not all cases of perforation require surgical intervention and select cases may be managed with gut rest and intravenous antibiotics; however, a significant fluid leak on CT will usually require drainage.

Pancreatitis

Prophylactic PD stenting is associated with a marked decrease in the risk of postampullectomy pancreatitis [10] and is the accepted standard. Prompt placement of a PD stent immediately after ampullectomy is necessary as brisk bleeding may swiftly ensue, making PD localization difficult. Prior MRCP may demonstrate pancreas divisum, in which case PD stenting is usually not necessary. Management of postampullectomy pancreatitis is generally the same as post-ERCP pancreatitis. Unexpected pancreatitis should prompt a swift X-ray to ensure that the PD stent has not migrated distally, in which case prompt endoscopic replacement (within a few hours) may ameliorate the severity.

Conclusion

The optimal technique for endoscopic ampullectomy is dependent on the lesion's size and the presence and extent of extrapapillary extension. Lesions confined to the papilla should be resected en bloc. The endoscopist must be mindful of both early and delayed complications and in particular the importance of early placement of a PD stent.

Endoscopic ampullectomy is a safe and effective therapy for papillary adenomas, LST-P, and some submucosal ampullary lesions when performed by experienced endoscopists. However, there is a substantial incidence of moderate to severe complications that the patient must be consented to and the endoscopist must be prepared to identify and manage. It is an advanced technique that requires optimal endoscopic expertise, appropriate equipment, and an experienced support team.

References

1 Adler DG, Qureshi W, Davila R, *et al.* The role of endoscopy in ampullary and duodenal adenomas. Gastrointest Endosc 2006; 64:849–54.

2 Manta R, Conigliaro R, Castellani D, *et al.* Linear endoscopic ultrasonography vs magnetic resonance imaging in ampullary tumors. World J Gastroenterol 2010; 16:5592–7.

3 Chen C-H, Yang C-C, Yeh Y-H, *et al.* Reappraisal of endosonography of ampullary tumors: Correlation with transabdominal sonography, CT, and MRI. J Clin Ultras 2009; 37:18–25.

4 Ito K, Fujita N, Noda Y, *et al.* Preoperative evaluation of ampullary neoplasm with EUS and transpapillary intraductal US: A prospective and histopathologically controlled study. Gastrointest Endosc 2007; 66:740–7.

5 Itoi T, Tsuji S, Sofuni A, *et al.* A novel approach emphasizing preoperative margin enhancement of tumor of the major duodenal papilla with narrow-band imaging in comparison to indigo carmine chromoendoscopy (with videos). Gastrointest Endosc 2009; 69:136–41.

6 Bassan M and Bourke MJ. Ampullectomy: A practical guide. J Interv Gastroenterol 2012; 2(1): 23–30.

7 Hopper AD, Bourke MJ, Williams SJ, Swan MP. Giant laterally spreading tumors of the papilla: Endoscopic features, resection technique, and outcome (with videos). Gastrointest Endosc 2010; 71:967–75.

8 The Paris endoscopic classification of superficial neoplastic lesions: Esophagus, stomach, and colon: November 30 to December 1, 2002. Gastrointest Endosc 2003; 58:S3–43.

9 Moss A, Bourke MJ, Metz AJ. A randomized, double-blind trial of succinylated gelatin submucosal injection for endoscopic resection of large sessile polyps of the colon. Am J Gastroenterol 2010; 105:2375–82.

10 Harewood GC, Pochron NL, Gostout CJ. Prospective, randomized, controlled trial of prophylactic pancreatic stent placement for endoscopic snare excision of the duodenal ampulla. Gastrointest Endosc 2005; 62:367–70.

11 Kim JH, Moon JH, Choi HJ, *et al.* Endoscopic snare papillectomy by using a balloon catheter for an unexposed ampullary adenoma with intraductal extension (with videos). Gastrointest Endosc 2009; 69:1404–6.

12 Norton ID, Gostout CJ, Baron TH, *et al.* Safety and outcome of endoscopic snare excision of the major duodenal papilla. Gastrointest Endosc 2002; 56:239–43.

13 Fahrtash-Bahin F, Holt BA, Jayasekeran V, *et al.* Snare tip soft coagulation achieves effective and safe endoscopic hemostasis during wide field endoscopic resection of large colonic lesions. Gastrointest Endosc 2013; 78:158–163.e1.

14 Moss A, Bourke MJ, Williams SJ, *et al.* Endoscopic mucosal resection outcomes and prediction of submucosal cancer from advanced colonic mucosal neoplasia. Gastroenterology 2011; 140:1909–18.

15 Yamao T, Isomoto H, Kohno S, *et al.* Endoscopic snare papillectomy with biliary and pancreatic stent placement for tumors of the major duodenal papilla. Surg Endosc 2010; 24:119–24.

16 Moon JH, Cha SW, Cho YD, *et al.* Wire-guided endoscopic snare papillectomy for tumors of the major duodenal papilla. Gastrointest Endosc 2005; 61:461–6.

17 Irani S, Arai A, Ayub K, *et al.* Papillectomy for ampullary neoplasm: Results of a single referral center over a 10-year period. Gastrointest Endosc 2009; 70:923–32.

18 Fanning SB, Bourke MJ, Williams SJ, *et al.* Giant laterally spreading tumours of the duodenum: Endoscopic resection outcomes, limitations and caveats. Gastrointest Endosc 2012; 75(4):805–12.

ASGE practice guidelines

The role of endoscopy in the evaluation and treatment of patients with biliary neoplasia, 2013.

The role of endoscopy in ampullary and duodenal adenomas, 2006.

CHAPTER 12

The Radiology of ERCP

Derrick F. Martin

Wythenshawe Hospital, Manchester, UK

Department of Radiology, University Hospital of South Manchester, Manchester, UK

KEY POINTS

- ERCP is a collaborative radiological–endoscopic procedure performed when less invasive imaging and other techniques have identified a condition requiring endoscopic treatment.

- Good results depend on having appropriate radiological equipment and knowledge of its optimal use.

- Reporting radiological images obtained at ERCP should be done with access to the endoscopy report.

- The risks of radiation for patients and practitioners can and should be minimized.

Emerging from the gloom

It seems that *Apollo 11*'s guidance computer was less powerful than today's mobile phone. Edmund Hillary's cotton jacket would struggle to keep you warm in England in winter, but these pioneers succeeded in their missions. Endoscopic retrograde cholangiopancreatography (ERCP) in the 1970s was not quite such a challenge as the Moon or Everest but there was no computed tomography (CT) or ultrasound scanning, and magnetic resonance cholangiopancreatography (MRCP) wasn't even thought of. ERCP was a voyage of discovery for the endoscopist, radiologist, and patient alike, and, given the fiberoptic endoscopes, accessories (reusable), and available fluoroscopy, it was sometimes very risky. Like the mobile phone and protective clothing for climbers, ERCP has moved on with developments on all fronts and advances in radiological techniques and equipment have combined to allow the current sophisticated clinical practice of ERCP.

In the early days, ERCP was an exciting procedure for radiologists, who attended the sessions and contributed both to interpretation and to development. However, most radiologists have plenty of other primary interests, so that ERCP endoscopists tend to function with only a radiographer/technician who may or may not be very familiar with the technique.

ERCP: The Fundamentals, Second Edition. Edited by Peter B. Cotton and Joseph Leung.
© 2015 John Wiley & Sons, Ltd. Published 2015 by John Wiley & Sons, Ltd.
Companion Website: www.wiley.com\go\cotton\ercp

These comments are intended to help endoscopists maximize the value of their procedures, while also reducing the risks.

Diagnostic radiology and ERCP

It is impossible to know how many ERCPs are undertaken annually worldwide, but with increasing obesity and an ageing population, gallstone disease is unlikely to decline. There seems little that can be done to ameliorate the risk factors for obstructing malignancy, and so the need for biliary drainage will remain.

ERCP has its own risks; the only way to avoid risk completely is not to do the procedure. It is best to use imaging to define the problem before ERCP and never before has the endoscopist been in the fortunate position of being able to know what ERCP will demonstrate and what should be done. In the past, we have all been in the position of undertaking a procedure only to discover something unexpected and to wish that, at that moment, we were elsewhere.

Ultrasound

The role of ultrasound (US) in the management of obstructive biliary disease has not altered. US is excellent at demonstrating bile duct dilatation and gallbladder stones. It is less good at demonstrating the level of obstruction or the presence of stones in the bile duct, which lies in the shadow of gas in the stomach or duodenum. It is said that US is operator dependent. This is a misunderstanding and it is clear that every procedure, diagnostic or therapeutic, is operator dependent. Not every radiologist will appreciate the subtleties of an imaging examination except perhaps in retrospect, and not every endoscopist is able to cannulate the desired duct.

Other roles for US are detection of parenchymal liver disease, generalized or focal, and the evaluation of focal liver lesions seen on other imaging. Despite its limitations, US should be undertaken on every patient suspected of biliary or pancreatic disease.

Computed tomography

Modern multidetector CT (MD CT) machines can scan the abdomen in seconds and rapidly reproduce 1–3-mm axial, coronal, and sagittal images (Figure 12.1). CT does not come without cost. Radiologists are anxious about intravenous contrast media (CM)–related anaphylaxis, but this risk is insignificant compared with the risk of CM-induced acute kidney injury [1]. Referral for CT should be made with knowledge of the patient's renal status and the presence of comorbidities such as diabetes mellitus. Renal protective measures can be undertaken in those with borderline function.

Radiation dose from CT causes concern globally. For the elderly, the risk is low, but for young patients, the risk of long-term malignant complications is real and needs to be set against the anticipated benefits.

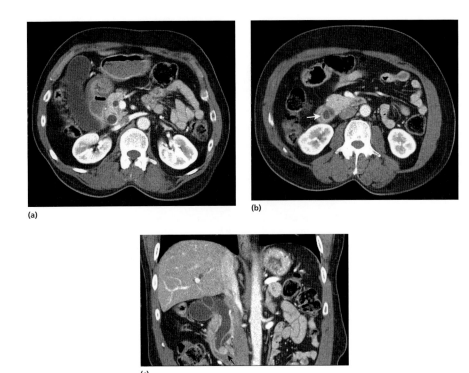

Figure 12.1 A 70-year-old man with painless jaundice. (a) Axial image showing dilated pancreatic and bile ducts with a distended gallbladder. (b) Confluence of the bile duct and pancreatic duct at the papilla bulging into the duodenum (arrow). (c) Coronal reformatted image showing an enhancing tumor of the papilla (arrow) with dilated bile duct and pancreatic duct above.

CT is best reserved for patients with suspected malignancy for diagnosis and staging. CT should always be undertaken before stenting.

Patients with gallstones may undergo CT when the diagnosis is unclear or when they have acute pancreatitis. The provision of clinical information to the radiologist who protocols the CT examination is important. The pattern of CT examination with regard to the administration of CM differs depending upon the clinical question; for example, a patient with suspected pancreatic cancer, another with acute pancreatitis, and another with focal liver lesions all need different CT examinations. Operator dependency also refers to the requesting physician or surgeon; ask the wrong question and don't be surprised if you get the wrong answer.

Magnetic resonance

Magnetic resonance (MR) is equivalent to CT for the investigation/staging of pancreatic cancer, but superior for the evaluation of hepatic and biliary disease. MRCP in particular is a rapid, noninvasive investigation that depicts the biliary

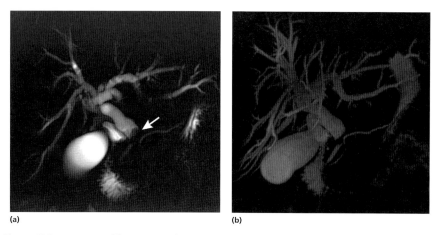

(a)   (b)

Figure 12.2 A 37-year-old woman with pain and jaundice. (a) A 20-mm-thick radial T2-weighted MRCP image showing a stone (arrow) impacted at the junction at the cystic duct and common duct. (b) Maximum intensity projection image in the same patient.

system exquisitely without the need for CM, using only the inherent contrast of bile on T2-weighted imaging (Figure 12.2). MRCP has equivalent sensitivity to endoscopic ultrasound (EUS) for the detection of bile duct stones. Physicians and surgeons referring for MR examination should be aware of the contraindications, which include the presence of a pacemaker. However, there are now MR-friendly pacemakers and MRCP in patients with some types of pacemaker is possible after discussion with the patient's cardiologist and the MR imaging staff [2].

It is clear that before ERCP, some scanning techniques (US, CT, MRCP, and/ or EUS) should already have defined the nature of the disease and have guided a strategy for therapy. With modern imaging there need be no surprise, which might leave the endoscopist rueful [3].

A word about timing

Desperately urgent imaging or intervention is rarely needed in hepatobiliary and pancreatic disease. Even in severe acute cholangitis there is time and clinical need, to resuscitate the patient in order to optimize the outcome of biliary drainage. In acute pancreatitis and malignant obstruction, urgency is not an issue except for the patient and relatives to understand what is going on. Time for proper preparation and the development of a strategy of management should always be taken. A simple example for the need to consider timing is for the patient who presents with mild interstitial edematous gallstone pancreatitis. Such patients get better quickly and have usually passed the offending stone. ERCP is not indicated. Cholecystectomy may be planned and MRCP requested to assess the bile duct beforehand. MRCP showing a clear bile duct is of no value at the time of cholecystectomy a month later. Better to arrange MRCP a few days before cholecystectomy with ERCP provisionally booked so that cholecystectomy is not delayed if MRCP is positive. Careful thought to a

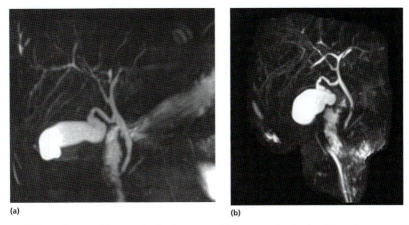

(a)   (b)

Figure 12.3 A 40-year-old man who had recovered from an episode of mild acute pancreatitis. (a) Preoperative MRCP showing a clear bile duct. (b) Same patient presented a short time later with painful jaundice repeat MRCP demonstrating a bile duct stone.

management strategy for any individual patient should be given in order to optimize the imaging plan (Figure 12.3).

Percutaneous transhepatic cholangiography

Percutaneous transhepatic cholangiography (PTC) with external or internal/external drainage and stenting is still widely practiced. Emerging EUS-based techniques for intervention are interesting but not yet widely practiced or available [4]. Randomized studies are lacking. Endoscopic biliary drainage techniques for the growing number of patients with Roux-en-Y gastric bypass are likely to develop but will surely only be for the endoscopic heroes. Percutaneous techniques will need to be maintained. Despite single-center excellence the generality of practice shows that PTC is a procedure with significant morbidity and mortality even in benign disease. Its main use is likely to remain the management of patients with obstructive biliary disease where endoscopic access has failed or is impossible. For patients with malignant disease transhepatic metal stenting has removed the need for combined endoscopic and percutaneous procedures. This is now reserved for the patients with bile duct stones where endoscopic access is impossible usually because of a large periampullary diverticulum.

Arguments regarding the preference of endoscopic or percutaneous drainage of complex hilar malignancy have never been resolved and will continue, practice depending upon local skills and availability.

Radiology of ERCP

Radiographic equipment

Many ERCPs are done in radiology suites, where the equipment is usually of reasonable quality. This is less obviously the case when C-arm units are installed in endoscopy units. No national guideline relating to ERCP training and practice makes any stipulation about the quality or standards of hardware. Interestingly, this is so for endoscopes as well as for radiographic equipment. Endoscopists are interested in endoscope technology, and endoscopes are relatively inexpensive; therefore most units have good stock. This cannot be said for radiographic equipment, which is expensive and has to last for years. The more expensive it is, the more it needs to be used, to maximize return on investment and the cost of maintenance.

With radiographic equipment you get what you pay for. Radiologists are interested in image resolution, contrast, brightness, lesion conspicuity, image noise, and so on, and for image-guided intervention, radiologists demand the highest quality to ease interpretation of pathology and guide intervention. Why should endoscopists be different? Some ERCP units work with old or inexpensive mobile or fixed fluoro units, either because that is all they can afford or because that is all that their radiology department can allow. Graduation to a state-of-the-art fluoroscopy system can bring a revelation similar to that experienced when you put on your first pair of reading glasses and realize what you have been missing for the last 5 years. Good solid scientific evidence that supports this philosophy is obviously lacking but it is intuitively true. The endoscopist who operates with poor-quality fluoroscopy has one hand tied behind their back and not only chances their reputation and livelihood but risks their patients as well. The choice is not about the mobile C-Arm or the all-singing, all-dancing fixed fluoro unit, but is about image quality. Go for the best you can possibly get and do not compromise.

Room design

For radiology rooms, such as installations for interventional radiology (IR), there are clear national guidelines in most countries, which relate particularly to radiation protection. In undertaking ERCP, operators are advised to make certain that they are aware of their institution's as well as their national guidelines.

When installing a unit, it is essential to make sure that the design allows optimal access for the endoscopist and the anesthesia/sedation provider.

Image recording

The digital camera has revolutionized family photography. Most of us have thousands of images on computer, quite different from the couple of shoeboxes full of old photos kept under the stairs by our parents. The same is true of digital radiography. Static images and video loops can be easily recorded and kept for review, the only limitations being radiation dose and image storage capacity. Even the latter will eventually be limitless. The ERCP fluoro unit should be connected to the hospital Picture Archiving and Communication System (PACS) so that images are available for team review locally or remotely. Radiographic film–based imaging systems are years out of date and lack the immediacy and availability of digital systems.

Contrast media

The days of ionic CM are gone and now all iodine-based water soluble CM are either hypotonic or isotonic with blood. These have greater acceptability when given intravascularly and maximize comfort during intervention. There is no evidence for the preference of any CM in terms of complications of ERCP, particularly pancreatitis [5]. However, there are simple tips that make life easier. Use two different concentrations of CM. One concentration should be 300–350 mg of iodine/ml, which is dense. Before an initial attempt at cannulation is made, the cannulation device should be primed with this dense CM. On injection only a small volume is necessary to confirm entry into a duct system. If the biliary system is preferred and the pancreatic duct is to be avoided, inadvertent cannulation of the pancreatic duct is immediately evident with the denser CM. Dense CM is also more viscous, making it more difficult to overfill the pancreatic duct rapidly, perhaps reducing the risk of inducing pancreatitis. If the dense CM is contained within a larger diameter syringe the protection is even greater, since the injection force is reduced. If the bile duct is cannulated and cholangiography is required then the dense CM should be changed or a less dense medium containing approximately 150 mg of iodine/ml. This lower-density CM is less likely to obscure small stones within a dilated system. If intrahepatic duct cholangiography for the demonstration of small duct disease is necessary then it is wise to revert to the dense CM to improve image resolution, perhaps also using balloon occlusion cholangiography.

Contrast media reactions—prevention and treatment

As with all procedures involving CM administration, a preprocedural check for allergies should be made. CM reactions during ERCP are vanishingly rare, but all endoscopists should familiarize themselves with their local and national guidelines regarding prophylaxis and treatment of acute allergic reactions.

Who owns the fluoro button?

Radiation dose protection for staff and patients is paramount and most institutions have guidelines and training facilities for endoscopists to undertake fluoroscopy. In many units the radiology technician/radiographer is asked to operate the fluoro whilst the endoscopist views the image. Very clear principles need to be established between the endoscopist and the radiographer regarding this. There is a tendency for the endoscopist to ask for the radiographer to "screen" or "fluoro" but then forget to say "stop." Equally, if the endoscopist operates the fluoro with a foot switch it is crucial that brain and foot communicate so that when the endoscopist stops looking at the fluoro image, the foot is lifted. Clear local institutional training should be provided.

How to improve image quality and aid accurate interpretation

Except during cholangioscopy, ERCP is a radiological procedure with immediate interpretation of the findings and decisions regarding therapy being made in the light of preprocedural information and imaging findings. It is therefore helpful to take all possible steps to improve image quality. The use of CM in order to do this has been explained earlier.

Patient position

It is best to lay the patient prone. Although many elderly people state that they have not lain prone for years, once they get into position with help they are normally very comfortable, particularly if stiff necks, shoulders, and hips are padded with pillows. The prone position gives stability and provides good endoscopic and airway access. From a radiographic standpoint a vertical fluoro setup gives good anteroposterior (AP) imaging. Thus image interpretation of relative anatomy is easier but also, because the AP diameter of the patient is normally less than the lateral diameter, this position reduces radiation scatter and image noise and improves image resolution. It also reduces radiation dose. If a patient cannot lie prone, then get them as near as possible and then rotate the fluoro unit in order to achieve an AP position. For some with severe lung disease or who are intubated and ventilated and those for whom the prone position is not physiologically appropriate, supine ERCP is straightforward although slightly more tricky for the endoscopist.

Which way is up?

In the days of abdominal fluoroscopy for small bowel studies or barium enema, the patient lay supine on the table and images were projected and recorded conventionally, so that the patient's right side was on the left of the image as viewed. The same is so for the standard chest radiograph.

If the patient lies prone then convention is that the patient's right side is on the right side of the image, which is much more obvious. Many ERCP images are therefore incorrectly displayed with the patient's right side on the left of the image as if the patient was lying supine. Does it matter? Not if you know what your local convention is and as long as you are consistent. The obvious advantage is the easy comparison with MRCP images, normally displayed with the patient supine (Figure 12.4).

Preliminary image

Before or after the insertion of the endoscope, it is useful to take a plain film before the injection of CM; this can show gas in the bile duct and calcification in stones. It also allows assessment of calcification of costal cartilages, a common irritant that can cause debate as to the presence of stone or bile duct leak if contrast has been injected without a preliminary image for comparison. Always try to clear the field of artifacts, monitoring cables, buttons, and so on (Figure 12.5).

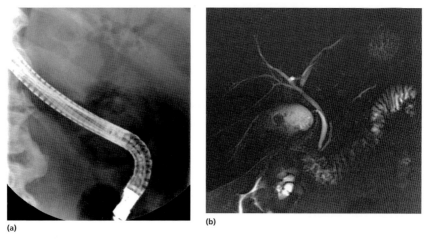

(a)

(b)

Figure 12.4 (a) Radiographically correct projection of ERCP image showing an air choloangiogram. (b) Radiographically correct projection of an MRCP image.

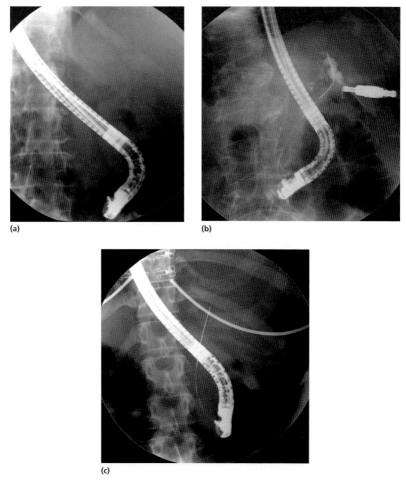

(a)

(b)

(c)

Figure 12.5 (a) A correctly projected and collimated plain film before contrast injection. (b and c) Imaging field cluttered by extraneous artifacts, which could lead to confusion.

Further imaging

There is no set rule regarding image recording. It is wise to document findings at relevant points during the procedure; for example, when pathology is first demonstrated; when CM is injected through a stricture to delineate its margins; after intervention, for example, stone removal or stent placement and to document any complication. It is also helpful to have a completion image as a record of what was achieved. This image is also useful to evaluate the presence of retroperitoneal perforation.

Contrast injection

Most endoscopists now cannulate using a sphincterotome and guide wire injecting CM once the bile duct has been entered and bile is seen in the cannula. However, occasionally if the wire will not run freely a short puff of CM to open the biliary sphincter will allow the wire to pass. Once the cannulation device is in the bile duct it is only necessary to inject enough CM to determine that you are in position and what the next step in therapy should be. If there are known gallstones in the bile duct, sphincterotomy can be undertaken and full cholangiography performed using an extraction balloon or basket subsequently. If a stricture is encountered CM should be injected below the stricture and then above after the passage of a guide wire in order to delineate its extent.

When injecting CM into the bile duct it is wise to be aware of the effects of flow. CM injected into the distal bile duct will cause stones to migrate proximally, even into the intrahepatic ducts, possibly leading to misinterpretation. CM injected at the level of the confluence of the hepatic ducts will cause any stone to be washed distally and therefore more easily seen.

Image size and magnification

The area to be imaged should not normally extend beyond the right upper quadrant, an anticipated area to encompass the gallbladder laterally, the body of the pancreas medially, the right costophrenic sulcus superiorly, and the third part of the duodenum inferiorly. An image that shows an endoscope isolated in a view of the whole abdomen is to be deprecated as bad practice. Such images reduce diagnostic image quality, waste radiation dose, and demonstrate poor technique.

Most fluoro units have a range of three or four levels of magnification. Always choose the level of magnification to suit the task in hand. For example, during cannulation of the bile duct, magnify the image maximally in order to be able to see the tip of the cannulation device and assess the passage of the guide wire into the duct system. Once access has been achieved, the level of magnification can be reduced in order to demonstrate the relevant duct system (Figure 12.6).

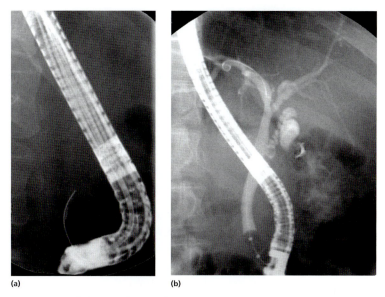

(a)   (b)

Figure 12.6 (a) Magnified image during sphincterotome and wire-guided cannulation of the bile duct. (b) Correct magnification for imaging of the whole biliary system.

Collimation (coning)

All fluoro systems have movable symmetrical collimators, which reduce the visible image size for any magnification. All systems have an automatic exposure device similar to the automatic iris in a video endoscope. This alters the brightness of the image depending upon the level of radiation hitting a sensor. If this level is high, for example, if the base of the lungs is included on the image, the system will reduce the level of radiation thereby reducing the clarity of a cholangiogram. If the collimators are drawn in, the level of radiation will be more appropriate and image quality improves. Also, collimation of the X-ray beam reduces scattered radiation, reduces image noise, and improves image resolution. You can see more clearly (Figure 12.7).

Tricky imaging situations

Is there a stone?

It is a common occurrence when the history or preprocedural imaging indicate a bile duct stone, that a stone is not visible on cholangiography. Stones pass spontaneously. It is also not uncommon for an invisible stone to be extracted after sphincterotomy. There are of course circumstances where it would be better to avoid sphincterotomy if the ducts can be shown to be clear with confidence. Cholangiography is a dynamic situation. It is possible to inject and aspirate CM in an attempt to reveal the elusive stone. Avoid overfilling the ducts

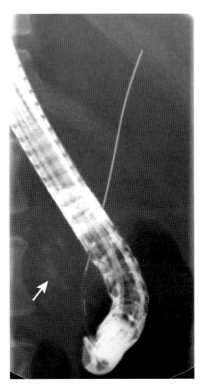

Figure 12.7 Tight collimation of the magnified image allows clear definition of faint pancreatic calcification in the head of the gland (arrow).

as this causes patient discomfort and increases the risk of cholangitis but, by exploring the duct with a catheter, injecting and aspirating CM, better-quality cholangiography can be achieved. Using an inflated balloon drawn down the duct can suck stones out of the intrahepatic ducts.

Bubbles

Care should be taken to avoid bubbles in the cannulation device and injecting syringe, but bubbles sometimes appear. There is no failsafe method of distinguishing bubbles from stones on simple imaging alone. Placement of the cannulation device alongside what looks like a bubble and aspirating may make it disappear. Sucking with a balloon may work. Turning the patient or tilting the table is disappointing.

Clarifying difficult anatomy

Conventional biliary anatomy is as follows: two right-sided anterior segments drain into an anterior sectoral duct and fuse with a similar posterior right-sided sectoral duct to form the right hepatic duct. Segments 2, 3, and 4 join to form the left hepatic duct. The right and left hepatic ducts converge into the

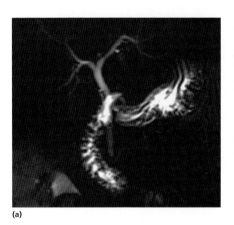 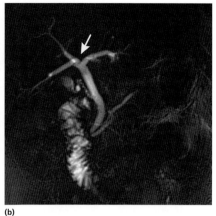

(a)   (b)

Figure 12.8 (a) Normal confluence of sectoral and hepatic ducts. (b) A normal variant in which the anterior and posterior right ducts join at their confluence with the left hepatic duct.

common hepatic duct, which joins the cystic duct to form the common bile duct. This conventional anatomy occurs in less than two-thirds of the normal population. There is an array of biliary anatomical variants. Thankfully for the endoscopist, most of these are easily and safely interpreted on magnetic resonance cholangiography. However, it is helpful for the endoscopist to understand a few of the more common variants. Radiologists should report anatomical variants on MRCP (Figure 12.8).

Cystic duct

The cystic duct can enter the common duct laterally, medially, high, or low. Difficult circumstances can arise when inadvertent entry into the cystic duct is not appreciated. This is particularly so when stent placement is planned. Entry into the common hepatic duct or the intrahepatic duct system in such circumstances should always be confirmed by the presence of a guide wire in the intrahepatic duct system or the injection of CM to confirm position.

Right posterior sectoral duct

This can be a problem duct for two reasons. In about 15%, the right posterior sectoral duct (RPSD) drains into the left hepatic duct (Figure 12.9). This clearly has an influence on the result of attempted right-sided drainage in a patient with a hilar lesion. A stent placed in the right hepatic duct would only drain two segments of the liver.

A second problem is that the RPSD can enter the common hepatic duct below the level of the hilum of the liver. The RPSD can enter close to the cystic duct and these can be confused particularly at dissection during laparoscopic cholecystectomy. Injury to the RPSD under such circumstances is a well-recognized

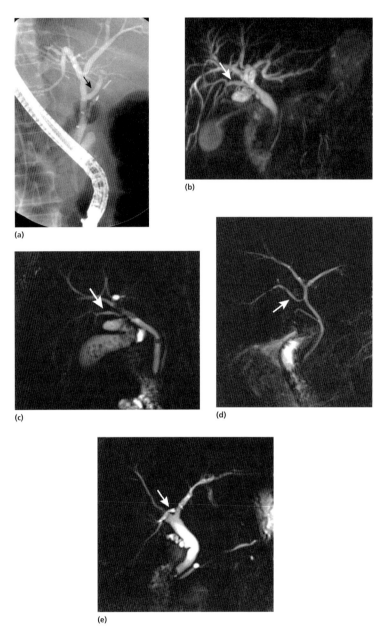

Figure 12.9 The right posterior sectoral duct. (a) ERCP in a patient after cholecystectomy shows how close the surgeon was to this low-lying right posterior sectoral duct. (b, c, and d) Shows other patterns of low-lying right posterior sectoral duct insertion. (e) The right posterior sectoral duct inserted into a left hepatic duct.

problem [6]. To make life even more complicated, the RPSD can drain into the cystic duct or the cystic duct can drain into the RPSD. These variants need to be understood and recognized as a misunderstanding of the anatomy can be disastrous.

Because of the great variety in biliary anatomy a planning MRCP is an essential component of preprocedural assessment of biliary tumors.

Stricture assessment

If there is a complex stricture in a duct system, particularly the biliary system, the two-dimensional fluoroscopic representation of the three-dimensional duct system can make it difficult to understand the relative anatomy. This is needed in order to place stents correctly. To gain an understanding of the three-dimensional anatomy, rotation of the patient or the fluoro unit will help. Remember parallax. Two structures close together will maintain their relative positions with rotation. Two structures distant from one another will not maintain this relationship; rotating a prone patient to the right will make an anterior structure move medially and a posterior structure move laterally. It is easier to swing the tube than to move the patient.

Radiation risk and protection

For the patient ERCP brings the necessity for radiation exposure. For the endoscopist and staff attending the patient a degree of radiation exposure is inevitable because of their necessary proximity to the radiation source.

Particularly because of the inexorable rise in the use of CT, radiologists and radiation protection authorities are increasingly anxious about the radiation burden being borne by patients, especially the young. Worrying figures of cancer risk can be found in the literature and on the Internet and whilst accuracy regarding risk is debatable there is no doubt that the higher the radiation dose, the greater the risk of adverse occurrence. This risk is not just about cancer. Studies of IRs demonstrate a significant risk of cataract and perhaps brain tumors, in long-term operators, risks to which endoscopists too are exposed.

Endoscopists may feel that measures to protect elderly patients, particularly those with malignant disease, from risk from radiation-induced harm are less necessary because of the patient's limited longevity and because of clear benefit versus low risk. However, endoscopists should remember that their source of irradiation is scattered radiation from the patient and therefore any measure that reduces radiation dose to the patient also diminishes dose to staff.

How can we minimize radiation dose?

1 Planning—ERCP should only be undertaken as a therapeutic maneuver in a defined clinical situation where preliminary imaging has shown the need. In radiation protection terms this is "justification" for the use of ionizing radiation and is a legal requirement.

2 Optimization—This means having the best possible circumstances in order to undertake the procedure successfully in the shortest time. Naturally this depends on the skill of the team; an extremely skilled team will probably complete an interventional procedure more quickly. Nonetheless, despite the level of skill, the situation should always be optimal. Optimization involves using the best fluoroscopic equipment available on a patient who is properly positioned and comfortably sedated or anaesthetized and paying attention to radiographic technique.

3 Limitation—Limitation of radiation dose is not just about keeping your foot off the fluoro switch. It involves a number of measures all of which combine to limit radiation dose to patient and staff.

Fluoroscopy unit

A unit with the tube beneath the table has inherently lower radiation exposure for operators than an over-table tube because of the physics of scattered radiation.

All fluoroscopy units have electronic and mechanical dose-saving aspects. With the expansion of IR, equipment manufacturers have increasingly sophisticated dose-saving protocols. Those available on every fluoroscopic unit include automatic exposure devices, which set tube voltage and tube current to optimum levels. All fluoroscopy units have intermittent fluoroscopy settings. This means that the operator can set the emission rate of radiation from being permanently on when the foot switch is activated to pulsed radiation a few times a second. Clearly, if the fluoroscopy unit pulses radiation for a total of half a second every second then there is as 50% dose saving compared with continuous fluoroscopy. Perfectly adequate imaging can be achieved with lower pulse settings.

Collimation of the X-ray beam has already been described as a maneuver to improve image quality. A tightly collimated X-ray beam reduces scattered radiation from the patient thereby reducing patient and operator dose. Collimate the beam as tightly as you can to see what you want to achieve.

Mechanical devices

Most fluoroscopy units come with table-mounted lead-glass or lead-rubberized protection screens. Surprisingly, the endoscopist's legs receive a significant radiation dose during ERCP, which can be controlled with the use of such screens. Eye dose and thyroid dose can be reduced by interposing a ceiling-mounted lead-glass screen between the radiation source and the operator.

Personal protection

Radiation dose is dependent on the inverse square law. The further you are from the patient the lower the radiation dose as a function of the square of that distance. Endoscopists inevitably have to stand close to their patient, so protective clothing is essential. Manufacturers of lead gowns now have materials that are quite light in weight but have significant protective properties. A properly fitting gown should be worn that covers the entire red marrow–containing skeleton, the shoulder girdle, spine, pelvis, sternum, and femora. Gowns should not be open at the side; endoscopists may stand sideways on to the table rendering open gowns ineffective. Thyroid shields should be worn, as should lead-glass spectacles. Spectacles should shield laterally as well. Lead-rubberized shin and foot protectors are also advisable for high-dose operators. Staff supporting the endoscopist should wear similar personal protection. Radiation dose monitoring for all is mandatory and should be regular.

Pregnant patients

ERCP is occasionally necessary in pregnant ladies with bile duct stones. It is possible to undertake ERCP after preliminary MRCP assessment. If bile duct access if easy and confirmed by the aspiration of bile, sphincterotomy and stent placement can be undertaken without any radiation exposure, further treatment being delayed until after the pregnancy. If fluoroscopy is required then the patient can wear the skirt of a two-piece lead gown, which gives 360° protection to the fetus in AP and lateral directions. An additional lead gown can be placed on the table under the patient's abdomen for extra protection. It is important also to protect the patient's breasts from ionizing radiation, as the breast is particularly sensitive to radiation during pregnancy. Naturally, all other dose-saving measures should be undertaken, keeping fluoroscopy time to an absolute minimum and avoiding exposures for permanent images. All fluoro units have the ability to image grab the final frame of a fluoroscopy burst and keep this stored.

Interestingly, most of the measures designed to reduce radiation dose also improve image quality and therefore diagnostic and therapeutic success.

Endoscopists should see radiation protection measures, not as a tedious irrelevance but as a quality aspect of their service.

References

1 Anathhanam S, Lewington AJ. Acute kidney injury. J R Coll Physicians Edinb 2013;43: 323–329.
2 Viera MS, Lazoura O, Nicol E, *et al.* MRI in patients with implantable electronic devices. Clin Rad 2013;68;928–934.

3 Akisik MF, Jennings SG, Aisen AM, *et al.* MRCP in patient care: a prospective survey of gastroenterologists. Am J Roentgenol 2013;201:573–577.

4 Bapaye A, Dubale N, Aher A. Comparison of endosonography-guided vs. percutaneous biliary stenting when papilla is inaccessible for ERCP. United European Gastroenterol J 2013;1: 285–293.

5 Ogawa M, Kawaguchi Y, Kawashima Y, *et al.* A comparison of ionic, monomer, high osmolar contrast media with non-ionic, dimer, iso-osmolar contrast media in ERCP. Tokai J Exp Clin Med 2013 Sep 20;38(3):109–113.

6 Wojcicki M, Patkowski W, Chmurowicz T, *et al.* Isolated right posterior bile duct injury following cholecystectomy: report of two cases. World J Gastroenterol 2013;19:6118–6121.

CHAPTER 13

ERCP reporting and documentation

Lars Aabakken

Oslo University Hospital—Rikshospitalet, Oslo, Norway

KEY POINTS

- The endoscopic report is the main tool to document and convey the endoscopic retrograde cholangiopancreatography (ERCP) procedure and the result.

- Differentiated reports may be needed for different readers; patients need special adaptions to appreciate the report.

- Structuring the report and including compulsory items facilitates quality assurance work and helps track the performance of the unit.

- Structured description of findings based on MST and standard definitions helps develop a common language.

- Image documentation is crucial to ERCP but standardization is needed even here, as well as good communication with the radiologists.

While most endoscopists aspiring to master ERCP will focus on intubation, cannulation, and therapeutic techniques, the issue of accurately reporting what was done is an indispensable element of a successful procedure. An accurate report is crucial for the referring doctor, but it has several other practical, administrative, and legal applications as well.

Previously, endoscopic reports, like most doctors' notes, were nonstructured narrative descriptions of findings, conclusions, and recommendations. Increasingly, however, structure, minimal requirements, and standardized language are becoming ubiquitous features of medical documentation. This applies to endoscopic reports as well, and good structured reporting should be an integral element of ERCP training.

Structured reporting

When you read a textbook chapter or a scientific report in a medical journal, you expect a defined structure, with certain elements appearing at standard places. Similarly, a standardized structure will aid those who receive endoscopy reports.

ERCP: The Fundamentals, Second Edition. Edited by Peter B. Cotton and Joseph Leung.
© 2015 John Wiley & Sons, Ltd. Published 2015 by John Wiley & Sons, Ltd.
Companion Website: www.wiley.com\go\cotton\ercp

This goes partly for what components are included, their internal order, as well as the content and internal structure of each component. As for reporting findings, the "Minimal Standard Terminology" of gastrointestinal endoscopy [1] offers a framework for the description of lesions. This system offers a limited number of core terms that can be used to describe the most frequent findings. A number of required attributes with possible attribute values are presented for each term/lesion. In addition, a backbone of definitions for these terms is available [2] guiding the correct use of the individual terms. This system was originally developed for luminal endoscopy, and thus easiest to implement for these modalities. However, ERCP and endoscopic ultrasound (EUS) have been included in the later version—MST 3.0 [3]. Thus, the description of ERCP findings can mostly be performed in adherence to the MST systems, while other technical elements or details of therapeutic maneuvers are less well implemented at the present time.

Report content

The structure of the ERCP report should mirror the reports of other endoscopic modalities as far as possible. This is one of the utilities of the standardized recommendations offered by a recent Working Party Report of the World Endoscopy Organization (WEO) [4], and the structure described later relates to these recommendations. However, it must be noted that this document is a minimal guidance, and most centers will opt for additional details or options based on local needs, repertoire, and scientific interest.

Administrative data
- Endoscopy facility
- Patient identifier (name, medical record number, date of birth)
- Date, time, location
- Endoscopic procedure (main category)
- Elective/emergent procedure
- In-/outpatient
- Endoscopist(s)
- Endoscopy nurse(s)
- (Anesthetist/nurse)
- Referring doctor, additional addressees

Comments. Most endoscopic facilities will likely present their endoscopy reports in a special format including letterheads, logos, typographic specifics, and structure. All the elements of the administrative data would be similar for all endoscopic modalities and should be developed as a joint venture within the endoscopy unit, and probably also in keeping with hospital-wide standards. Adaptions would be likely; for example, the endoscopic procedure ("ERCP") might be presented in large letters at the top of the reports to identify this crucial piece of information right away. In other facilities, the patient ID might be given a more central position, and standardized toward other components of the general medical record of the hospital.

A listing of all recipients of the reports is important, to clarify the responsibilities of the reader. The referring physician will see which key consultants have been notified of the findings directly.

Clinical data

- Indication/reason for endoscopy (MST)
- Brief history including relevant family history
- Risk assessment: American Society of Anesthesiologists score, comorbidities, anticoagulation, infection risk, electromedical risk, other specific risk factors
- Information given/informed consent statement

Comments. The report should include the reasons for doing the procedure, and the considerations made to take this decision. These include the clinical situation, including relevant previous imaging, but also the alternatives, the risk profile of the patient and explicit statements about the patient's informed consent. While components of this information may be documented already in the general medical record of the patient, or in the referral letter, core items belong in the endoscopy report as well. This is especially important for ERCP, where the risk/benefit ratio is fundamentally different from simpler procedures.

MST 3.0 offers a core listing of indications for ERCP. However, most facilities will need to modify this list for local needs, expanding the list or adding subcategories for research or other purposes. The history should include pertinent details of previous ERCP procedures, including findings, therapy and technical issues, including specific problems, patient tolerance.

Technical information

- Sedation and other drugs
- Equipment (endoscope) used
- Quality of cleansing/visualization
- Extent of the examination
- Technical/procedural aspects (specific problems/solutions)
- Patient comfort/sedation quality

Comments. Although some of these details may be of minor interest to the referring physician, they might be vital to the recovery area personnel (e.g., amount and timing of sedation), or to the next endoscopist who could be greatly aided by knowing certain specifics of previous procedures.

Some of these aspects, including quality of the ductal imaging or patient comfort, would be relevant in a quality assurance program, together with other more explicit quality aspects.

The extent of the examination for ERCP would entail information about what level of ductal access was achieved, *relative to the intentions.* Pancreatic ductography may well be intended and even critical, but if opacification was accidental, this should be stated in the report. Thus, the success of the procedure is not as predefined and constant as, for example, in colonoscopy. Rather, the success is the relation between intentions and final results. For quality assurance, this aspect is important, but it requires objective reporting by the endoscopist.

In some training institutions, details on the relative contribution (and even times) by fellow and tutor are recorded. These data are not considered compulsory, but may be important, for example, to monitor the learning curve of the trainees.

Some patient metrics (e.g., blood pressure, oxygen saturation curves, and arrhythmias) may well be collected automatically from monitoring hardware. Some endoscopy software systems can incorporate these data, as well as tracking the specific endoscope used (and even its disinfection and storage history).

Statements on patient consent should be included. However, it is crucial that these reflect the reality of the consent process. Automated text entries at one click of a button may be misinterpreted, and software solutions must ensure that this information is entered correctly.

Procedural details

• Duodenal intubation and pertinent luminal findings
• Cannulation details and accessories
• Ductographic findings
• Sampling or therapeutic procedures including results
• In-procedure events

Comments. This section differs somewhat from the template for luminal procedures, since additional details of how things are performed is often of interest, not just end results.

Positioning of the patient should be noted, as well as details of the intubation and positioning in the second part of the duodenum. Depending on the clinical context, luminal findings outside of the periampullary may be of interest, for example, esophageal varices in patients with liver disease, strictures of the esophagus, duodenal ulcerations. In these cases, additional dedicated upper endoscopy should be considered. Relevant periampullary anatomical variations should be noted, for example, mucosal swelling, strictures, or diverticula. Even relevant negative findings should be explicit in the report, for example, "no esophageal varices" or "no sign of leakage" or of previously seen pathology.

The method of ductal access as well as specific issues of papillary cannulation should be noted, to acknowledge an increased risk of pancreatitis or other complications. Ductographic findings should be described according to standardized terminology (MST 3.0), to ensure accurate descriptions and avoid ambiguous terms. Measurements should be presented in millimeters or centimeters insofar as possible. Anatomical terms should also be standardized (Figure 13.1).

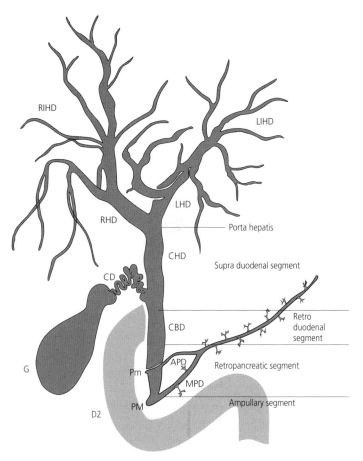

Figure 13.1 Standardized terminology of the pancreatobiliary ductal anatomy. APD, accessory pancreatic duct (ductus pancreaticus accessorius); CBD, common bile duct (ductus choledochus); CD, cystic duct (ductus cysticus); CHD, common hepatic duct (ductus hepaticus communis); D2, descending part of the duodenum; G, gall bladder; LHD, left hepatic duct (ductus hepaticus siniter); LIHD, left intrahepaticus ducts (ducti intrahepaticus sinistri); MPD, main pancreatic duct (ductus pancreaticus major); PM, papilla duodeni major; Pm, papilla duodeni minor; RHD, right hepatic duct (ductus hepaticus dexter); RIHD, right intrahepatic ducts (ducti intrahepaticus dextri). Source: Waye 2013 [2] Reproduced with permission of Normed Verlag.

Sampling procedures must be noted, including what analyses will be done. Therapeutic measures should be described in detail, for example, caliber of dilating catheters, length and size of balloons and stents, duration of dilation procedures. End results should be stated, in relation to starting point where relevant.

In-procedure unplanned events should be described, with measures taken to remedy the situation, and the outcome at the end of the procedure. It should also be stated whether the event changed the outcome or results of the procedure per se. These facts will determine whether the event reaches threshold for a countable "adverse event," as recently defined [5].

Summary and recommendations

For many readers of ERCP reports, the summary and recommendations will be the main items of interest. This section should include core information of the procedure including the diagnostic and therapeutic aspects of the ERCP and the end result. Recommendations should be made as to immediate monitoring, but also about the interpretation of findings, repeat procedures, or other follow-up. A clear statement should made as to the responsibility for follow-up aspects.

Imaging

Image documentation of endoscopic procedures is a natural part of the report [6]. For ERCP, the radiology images have for a long time been a component of the ERCP output, but with the image storage and reporting systems residing within the radiology department in most hospitals, the "endoscopic" and "radiological" reporting aspects have had a tendency to live separate lives. Easily accessed storage of endoscopic images has been scarce, partially due to lack of suitable hardware, difficulties to integrate medical record systems in general, and also because of the focus on the X-ray images. The radiology images tend to live in the world of radiology, with separate protocols, hardware, and storage mechanisms and even networks.

Reading and reporting the X-ray images, often suboptimally captured by the endoscopist, is difficult for radiologists who are usually not present during the procedure [7, 8]. This is unfortunate, and it would be good to strive for a more joint documentation mechanism in the future. Making sure that the radiologist receives a copy of the endoscopy report is essential. Hopefully, integrated electronic medical record systems may remedy this dysfunctional dualism.

Radiology imaging

Recommendations and advice for optimal radiological documentation are largely lacking in the endoscopic domain. Standards are now slowly emerging (in press), but they can only serve as a rough guidance, given the diversity of ERCP and the variable need for specific images.

However, some general principles can help to optimize the quality (and quantity) of radiographic imaging [8]. More details are given in Chapter 12.

1 Make sure the patient is correctly identified on the X-ray monitor. This should be a part of your compulsory start-up routine together with checking all of the equipment and X-ray shielding.

2 Before exposure, position your X-ray tube at an optimal position, and screen the edges of your image inasmuch as possible, to improve image quality and reduce radiation. Usually, a direct anteroposterior angle is preferable, although other angulation may occasionally be useful.

3 If you struggle approaching the ampulla, especially in the setting of duodenal strictures and dilation, imaging of this procedure should be done. This is particularly important in the unlikely event of adverse events, for example, perforations.

4 Capture a scout picture with your endoscope in cannulating position, before any contrast is injected. Make sure any foreign bodies (cables, cloth details, piercings) are removed from the field of interest. Without this, calcifications in ribs or vessels, and recent contrast imaging, may cause much confusion.

5 Initial guide wire positions need not be documented, but the initial contrast injections must be very accurately recorded. Frequently, these first images with limited contrast saturation are the most instructive, particularly to delineate hilar anatomy or reveal the location of leaks. Small stones will also drown in overfilled ducts.

6 Complete filling of the pertinent ductal system should be shown. This may require balloon occlusion, in particular in the setting of narrow or obstructed intrahepatic ducts, to avoid preferential overfilling of the gallbladder or contrast leak through a papillotomy. Angulation of the imaging or temporary repositioning of the endoscope may be necessary to capture the key elements.

7 Any pathological (or suspicious) lesions, as well as relevant anatomical aberrations, should be documented. Good understanding of the ductal anatomy and their variations is critical.

8 Relevant phases of therapeutic maneuvers are shown, in particular the end result (stent in place, stones cleared, balloon at end of dilation period).

9 Any adverse events must be shown (basket impaction, contrast leakage or submucosal filling, pancreatic acinarization or free air).

10 Final images are taken after removing the endoscope. Emptying dynamics of the intraductal contrast may be important, and sometimes additional imaging in the supine position may add useful extra information, particularly in terms of better right-sided filling. Similarly, raising the head may facilitate gallbladder filling.

Endoscopic imaging

Recording images of the endoscopic appearances is less important than for other endoscopic modalities. However, any pathology or aberrations should be captured, for example, a duodenal ulcer, suspected invasive cancer, strictures or periampullary diverticula, or any pathological appearance of the ampulla.

Images of the papilla should be captured before and after any treatment (e.g., papillotomy). Important phases of therapeutic procedures (e.g., stone extraction or multiple stenting) may be of interest. However, therapeutic procedures are often better conveyed with video, and the utility of video storage is likely to increase in the future as this format is more easily transferred across networks and computer systems.

In the situation of an ampullary tumor, it is crucial to document the status before and after ampullectomy—this disease is poorly shown radiologically. In lesions deemed nonresectable by endoscopy the imaging is important to the surgeon (or for the palliative strategy as a starting point).

Postprocedure data

The endoscopic report is normally recorded shortly after the procedure and contains data up to that point. However, certain later items of information are highly relevant, and thus belong at least connected to the ERCP report. The most important of these are delayed adverse events, outcomes of already recorded intraprocedural events, and pathology reports. With a broader perspective, outcomes of the procedure are also of interest, but this information may be better traced in the context of the general medical record system.

Adverse events

The appropriate recording of adverse events is an important aspect of ERCP practice. While intraprocedure events are a natural component of the endoscopy report, delayed events are a more difficult issue. An American Society for Gastrointestinal Endoscopy (ASGE) working party devised a system for recording adverse events in terms of types, severity, outcomes, and attribution [5], and it is recommended to relate to this structure, which is also included in the MST system [3]. It is important to realize that the reporting of adverse events does not imply "guilt" or "mistakes" on the part of the endoscopist. While the responsible endoscopist may indeed be to blame, the adverse events reporting must be done independently of this aspect.

Pathology reports

Sampling performed during ERCP has no value without the corresponding pathology report. Ideally, the endoscopy report should be updated when the pathology reading is ready, and some software systems allow this. If not, the general medical record system must somehow cater for linking the two, and any resulting new diagnoses and recommendations.

Report output

The traditional format of the ERCP output is a sheet of paper sent to the referring physician and interested parties. While this still has a great utility and will still be a core element of the documentation, other output modalities are increasingly recognized, particularly as most of the reports are now generated from database-recorded information. Thus, adapted formats are conceivable, for example, a more general format for the referring GP with focus on the interpretations and recommendations, and a more technically oriented format for the ERCP expert or perhaps the collaborating surgeon who needs more specifics on the procedure. For immediate use, a report format for the recovery room personnel would be of importance, perhaps more formatted for anesthesiologists in the context of deep sedation or general anesthesia, where extended monitoring is warranted.

Patients will likely increasingly want their own report of the procedure. Some endoscopists give them a copy of the report going to the referring physician, but a more focused version is preferable. This should include the important findings and conclusions, but in layman terms, and probably with somewhat more elaborate explanations and perhaps some pertinent sketch drawings. The report might also preferably include or be combined with pertinent disease descriptions, more elaborate anatomical explanations, or links to additional reading material on the Internet.

Finally, cumulated reports are needed for other purposes, for example, quality assurance programs, financial purposes, or hospital statistics. Thus, the output information is no longer strictly linked to what information is entered, and diverse reader categories can be addressed more to the point.

Cumulative, or at least anonymized, data may also be fed into joint data repositories for multicenter quality assurance purposes. Some such networks exist already, and there is an increasing demand for transparency as well as quality metrics from units offering ERCP.

Endoscopy reporting software

Some units still dictate their endoscopic procedures in a narrative way for subsequent transcription. Increasingly, however, the diverse needs for documentation noted earlier call for dedicated databases that will generate the appropriate reports. A number of such systems are commercially available, variably integrated in hospital-wide databases.

The main challenge of the software vendors is to develop an interface that presents the required structure of the database in a format that is acceptable for the user. There is a natural conflict between necessary structure on one side and the endoscopist need for flexibility and natural language on the other. Unless this dilemma is solved, the quality of the structured input data will suffer, and the data collected will not accurately convey the reality of the endoscopic activity.

The structure *standards* presently being recommended may offer an important input for the software companies. The recommendations for terms, attributes, and components of the endoscopy report should form at least default templates for the various software solutions. While these may obviously be amended or expanded, such a common platform still presents a joint basis that will help standardize endoscopic reporting throughout the world.

References

1 Crespi M, Delvaux M, Schaprio M, *et al.* Working Party Report by the Committee for Minimal Standards of Terminology and Documentation in Digestive Endoscopy of the European Society of Gastrointestinal Endoscopy. Minimal standard terminology for a computerized endoscopic database. Ad hoc Task Force of the Committee. Am J Gastroenterol 1996;91(2):191–216.

2 Digestive Endoscopy:Terminology with Definitions and Classifications of Diagnosis and Therapy and Standardized Endoscopic Reporting. Waye JDM, Z. Armengol-Miro, JR, editors. Bad Homburg: Normed Verlag; 2013. 238 pp.

3 Aabakken L, Rembacken B, LeMoine O, *et al.* Minimal standard terminology for gastrointestinal endoscopy—MST 3.0. Endoscopy 2009;41(8):727–8.

4 Aabakken L, Barkun AN, Cotton PB, Fedorov E, Fujino MA, Ivanova E, Kudo SE, Kuznetzov K, de Lange T, Matsuda K, Moine O, Rembacken B, Rey JF, Romagnuolo J, Rösch T, Sawhney M, Yao K, Waye JD. Standardized endoscopic reporting. J Gastroenterol Hepatol. 2014 Feb;29(2): 234–40

5 Cotton PB, Eisen GM, Aabakken L, *et al.* A lexicon for endoscopic adverse events: report of an ASGE workshop. Gastrointest Endosc 2010;71(3):446–54.

6 de Lange T, Larsen S, Aabakken L. Image documentation of endoscopic findings in ulcerative colitis: photographs or video clips? Gastrointest Endosc 2005;61(6):715–20.

7 Khanna N, May G, Bass S, *et al.* Postprocedural interpretation of endoscopic retrograde cholangiopancreatography by radiology. Can J Gastroenterol 2008;22(1):55–60.

8 Kucera S, Isenberg G, Chak A, *et al.* Postprocedure radiologist's interpretation of ERCP X-ray films: a prospective outcomes study. Gastrointest Endosc 2007;66(1):79–83.

SECTION 3
Clinical applications

CHAPTER 14

ERCP in acute cholangitis

Wei-Chih Liao & Hsiu-Po Wang

Department of Internal Medicine, National Taiwan University Hospital,
National Taiwan University College of Medicine, Taipei, Taiwan

---

KEY POINTS

- Endoscopic retrograde cholangiopancreatography (ERCP) is the preferred first-line modality for biliary decompression, the most important task in treating acute cholangitis.

- The major goal of ERCP in acute cholangitis is to relieve biliary obstruction, either by treating the cause of obstruction (mostly stones) or by inserting a nasobiliary drainage tube or a plastic stent.

- The timing of ERCP and the procedure to be performed should be determined considering the cause/site of biliary obstruction and the condition of the patient.

- Other modality for biliary decompression such as percutaneous transhepatic biliary drainage (PTBD) remains a valuable alternative when ERCP is high-risk, technically difficult, or unsuccessful.

Background

Acute cholangitis is one of the most common indications for ERCP. It results from bile duct obstruction and subsequent bacterial superinfection of the stagnant bile [1]. The classic presentation of acute cholangitis includes right upper quadrant pain, jaundice, and fever (Charcot's triad), but not every patient presents with all three symptoms [1]. Pain may be transient or mild, and jaundice may be mild if the ductal obstruction is of recent onset or incomplete. The occurrence of altered mental status and shock together with Charcot's triad constitute the *Reynolds'* pentad, which indicates acute suppurative cholangitis. This condition carries a significant risk of rapid deterioration and mortality, requiring aggressive resuscitative measures (fluid, broad-spectrum antibiotic, and intensive care) and urgent drainage of the obstructed and infected bile duct [2].

ERCP: The Fundamentals, Second Edition. Edited by Peter B. Cotton and Joseph Leung.
© 2015 John Wiley & Sons, Ltd. Published 2015 by John Wiley & Sons, Ltd.
Companion Website: www.wiley.com\go\cotton\ercp

Etiology of acute cholangitis

Choledocholithiasis is the most common cause of acute cholangitis. Other common causes include various benign biliary strictures (e.g., chronic pancreatitis, postsurgical stricture), Mirizzi's syndrome, and, less commonly, malignant biliary strictures [3]. An indwelling biliary stent predisposes to bacterobilia, and blockage of the stent often leads to acute cholangitis. Similarly, a previous sphincterotomy causes duodenobiliary reflux and bacterobilia and may lead to cholangitis or stone recurrence [4]. Acute cholangitis occurs less frequently spontaneously in malignant biliary obstruction because the more complete obstruction prevents ascending spread of bacteria, unless contrast has been injected into the duct in a previous ERCP attempt that failed to achieve biliary drainage.

Pathophysiology

Bacteria can enter the normally sterile biliary system either via the ampulla of Vater (as in ascending cholangitis) or via translocation from portal bacteremia [5]. Because of protection from the flushing effect of normal bile flow and the antibacterial effects of bile salts and biliary IgA, bacterobilia alone does not necessarily cause acute cholangitis [5]. However, in cases of biliary obstruction, the resultant reduced bile flow and impaired Kupffer cell function lead to acute cholangitis [6, 7]. Furthermore, obstruction raises intraductal pressure, which leads to spread of bacteria from bile into the systemic circulation and impairs excretion of antibiotic into bile [6, 8]. Cholangitis has been caused by ERCP when equipment reprocessing methods have failed.

Bacteriology

Enteric Gram-negative bacteria are the most common bacteria causing acute cholangitis, including *Escherichia coli*, *Klebsiella*, *Citrobacter*, *Enterobacter*, and *Proteus* spp.[9] Sometimes Gram-positive enterococci and anaerobes are also isolated from bile in acute cholangitis [1, 9].

Management for acute cholangitis

General management and antibiotic treatment

In addition to general resuscitative measures, blood cultures should be obtained immediately and followed by empirical antibiotic treatment to cover the common pathogens as soon as possible.

For the selection of antibiotic, the Tokyo guidelines [10] recommended that mild acute cholangitis can be treated for as short as 2–3 days with a first- or second-generation cephalosporin or penicillin with a β-lactamase inhibitor. Moderate to severe acute cholangitis should be treated with a minimum of 5–7 days with penicillin and a β-lactamase inhibitor, a third- or fourth-generation cephalosporin, or a monobactam with or without metronidazole for anaerobic coverage. Fluoroquinolones such as ciprofloxacin have good bile penetration and Gram-negative coverage and are good alternatives when the first antibiotic is ineffective or favored by sensitivity results [11]. However, antibiotic selection should also consider the local bacteriology and drug sensitivity patterns, and should be reevaluated once the results of blood culture or bile culture and sensitivity tests are available.

Relief of bile duct obstruction

As increased ductal pressure from obstruction causes systemic bacterial spreading and impairs penetration of antibiotic into bile, biliary decompression and drainage of the infected bile/pus plays a central role in treating acute cholangitis, usually with rapid symptom improvement and stabilization. While this can be achieved by ERCP, PTBD, or surgery, ERCP is the preferred first-line treatment.

In a randomized controlled trial (RCT) comparing ERCP versus emergency surgery, ERCP was associated with a lower risk of morbidity and mortality [12]. In cases due to stones, definitive treatment (i.e., removal of stones) can also be achieved by ERCP in most cases. There is no head-to-head RCT comparing ERCP and PTBD. The success rate of PTBD to provide drainage in acute cholangitis is similar with ERCP (>90%). PTBD has the advantage that it does not require anesthesia and can be performed in patients in whom ERCP is considered high-risk, but puncturing the liver carries the risk of bleeding and bile leak/peritonitis, especially in patients with severe septicemia and thrombocytopenia/disseminated intravascular coagulation (DIC). Therefore, PTBD is generally reserved for patients who are too frail to undergo ERCP, or when ERCP has failed or is technically difficult (e.g., surgically altered anatomy such as Billroth II, Roux-en-Y choledo-chojejunostomy or gastric bypass, and Bismuth type III or IV hilar strictures). Subsequent definitive treatment can be achieved after stabilization of the patient by ERCP, percutaneous approaches, or their combination.

Timing of biliary decompression

About 80–90% of patients improve within 6–12 h after antibiotic and resuscitative measures, with defervescence and decreased leukocyte count in the following 2–3 days. For these patients, ERCP can be scheduled electively. In about 10% of patients who have not improved after 6–12 h of initial treatment, and for those with Reynolds' pentad or altered mental status and shock on presentation, urgent biliary decompression is needed to relieve ductal pressure and associated bacteria dissemination/septicemia.

ERCP techniques in acute cholangitis

While ERCP is effective in demonstrating the site and cause of bile duct obstruction, diagnostic ERCP has largely been replaced by less invasive diagnostic studies such as sonography, computed tomography (CT), MRCP, or endoscopic ultrasound (EUS). The role of ERCP is mainly therapeutic, achieving drainage and possible definitive treatment for the underlying cause.

Pre-ERCP evaluation

An assessment of the patient's condition and relevant history and informed consent are essential before ERCP. Understanding the likely cause and location of biliary obstruction by imaging studies is possible in most cases and is very helpful in planning the ERCP procedure. Significant bleeding diathesis should be corrected if possible, and antithrombotic agents may have to be withheld if feasible (see discussion on endoscopic papillary balloon dilation (EPBD) versus endoscopic sphincterotomy (EST) and Chapter 2 on patient preparation).

Cannulation and cholangiogram

As in routine ERCP procedure, the first step is to achieve selective cannulation of bile duct and insert a guide wire to allow exchange of accessories for subsequent therapies. In the case of cholangitis, cannulation is usually easier, because the duct is often dilated and the orifice may have been enlarged from previous spontaneous passage of stone fragments. When cannulation cannot be easily accomplished, carefully injecting a small amount of contrast may allow opacification of the distal bile duct or pancreatic duct, serving as a landmark to facilitate cannulation of bile duct. Cannulation with cannula or guide wire may be difficult when the stone is impacted at the biliary orifice. In such cases, cutting the roof of the papilla over the underlying stone with a needle knife offers easy access into the bile duct, often with dislodgement of the impacted stone (Figure 14.1).

After selective cannulation of bile duct, care should be taken to aspirate the infected bile or pus to decompress the bile duct before injecting contrast to avoid further increase in ductal pressure and further spread of bacteria. The aspirated

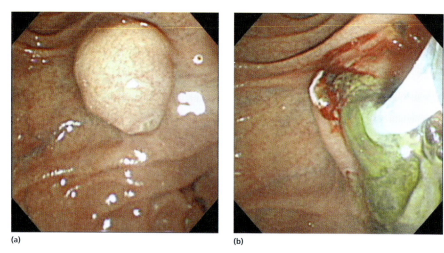

(a)   (b)

Figure 14.1 (a) Stone impaction at papilla. (b) Exposure of the impacted stone and drainage of pus after cutting over the underlying stone with a needle knife.

bile can be sent for culture and/or cytology as necessary. Minimal contrast is then injected to confirm successful cannulation and demonstrate the cause (e.g., stone, stricture) and site of obstruction. In cases with complicated hilar strictures, the duct(s) to be drained should be planned before ERCP with the guidance of MRCP, and only the segments of the ductal system attempted for drainage should be opacified with contrast to avoid incomplete drainage of all filled segmental ducts and worsening of infection after ERCP [13].

Cholangitis caused by stones

Aside from biliary decompression using stents or a nasobiliary catheter, extraction of the bile duct stone(s) also provides adequate drainage of the bile duct. However, attempted stone extraction may result in a prolonged procedure and should only be considered in a relatively stable patient to avoid unnecessary complications. To extract the stone the biliary orifice must be enlarged and this can be achieved by EST or endoscopic balloon sphincteroplasty (EPBD or endoscopic papillary large balloon dilation (EPLBD)).

Endoscopic sphincterotomy

The sphincterotome is advanced over the guide wire and placed across the biliary orifice. The cutting wire of the sphincterotome is then bowed to maintain contact with the roof of the papilla, and cutting is performed by maintaining contact between the distal tip of the wire and the papilla using either the endocut mode or a blended current consisted of high cutting and low coagulation current (Figure 14.2) [14, 15]. The cutting should be made along the ridgeline of the papillary bulge, usually at the 11–12 o'clock direction, in a stepwise, controlled manner. As the sphincterotome tends to deviate toward the right upon bowing, shaping of its tip is often helpful to avoid a deviated cut, which increases the risk of complications [16]. The optimal size of the sphincterotomy depends on the size of the stones as well as the size of the papilla, with the junction of

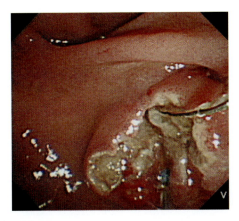

Figure 14.2 Endoscopic sphincterotomy.

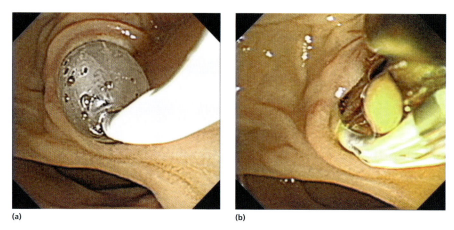

(a)   (b)

Figure 14.3 (a) Endoscopic papillary balloon dilation using a 10-mm-diameter balloon. (b) Spontaneous passage of stones from enlarged papillary orifice after deflation of the balloon.

the papillary bulge and duodenal wall as the limit. This can often be noted as a horizontal mucosal fold at the oral end of the papilla. Avoid excessive bowing of the cutting wire, as it will cause the wire to deviate toward the right and may cause an uncontrolled zipper cut. After EST, the stones can be extracted with an extraction balloon, basket, or mechanical lithotripter if needed.

Endoscopic balloon sphincteroplasty (EPBD or EPLBD)

In stable patients where stone extraction is performed, EPBD can be used as an alternative to EST for stone extraction. It uses a contrast-filled dilation balloon (6- to 10-mm diameter) to dilate the biliary sphincter (Figure 14.3) [17]. In general, up to 10-mm balloons are used for EPBD. The balloon is advanced over the guide wire and placed across the biliary orifice and then slowly inflated to the recommended pressure by the manufacturer. Successful dilation is confirmed by disappearance of the balloon waist on fluoroscopy. The balloon is kept inflated for 3–5 min (instead of the usual 1 min), to achieve adequate dilation [18, 19]. This prolonged dilation reduces the risk of PEP from compartment syndrome. Stones ≤ 1 cm in size can be removed but larger stones may require mechanical lithotripsy to achieve complete ductal clearance.

Endoscopic papillary large balloon dilation

There is a growing trend in performing endoscopic papillary large (12–20 mm) balloon dilation following a limited (small to medium)-sized EST (Figure 14.4) [20]. This method is used in patients with a dilated distal bile duct and allows extraction of larger stones without lithotripsy [21]. However, the potential risks of severe bleeding and perforation may increase.

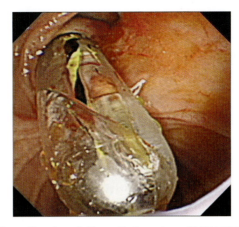

Figure 14.4 Endoscopic papillary large balloon dilation using a 12/13.5/15 mm diameter balloon.

EPBD versus *EST*

EST and EPBD are comparable in terms of overall success rate of stone extraction [22, 23]. Early studies with EPBD were associated with a higher risk of pancreatitis [24], and is less commonly used especially in the United States except in patients with coagulopathy. EST is still considered the standard treatment for bile duct stones [22]. However, more recent studies show that EPBD actually has a lower overall post-ERCP complication rate if adequate dilation duration is used [18, 19]. Furthermore, EPBD has a lower stone recurrence rate than EST. The sphincter function is more likely to be preserved after EPBD [4] than after EST, which ablates the sphincter and predisposes to subsequent duodenobiliary reflux/bacterial colonization and recurrent stone formation.

A recent meta-analysis showed that a longer dilation duration (5 min) of EPBD is associated with a lower risk of bleeding and overall complications without increasing the risk of pancreatitis compared with EST [19].

The risk of bleeding after EST is higher in patients with bleeding diathesis (liver cirrhosis, uremia, thrombocytopenia/DIC from septicemia) or taking antithrombotic medications. Current guidelines recommend discontinuation of antithrombotic agents for 5–10 days before EST, which may cause delayed treatment and prolonged admission [25, 26], and the interruption of antithrombotic therapy can cause devastating thromboembolic events [25]. By contrast, EPBD can be safely performed with continued antithrombotic therapy [26].

EPBD with adequate dilation duration has lower post-ERCP and long-term complication rates than EST and may be used as the first-line treatment for bile duct stones while EST can be used as a rescue procedure for failed stone extraction. EPBD is also easier to perform in cases with surgically altered anatomy [27].

Drainage of bile duct

If the cause of bile duct obstruction cannot be treated by ERCP, adequate drainage of the bile duct can usually be achieved by inserting a biliary stent or endoscopic naso-biliary drainage tube to resolve the cholangitis. Such scenarios include an inability to remove all stones in the first ERCP session due to large/difficult stones or critical condition of the patient, or obstruction caused by benign or malignant strictures that require repeated endoscopic treatments or surgery. Occasionally, ampullary edema after ERCP with prolonged manipulation or after injection therapy to control post-EST bleeding may also cause transient obstruction after ERCP and require drainage.

Nasobiliary drainage versus stenting

Insertion of a nasobiliary drainage tube or a plastic stent provides effective drainage of the obstructed bile duct in the short term. Stenting is usually preferred over naso-biliary drainage because it is more comfortable and less susceptible to inadvertent removal. However, nasobiliary drainage has the advantages of being able to monitor the drain amount, repeat cholangiogram, and removal without a second endoscopic procedure. Two RCTs comparing nasobiliary drainage and stenting for treating patients with acute cholangitis found that these two treatments are equally safe and effective [28, 29]. The authors' preference is to use a plastic stent for this purpose. However, if the cholangitis is caused by an inoperable malignant stricture and the patient has a life expectancy greater than 6 months, a self-expandable metal stent (SEMS) may be better than a plastic stent because of its longer patency, which reduces the risk of recurrent obstruction and the need for repeat ERCPs [30].

Drainage as a treatment for difficult stones

In cases of difficult stones, temporary biliary stenting can also be a quick alternative to lithotripsy or EPLBD, as partial stone dissolution occurs in 50% or more of cases after a period (e.g., 3 months) of stenting, making subsequent stone extraction easier [31]. However, this should be used only as a temporary measure, and the patient should be followed for possible stent blockage and recurrent cholangitis in the meantime.

Care after ERCP for acute cholangitis

As in ERCP for other indications, the patient should be followed for possible post-ERCP complications, such as bleeding, pancreatitis, perforation, or worsening cholangitis. For patients considered to be at high-risk for PEP because of patient- and/or procedure-related factors (e.g., past history of PEP, repeated pancreas injection, difficult cannulation), rectal administration of 100 mg indomethacin immediately after the procedure is warranted, which reduced the risk of PEP by 46% in an RCT [32].

Acute cholangitis usually responds rapidly to successful biliary decompression, usually with resolution of symptoms (fever, pain, hypotension) and improving laboratory abnormalities (hyperbilirubinemia, leukocytosis) within 24 h [2]. If the patient does not improve after ERCP, the possibility of incomplete drainage should be considered. This may be caused by residual bile duct stone, stent malfunction (due to blockage, migration, or inadequate stent length), incomplete drainage of opacified segmental ducts in hilar strictures, or unrecognized Mirizzi's syndrome in the first ERCP. Sonography is a convenient study to assess the adequacy of biliary drainage after ERCP, and persistent bile duct dilation after ERCP indicates incomplete drainage, which requires a second ERCP or PTBD. In cases of persistent fever after ERCP, other sources of infection such as liver abscess or aspiration pneumonia should be sought, and adjustment of antibiotic regimen should be considered.

Conclusion

As the method of choice for biliary decompression and choledocholithiasis, ERCP plays a central role in the management of acute cholangitis. It should be remembered that the major goal of ERCP in acute cholangitis is to relieve biliary obstruction, though in patients with acute cholangitis caused by choledocholithiasis both drainage and definitive treatment can usually be achieved in the first ERCP session by removing the stones. The timing of ERCP and the procedure to be performed should be determined considering the cause and site of biliary obstruction, the severity of infection, and the condition and comorbidity of the patient. While ERCP has a high success rate, other modalities for biliary decompression such as PTBD remain a valuable alternative when ERCP is considered high-risk, technically difficult, or unsuccessful.

TIPS AND TRICKS

- In acute cholangitis, aspirate infected bile or pus after deep cannulation before injecting contrast to avoid further increase in ductal pressure and spread of bacteria.

- With stone impaction and failed cannulation, needle-knife precut sphincterotomy over the impacted stone improves access into the bile duct, often with spontaneous dislodgement of the impacted stone.

- Avoid a full cholangiogram in complicated hilar strictures. Plan ahead with magnetic resonance cholangiopancreatography (MRCP). Only injecting contrast into the segments of the ductal system intended for drainage will prevent infection after ERCP.

- With EPBD, maintain full inflation of the balloon for 3–5 min to reduce the risk of post-ERCP pancreatitis (PEP).

- With large/difficult stones obstruction, biliary decompression with an indwelling stent or stents is a quick temporary alternative to stone extraction. Partial stone disintegration can occur after a period (e.g., 3 months) of stenting, making subsequent stone extraction easier.

References

1 Wang Q-H, Afdhal NH. Gallstone disease. In: Feldman MFL, Brandt LJ, eds. Sleisenger and Fordtran's Gastrointestinal and Liver Disease. 9th ed. Philadelphia, PA: W.B. Saunders, 2010:1089–20.

2 Leung JC, Sung JY, Chung SS, *et al*. Urgent endoscopic drainage for acute suppurative cholangitis. The Lancet 1989;333:1307–9.

3 Stockland AH, Baron TH. Endoscopic and radiologic treatment of biliary disease. In: Feldman MFL, Brandt LJ, eds. Sleisenger and Fordtran's Gastrointestinal and Liver Disease. 9th ed. Philadelphia, PA: W.B. Saunders, 2010:1185–98.

4 Yasuda I, Fujita N, Maguchi H, *et al*. Long-term outcomes after endoscopic sphincterotomy versus endoscopic papillary balloon dilation for bile duct stones. Gastrointest Endosc 2010;72:1185–91.

5 Sung JY, Costerton JW, Shaffer EA. Defense system in the biliary tract against bacterial infection. Dig Dis Sci 1992;37:689–96.

6 Lee JG. Diagnosis and management of acute cholangitis. Nat Rev Gastroenterol Hepatol 2009;6:533–41.

7 Parks RW, Clements WD, Smye MG, *et al*. Intestinal barrier dysfunction in clinical and experimental obstructive jaundice and its reversal by internal biliary drainage. Br J Surg 1996;83:1345–9.

8 Huang T, Bass JA, Williams RD. The significance of biliary pressure in cholangitis. Arch Surg 1969;98:629–32.

9 Brook I. Aerobic and anaerobic microbiology of biliary tract disease. J Clin Microbiol 1989;27:2373–5.

10 Tanaka A, Takada T, Kawarada Y, *et al*. Antimicrobial therapy for acute cholangitis: Tokyo Guidelines. J Hepatobiliary Pancreat Surg 2007;14:59–67.

11 Sung JJ, Lyon DJ, Suen R, Cheung SCS. Intravenous ciprofloxacin as treatment for patients with acute suppurative cholangitis: a randomized, controlled clinical trial. J Antimicrob Chemother 1995;35:855–64.

12 Lai EC, Mok FP, Tan ES, *et al*. Endoscopic biliary drainage for severe acute cholangitis. N Engl J Med 1992;326:1582–6.

13 Hintze RE, Abou-Rebyeh H, Adler A, *et al*. Magnetic resonance cholangiopancreatography-guided unilateral endoscopic stent placement for Klatskin tumors. Gastrointest Endosc 2001;53:40–6.

14 Verma D, Kapadia A, Adler DG. Pure versus mixed electrosurgical current for endoscopic biliary sphincterotomy: a meta-analysis of adverse outcomes. Gastrointest Endosc 2007;66:283–90.

15 Perini RF, Sadurski R, Cotton PB, *et al*. Post-sphincterotomy bleeding after the introduction of microprocessor-controlled electrosurgery: does the new technology make the difference? Gastrointest Endosc 2005;61:53–7.

16 Leung JW, Leung FW. Papillotomy performance scoring scale—a pilot validation study focused on the cut axis. Aliment Pharmacol Ther 2006;24:307–12.

17 Bergman JJ, Rauws EA, Fockens P, *et al*. Randomised trial of endoscopic balloon dilation versus endoscopic sphincterotomy for removal of bileduct stones. Lancet 1997;349:1124–9.

18 Liao WC, Lee CT, Chang CY, *et al*. Randomized trial of 1-minute versus 5-minute endoscopic balloon dilation for extraction of bile duct stones. Gastrointest Endosc 2010;72:1154–62.

19 Liao WC, Tu YK, Wu MS, *et al*. Balloon dilation with adequate duration is safer than sphincterotomy for extracting bile duct stones: a systematic review and meta-analyses. Clin Gastroenterol Hepatol 2012;10:1101–9.

20 Ersoz G, Tekesin O, Ozutemiz AO, Gunsar F. Biliary sphincterotomy plus dilation with a large balloon for bile duct stones that are difficult to extract. Gastrointest Endosc 2003;57:156–9.

21 Teoh AY, Cheung FK, Hu B, *et al*. Randomized trial of endoscopic sphincterotomy with balloon dilation versus endoscopic sphincterotomy alone for removal of bile duct stones. Gastroenterology 2013;144:341–5.

22 Baron TH, Harewood GC. Endoscopic balloon dilation of the biliary sphincter compared to endoscopic biliary sphincterotomy for removal of common bile duct stones during ERCP: a metaanalysis of randomized, controlled trials. Am J Gastroenterol 2004;99:1455–60.

23 Weinberg BM, Shindy W, Lo S. Endoscopic balloon sphincter dilation (sphincteroplasty) versus sphincterotomy for common bile duct stones. Cochrane Database Syst Rev 2006: CD004890.

24 Disario JA, Freeman ML, Bjorkman DJ, *et al*. Endoscopic balloon dilation compared with sphincterotomy for extraction of bile duct stones. Gastroenterology 2004;127:1291–9.

25 Anderson MA, Ben-Menachem T, Gan SI, *et al*. Management of antithrombotic agents for endoscopic procedures. Gastrointest Endosc 2009;70:1060–70.

26 Boustiere C, Veitch A, Vanbiervliet G, *et al*. Endoscopy and antiplatelet agents. European Society of Gastrointestinal Endoscopy (ESGE) Guideline. Endoscopy 2011;43:445–61.

27 Liao WC, Huang SP, Wu MS, *et al*. Comparison of endoscopic papillary balloon dilatation and sphincterotomy for lithotripsy in difficult sphincterotomy. J Clin Gastroenterol 2008;42:295–9.

28 Lee DW, Chan AC, Lam YH, *et al*. Biliary decompression by nasobiliary catheter or biliary stent in acute suppurative cholangitis: a prospective randomized trial. Gastrointest Endosc 2002;56:361–5.

29 Sharma BC, Kumar R, Agarwal N, Sarin SK. Endoscopic biliary drainage by nasobiliary drain or by stent placement in patients with acute cholangitis. Endoscopy 2005;37:439–43.

30 Pfau PR, Pleskow DK, Banerjee S, *et al*. Pancreatic and biliary stents. Gastrointest Endosc 2013;77:319–27.

31 Dumonceau JM, Tringali A, Blero D, *et al*. Biliary stenting: indications, choice of stents and results: European Society of Gastrointestinal Endoscopy (ESGE) clinical guideline. Endoscopy 2012;44:277–98.

32 Elmunzer BJ, Scheiman JM, Lehman GA, *et al*. A randomized trial of rectal indomethacin to prevent post-ERCP pancreatitis. N Engl J Med 2012;366:1414–22.

CHAPTER 15

ERCP peri-cholecystectomy

Paul R. Tarnasky

Methodist Dallas Medical Center, Dallas, USA

KEY POINTS

- Urgent preoperative indications for endoscopic retrograde cholangiopancreatography (ERCP) include cholangitis and severe acute biliary pancreatitis associated with biliary obstruction.

- Ability to predict the likelihood for choledocholithiasis (CDL) and available ERCP expertise are the most important factors when determining the potential need for and timing of elective ERCP before cholecystectomy (CCX).

- The prevalence of CDL is low (<5%) when the serum liver chemistries and bile duct diameter are both normal. ERCP is not indicated before planned CCX in those circumstances.

- The prevalence of CDL is high (>50%) when a stone is suspected by ultrasonography or when there is a combination of a dilated duct and jaundice or cholestasis. Elective ERCP before CCX is reasonable in that situation.

- Ancillary imaging such as EUS or MRCP may be helpful to determine the need for preoperative ERCP when the likelihood for CDL is intermediate (>5% but <50%).

- Intraoperative ERCP during CCX has logistical challenges, but can be highly successful and safe when a rendezvous technique is utilized.

- When ERCP expertise if high, it is reasonable to depend more on intraoperative cholangiography to determine the potential need for postoperative ERCP.

- Other indications for ERCP soon after CCX include suspected postoperative bile leaks and/or ductal strictures

---

Introduction

CDL is the most common reason for ERCP in the peri-cholecystectomy (CCX) setting. Often CDL manifests in the form of obvious and sometimes serious symptoms while at other times it may be discovered incidentally. Diagnosis and/or treatment of CDL with ERCP may be accomplished in the preoperative,

---

ERCP: The Fundamentals, Second Edition. Edited by Peter B. Cotton and Joseph Leung.

intraoperative, or postoperative settings. Less common scenarios whereby ERCP is utilized in the peri-CCX setting include postoperative ERCP to assist in management of complications such as bile leaks or duct injuries.

The utilization and timing of ERCP in the peri-CCX setting depends on the clinical setting and presenting symptoms, the likelihood of bile duct pathology, available equipment and expertise, and evolving techniques and their outcomes. Indications and appropriate timing for urgent ERCP are well established. As examples, urgent preoperative ERCP is indicated in the setting of symptomatic gallstones with cholangitis, and urgent postoperative ERCP may be indicated for evaluation and treatment of an uncontrolled bile leak. The appropriate use of elective ERCP is less well defined and ERCP may be reasonable before, during, or after CCX; this is particularly so for stable patients with suspected CDL with or without recent biliary pancreatitis. Potential indications for preoperative (Table 15.1), intraoperative (Table 15.2), and postoperative (Table 15.3) ERCP will be reviewed according to the particular clinical setting.

The goal is to review relevant data in order to provide reasonable recommendations regarding the appropriate use of preoperative, intraoperative, and postoperative ERCP. Details on general techniques and complications of ERCP are covered elsewhere in this book and will not be emphasized unless pertinent to the particular

Table 15.1 Potential indications for ERCP before cholecystectomy.

Urgent
Cholangitis
Biliary pancreatitis with suspected ongoing biliary obstruction
Elective
Resolved biliary pancreatitis and/or cholangitis:
Suspected retained bile duct stones
Suspected disrupted and/or obstructed pancreatic duct
Patent unfit or unwilling to undergo cholecystectomy
Significant delay before cholecystectomy
Biliary obstruction and concern for malignancy
Symptomatic biliary tract disease during pregnancy
Symptomatic gallstones and known or high suspicion for bile duct stone

Table 15.2 Potential indications for ERCP during cholecystectomy.

IOC demonstrates choledocholithiasis
Suspected difficult cannulation due to aberrant and/or difficult anatomy
Limited ERCP cannulation expertise
To eliminate risk for post-ERCP pancreatitis
To achieve single-stage procedure
Surgically altered anatomy

Table 15.3 Potential indications for ERCP after cholecystectomy.

IOC demonstrates choledocholithiasis
Suspected choledocholithiasis by clinical criteria
Bile leak
Operative bile duct injury
Complications of pancreatitis, e.g., peripancreatic fluid collections

setting being described. Paramount to the successful integration of ERCP and CCX is efficient multidisciplinary collaboration between the endoscopic, radiological, and surgical teams.

Preoperative ERCP for treatment of choledocholithiasis

Cholangitis

There is no dispute regarding the need for urgent ERCP in patients with gall-stones who present with acute cholangitis [1, 2]. The diagnosis is clear-cut, the techniques standard, and the clinical outcome is almost always good, as described in Chapter 14.

Biliary pancreatitis

More than half of all cases of acute pancreatitis are caused by gallstones and up to one-fourth of those cases can be severe, with significant mortality. The diagnosis is usually obvious, with stones in the gallbladder on ultrasonography, and abnormal liver chemistries (as well as amylase/lipase). A threefold elevation of serum alanine aminotransferase (ALT) is the most helpful laboratory predictor for a biliary etiology of pancreatitis [3].

ERCP appears logical to defuse the situation by removing the offending impacted ductal stones, to prevent progression of the disease, and results are good if performed early in the attack (within 24 h) [4, 5]. ERCP can fail in any case [6], but is often more difficult when delayed, due to periampullary edema, sphincter spasm, and/or stone impaction.

However, it is important to realize that most patients pass their stones and improve quickly without intervention [7]. Thus, the key to effective and efficient use of ERCP is to predict which patients have not already passed their stones, or are unlikely to do so. A dilated duct on ultrasonography and abnormal liver chemistries are good pointers. One prospective study found stones in only 36% of patients; importantly, none had retained stones if the liver chemistries had returned to normal and/or decreased to <50% [8].

When the situation is doubtful, endoscopic ultrasound (EUS) and magnetic resonance cholangiopancreatography (MRCP) are useful adjuncts.

Arguedas *et al.* reported a decision analysis regarding options of EUS, MRCP, intraoperative cholangiography (IOC), and ERCP in patients with resolved mild acute biliary pancreatitis (ABP) [9]. A policy of conservative care with IOC during CCX was most cost-effective for a low likelihood (<15%) of CDL while ERCP was the most cost-effective option when the likelihood for CDL was considered high (>45%). For an intermediate likelihood of CDL, EUS but not MRCP was recommended. A retrospective study of mild to moderate ABP compared strategies of selective preoperative ERCP followed by CCX to CCX plus IOC followed by postoperative ERCP if IOC showed CDL [10]. The authors suggested that an IOC approach is more cost-effective; however, the diagnostic yield for CDL was quite low in the IOC group (16%) compared to the preoperative ERCP group (71%). Had an IOC approach been used in all patients it would have been more costly due to the need for more postoperative ERCPs. A decision tree analysis with economic evaluation compared a standard approach of selective preoperative ERCP to routine preoperative EUS or MRCP in patients with ABP [11]. Using EUS first was deemed to be the most cost-effective approach when the frequency of preoperative ERCP was <45%.

The decisions regarding preoperative, intraoperative, or postoperative ERCP in the setting of resolved stable ABP are identical to that in patients with symptomatic gallstones without pancreatitis, and will be covered in more detail later.

It may be reasonable to consider elective ERCP with endotherapy after ABP in settings where CCX is either delayed (e.g., pregnancy) or considered too risky (e.g., medically unfit). Rarely, ERCP may be indicated before CCX in patients with suspected impaired pancreatic drainage and/or symptomatic fluid collections as sequelae from recent pancreatitis.

If no duct stones are found during ERCP in the context of biliary pancreatitis, it is reasonable to perform biliary sphincterotomy that will augment ductal (including pancreatic) drainage as well as reduce the likelihood of a recurrence prior to CCX.

Symptomatic gallstones with possible duct stones

Whether and when to perform an elective ERCP to diagnose and potentially treat CDL in patients with symptomatic gallbladder stones remains a challenging decision. Relevant issues include the frequency and clinical significance of CDL, diagnostic options, methods to predict the likelihood of CDL, outcomes of comparative treatment strategies, and technical expertise.

Frequency and clinical significance of CDL

Gallstones are not uncommon (15% of general population) but most commonly are asymptomatic [12–14]. Approximately one million CCX are performed each year in the United States, mostly laparoscopically [15]. The frequency of CDL among patients with symptomatic gallbladder stones is estimated to range from

10 to 18% but the prevalence increases with age [14]. Overt symptoms of CDL include cholangitis and biliary pancreatitis as described earlier. CDL may also be asymptomatic, or produce less obvious symptoms such as biliary colic that may be attributed to gallbladder stones, thus forming the foundation of the dilemma that looms large for both endoscopists and laparoscopic surgeons.

Some individuals with stones found incidentally may remain asymptomatic, and stones often pass spontaneously [16]. There was evidence of spontaneous migration in more than 25% of patients who underwent ERCP 6 weeks after a stone was demonstrated on IOC [17]. Another report described spontaneous migration rate in >20% within 1 month if stones were <8mm in diameter [18]. Tranter and Thompson estimated that nearly three-fourths of patients with symptomatic gallstone disease have a history of spontaneous stone migration [7]. Further, they reported that median gallstone size in patients with spontaneous migration is significantly smaller (3mm) in patients with ABP compared to those with a history of jaundice (10mm) but no pancreatitis. However, despite the tendency for spontaneous migration, the potential for stones (even small stones) to cause serious symptoms means that they should be removed if at all possible [19–21].

Diagnostic options and predictive factors for CDL

In patients with gallbladder stones being considered for CCX it is traditional to try to separate them into three groups (low, medium, and high risk) with regard to the likelihood of having ductal stones. ERCP is not indicated when the likelihood is low (<5%), and is usually recommended when it is high (>50%). For patients with medium risk (>5% and <50%) there are numerous diagnostic and predictive tools, several practical considerations, and a range of treatment approaches.

Predictors of low risk

Patients with normal-sized bile ducts and liver chemistries have been found to have only a 2–5% chance of harboring stones [22, 23]. A group of patients with that low-risk profile were followed for a mean of 20 months; only 1% developed biliary symptoms [24].

Predictors of high risk

There is no single clinical parameter that consistently proves the presence of CDL [25]. The most reliable (>80%) is observation of echogenic foci in the bile duct on imaging [25, 26]. Other information from ultrasonography such as bile duct diameter and the number and size of gallbladder stones may also be helpful. One report described a linear relationship between the degree of duct dilation and risk of stones [27]. The prevalence of CDL was <5% when bile duct diameter was ≤4mm but increased to 28 and 60% at >6 and 12mm, respectively. A large retrospective study reported that the risk of needing postoperative ERCP to treat retained CDL was highest in patients with an increased number (>3) of small (<7 mm) gallbladder stones [28].

Serum liver chemistries that indicate cholestasis are the most reliable laboratory predictors for duct stones [17, 29–31]. The trend of liver chemistries is also important. A study of patients strongly suspected to have CDL showed that only 13% had stones if their tests normalized over 24 h, compared to 94% when at least one test was increasing [8].

The combination of cholestasis and a dilated bile duct is the best predictor for ductal stones [21, 25, 26, 32–35]. A 2010 American Society for Gastrointestinal Endoscopy (ASGE) guideline categorized patients as high likelihood for CDL if either a bile duct stone is demonstrated on ultrasound or jaundice and/or cholangitis is present, or if both the bile duct is dilated (>6 mm) and bilirubin is elevated [36].

Patients at medium risk

There are more options, and decisions are more difficult when the likelihood of duct stones falls into an intermediate range (>5% but <50%) after standard investigations. The diagnostic situation can be clarified preoperatively with MRCP or EUS. Several analyses have suggested that EUS is a safer and more cost-effective option compared to ERCP with the likelihood for CDL being <50% [37–39]. The use of MRCP for detection of CDL is limited somewhat by its inferior sensitivity for small stones [40, 41]. While EUS and MRCP may be of benefit, there are data to suggest that a policy of selective IOC is the preferred strategy when there is an intermediate likelihood for CDL [41–43]. It is acceptable to proceed directly to CCX with IOC when ERCP expertise is high and can almost guarantee to remove any stones postoperatively [36].

Intraoperative cholangiography

IOC can play a central role in determining the best treatment strategy, but its use varies enormously. A survey of surgeons in 2008 reported that only about one-fourth performed IOC routinely and that they were more likely to be higher-volume surgeons [44]. When performed routinely in every case, IOC is usually successful, has excellent sensitivity and specificity for detection of stones, and is very seldom associated with complications [45]. While it can clarify biliary anatomy, there is debate as to whether it reduces bile duct injuries (see later). However, it adds operating time, costs, and radiation, and routine IOC is not considered cost-effective in cases where the chance of stone is low [26]. There are also the data that suggest that finding small stones at IOC may not require further intervention due to an expected benign course and/or frequent spontaneous stone migration [17, 33].

The best argument for using IOC selectively in higher-risk situations is that the yield is high enough to justify the effort, and that the remaining patients who are not selected have a benign course. In one prospective study, only 33%

of patients were selected for IOC; the yield for CDL in those was 39%, and <1% of those not selected for IOC developed biliary symptoms later [46]. Similar criteria for predicting likelihood of CDL as described earlier can be applied when deciding the need for selective IOC.

CCX can be performed without IOC when preoperative ERCP is utilized appropriately, effectively, and safely [47]. In a cohort of over 1100 consecutive cases, 20% underwent preoperative ERCP, 53% of whom were found to have stones. ERCP was successful in 97% and complicated by pancreatitis in <2% of cases. Further, <1% of the total cohort later developed symptoms from CDL during a mean follow-up of 46 months.

If appropriate selection criteria are utilized and acted upon with preoperative ERCP, there may be only a limited need for IOC during subsequent CCX as long as the interval between ERCP and CCX is not prolonged. Among a cohort of 425 consecutive CCX with IOC, preoperative ERCP and stone extractions were done after MRCP identified CDL in 56 (13%) patients. Only eight patients were found to have CDL on IOC of which seven had undergone preoperative ERCP with stone extractions but more than 12 days prior [48]. Another large study, however, suggested that IOC is of value even after preoperative ERCP due to the risk of interval stone migration. As many as 13% were found to have CDL on IOC, of which one-third had no evidence of CDL at the time of preoperative ERCP [49].

When and how to remove bile duct stones

There are several options if a patient is proven or strongly suspected to have ductal stones. ERCP can be done before, during, or after CCX; advantages and disadvantages of different timing options are listed in Table 15.4. Stones can also be removed intraoperatively, during open or (preferably) laparoscopic surgery. With the increased use of ERCP, complications after open surgical common bile duct exploration (CBDE) have increased while volume has decreased [50]. Also, a randomized controlled trial comparing open to laparoscopic CBDE reported similar success (>94%) but significantly longer length of stay with open procedures [51]. Thus, ERCP as treatment for CDL will be compared to only laparoscopic surgical options.

Preoperative ERCP

Surgeons might request preoperative ERCP to clarify whether ductal clearance can be obtained, especially where local ERCP expertise is suboptimal, because of the concern for the risk of a second surgery if ERCP is needed and fails postoperatively. However, a repeat attempt at ERCP, perhaps by a different endoscopist will almost always be successful (Figure 15.1). Some advocate preoperative ERCP to define biliary anatomy, and sphincterotomy to ensure distal duct drainage, and to reduce risk for leakage from the cystic duct stump. Preoperative ERCP can also clear distal cystic duct stones (Figure 15.2) that might otherwise

Table 15.4 Potential advantages and disadvantages according to timing of ERCP in patients undergoing cholecystectomy for symptomatic gallstones.

Timing of ERCP	Advantages	Disadvantages
Preoperative	Achieves certainty of ductal clearance	Difficult to predict CDL
	Clarifies ductal anatomy	Possibly unnecessary due to clinically insignificant CDL
	Sphincterotomy may decrease risk for bile leak	Risk of complications if unnecessary ERCP
	May decrease need for IOC	Need second ERCP if stone migration before or during CCX
	Prevent further symptoms of CDL if CCX is delayed or contraindicated	Higher conversion rate to open CCX
	May detect unsuspected pathology that is best treated at time of surgery	
Intraoperative	Single anesthesia	Increases operative time
	Certainty of bile duct access and decreased post-ERCP pancreatitis when using rendezvous technique	Requires coordination with endoscopic team
		Requires additional endoscopic equipment
		ERCP may be more difficult in supine patient
Postoperative	Certainty of indication and known therapeutic intent	More dependent on ERCP expertise
		Need second surgery if ERCP fails and referral not an option

be left behind after CCX. It may also be reasonable to consider preoperative ERCP to clarify abnormal imaging particularly when there is concern for other pathology, such as malignancy (Figure 15.3). Generally though, ERCP should be done preoperatively only if there is a very high likelihood for CDL [33, 52].

Preoperative ERCP has some potential disadvantages beyond the obvious that it may be technically unsuccessful and/or associated with complications. Even when there was thought to be a high probability of stones, the yield for CDL in some studies was <50% [53–56]. Also, stones may migrate or be dropped into the bile duct during CCX, requiring another ERCP after surgery. There are some data that suggest an increased need for conversion to open CCX after preoperative ERCP but that this risk is lessened if the interval between procedures is short [57].

It should be emphasized that successful clearance with preoperative ERCP does not preclude the need for CCX. In a prospective study, nearly half of the patients developed recurrent biliary symptoms and over one-third required CCX (>50% open CCX) among those randomly assigned to a "wait and see" approach following ERCP with duct clearance [58].

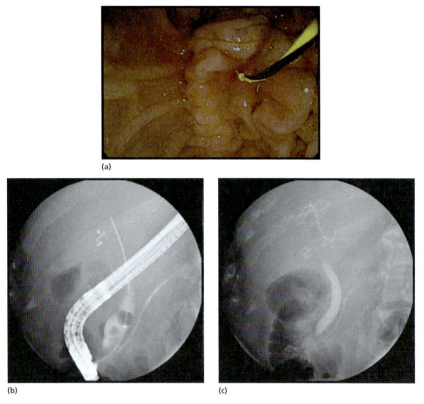

Figure 15.1 A 79-year-old female was referred for repeat ERCP. Intraoperative cholangiography had demonstrated retained stones but postoperative ERCP failed at the outside institution due to a difficult cannulation. Redundant periampullary folds (a) precluded biliary cannulation so an access sphincterotomy was performed after prophylactic pancreatic stenting. Cholangiography (b) confirmed CDL and clearance was achieved (c).

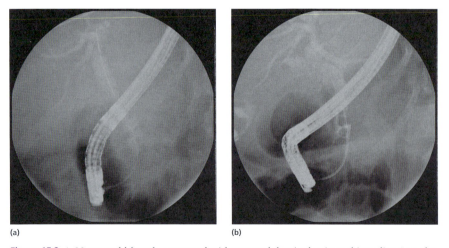

Figure 15.2 A 23-year-old female presented with upper abdominal pain and jaundice 4 weeks postpartum. Abdominal ultrasonography demonstrated a dilated bile duct and possible stones in both the bile and cystic ducts that was confirmed on ERCP (a). The gallbladder was cannulated with a guide wire (b) and clearance of both the bile and cystic ducts was achieved.

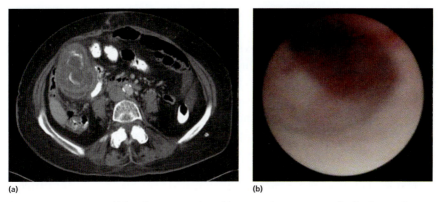

(a)   (b)

Figure 15.3 A 75-year-old female was transferred from another institution for further evaluation of jaundice and the possibility of gallbladder cancer. Computed tomography showed a large complex mass (a) and a dilated bile duct. ERCP revealed a dilated bile duct and there was evidence of hemobilia but cholangioscopy showed blood originating only from the cystic duct (b). Gallbladder pathology revealed acute cholecystitis without evidence of cancer.

Laparoscopic duct exploration

Single-stage laparoscopic treatment is conceptually attractive. Stones can be detected with IOC and then treated under the same anesthesia thus avoiding need for endoscopic expertise, sphincterotomy, and complications. An early decision analysis reported that laparoscopic CCX with IOC and/or CBDE was more cost-effective compared to either preoperative or postoperative ERCP [59]. A more recent analysis suggested that ERCP options were more cost-effective than laparoscopic CBDE [60]. Several prospective randomized trials comparing ERCP before or after CCX to CCX plus CBDE reported that the length of stay was longer in the ERCP groups [61–63]. The interval between ERCP and CCX being left to the discretion of the surgeon may be an explanation for this. A thorough review of prospective randomized controlled trials that compared laparoscopic approaches to preoperative ERCP (five trials), intraoperative ERCP (one trial), and postoperative ERCP (two trials) found no significant difference with regard to mortality, morbidity, and success [14].

Any true advantages of laparoscopic treatment for CDL may only be realized when it can be completed via a transcystic approach; postoperative ERCP is preferred over laparoscopic CBDE when a transcystic method fails or is not possible [57]. About two-thirds of laparoscopic CBDE are reported to be successful by transcystic exploration [64]. When there are many stones and/or if stones are relatively large compared to the cystic duct, a transductal CBDE may be required. One randomized controlled trial comparing laparoscopic treatment and transductal CBDE to preoperative ERCP was limited by including only patients with a dilated bile duct (>10 mm) [65]. The length of stay is longer and risk of complications is increased with transductal compared to transcystic exploration [66]. Also, transductal CBDE often requires T-tube placement, which adds complexity and potential for later complications [64]. Laparoscopic antegrade placement of a transpapillary biliary stent may be carried out to ensure drainage after transductal exploration but it requires endoscopic removal later [67]. Antegrade stenting might also be done either routinely or if transcystic CBDE fails [56, 68]. This approach obviates the need for an open CBDE, adds little operative time, facilitates postoperative ERCP without risk of post-ERCP pancreatitis, and does not require advanced laparoscopic skills.

Laparoscopic treatment of CDL has not become a standard approach outside of expert surgical centers. This could be due to the complexity of laparoscopic skills required and lack of training. From a survey of rural surgeons pertaining to treatment of CDL, 45% reported that they performed laparoscopic CBDE but most preferred ERCP compared to only 21% who preferred a laparoscopic approach [69]. Additional time required was cited as the most common reason for not performing laparoscopic CBDE. Ten years ago, one surgeon reported his very impressive results and suggested that "the role of ERCP has returned to its prelaparoscopic era" [70]. More recently it was acknowledged that successful reports of laparoscopic CBDE tend to originate from enthusiastic experts and that such results may not be transferable to other settings [56]. In reality, most surgeons wish to avoid the extra operative time required for laparoscopic treatment of CDL and prefer to pass the task to an endoscopist for postoperative ERCP. Practically then, the two-stage approach for treatment of CDL with CCX in conjunction with pre- or postoperative ERCP is preferred over a single-stage laparoscopic treatment [57]. Further, a cost-effective analysis comparing all possible options found that laparoscopic CCX with IOC and/or postoperative ERCP was the most cost-effective strategy [60]. It is too early to tell how the recent development of single-incision laparoscopic CCX with or without robotic assistance will affect outcomes related to laparoscopic cholangiography and/or CBDE [71, 72].

ERCP during cholecystectomy

Intraoperative ERCP is also a possible consideration when IOC is positive for CDL. Surgeons can place a catheter, basket, or guide wire via the cystic duct into the duodenum to facilitate ERCP access [73–75]. Intraoperative ERCP is almost always successful, with a low risk for pancreatitis. The principal advantage, like laparoscopic CBDE, is a single-stage procedure with only one anesthesia. This might also translate into a decreased length of stay if the need for postoperative ERCP is averted.

The disadvantages of intraoperative ERCP are mostly logistical. It requires additional endoscopic equipment and adds time to the operation. The surgical team must have endoscopic expertise; otherwise an endoscopist must be summoned thereby creating potential for delay and yet longer operative times. Most intraoperative ERCPs are performed in the supine position, which is not customary for gastroenterologists and can be more challenging.

Noel *et al.* recently described a 10-year experience in over 300 patients using the rendezvous technique for intraoperative ERCP [76]. Technical success of the rendezvous approach was 86%; standard ERCP cannulation was attempted in the operating room when it failed. Post-ERCP pancreatitis was low overall but occurred in 14% of cases when rendezvous access failed and conventional retrograde cannulation was required. They also summarized data on a total of nearly 700 rendezvous ERCP cases whereby stone clearance was initially achieved in 94% of cases with an overall post-ERCP pancreatitis rate of <1%. A prospective randomized trial performed by Lella *et al.* compared rendezvous intraoperative ERCP to postoperative ERCP to treat patients with CDL considered to be high risk for post-ERCP pancreatitis [77]. There was no post-ERCP pancreatitis in the intraoperative ERCP group compared to 10% pancreatitis in the postoperative ERCP group. Unintentional pancreatic duct injections occurred in about one-third of the postoperative ERCP group that included all of the patients who experienced pancreatitis. A meta-analysis of five trials reported significant differences between preoperative ERCP and intraoperative ERCP with respect to more cannulation failure (7.5% versus 0.3%), increased post-ERCP pancreatitis (4.4% versus 0.6%), and longer length of stay [78].

A variant option to intraoperative ERCP is to perform it immediately postoperatively while under the same anesthetic. This approach was first described by Sarli *et al.* whereby the patient was placed prone following completion of CCX and then a standard ERCP was performed in the operating room [79]. To avoid the logistical problems of performing ERCP in the operating room, an alternative is to simply transport the patient still intubated from the operating room to the endoscopy suite (Figure 15.4).

Patients with altered anatomy

Patients with surgically altered anatomy present additional technical and logistical challenges. An increasingly common scenario is the patient who has undergone a Roux-en-Y gastric bypass and then presents with symptomatic gallstones and possible CDL. With standard access to the papilla denied, other access approaches such as small bowel endoscopy techniques or creation of a gastrostomy are required. In situations where CCX is planned, a surgical gastrostomy can provide the conduit for passage of a duodenoscope into the excluded antrum to facilitate an intraoperative ERCP. As discussed earlier, one could argue for a surgical treatment of CDL with CBDE but the surgery-assisted ERCP technique seems to have gained the most traction [80]. Standard ERCP techniques are then possible. However, it can be more challenging due to a less maneuverable duodenoscope in a supine patient performed in a setting that is outside of the endoscopic team's comfort zone.

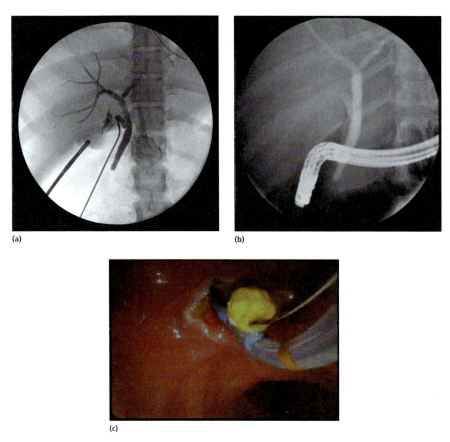

(a)

(b)

(c)

Figure 15.4 A 28-year-old female with a history of biliary colic presented for elective CCX. Preoperative serum liver chemistries were normal but she had visible jaundice on the day of CCX. An impacted stone was seen in IOC (a). She was transferred to the ERCP suite after CCX while still anesthetized and intubated. Scout ERCP radiography demonstrated a dilated duct filled with contrast (b). A bulging papilla was cannulated and the stone was removed after sphincterotomy (c).

Postoperative ERCP

ERCP is performed after CCX when an operative cholangiogram shows a stone (which has not been removed), and is usually successful. It may also be necessary when symptoms and signs of biliary problems appear soon after surgery. This is particularly troublesome for both the patient who had expected a good outcome and the surgeon who is concerned about a surgical complication. It is challenging for the endoscopist because stones, bile leaks duct injury, or a combination [81] can present similarly but may require different approaches.

Some indications for postoperative ERCP can be more challenging such as Mirizzi's syndrome (Figure 15.5). MRCP and biliary scintigraphy are valuable methods for defining the situation.

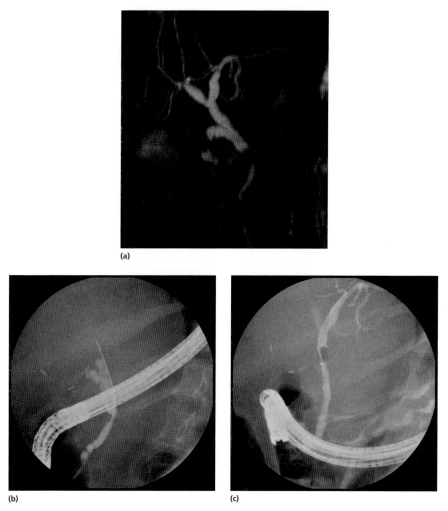

Figure 15.5 A 53-year-old female presented with upper abdominal pain and increased serum liver chemistries 6 weeks after CCX. An MRCP (a) demonstrated a stone with proximal dilation of both the bile duct and the cystic duct remnant consistent with Mirizzi's syndrome. Postoperative ERCP with cholangioscopy and intraductal laser lithotripsy (b) was successful and clearance was achieved.

Bile leak

A bile leak should be suspected when a patient has severe pain postoperatively (consistent with peritonitis), or if bile is present in a surgical drain. A duodenal injury may also result in bilious drainage via an external drain, but is far less likely. Biliary scintigraphy is usually the first step for diagnosis and it may also suggest the location of the leak. If a drain is not in place, it is prudent to consider additional imaging with either ultrasound or computed tomography to rule out a biloma. Percutaneous drainage either before or after ERCP should be considered if a biloma is symptomatic and/or large.

Most postoperative bile leaks are not related to ductal injury but simply due to impaired drainage via the papilla such that the pressure gradient promotes leakage from the cystic duct stump or from ducts of Luschka. Less commonly, a bile leak may be related to a major duct injury, a situation suggested by concomitant marked cholestasis.

A retrospective study of over 200 bile leaks during 10 years reported that about half are low-grade leaks, meaning that opacification of the intrahepatic ducts at ERCP was necessary before a leak could be demonstrated [81]. More than 90% of low-grade leaks without concomitant duct stones or strictures were successfully treated with sphincterotomy alone. Treatment with stenting and/or sphincterotomy was universally successful for high-grade leaks, for example, those that were demonstrated easily with contrast injection before intrahepatic duct opacification. Most bile leaks from the cystic duct can be successfully treated with a short transpapillary stent for 4–8 weeks without sphincterotomy [82, 83]. When that treatment fails, sphincterotomy and restenting is usually effective. Rarely it is necessary to apply suction with a nasobiliary drain. When scanning shows a bile leak and/or collection and careful ERCP is unrevealing, it means that the leak is coming from an aberrant intrahepatic duct.

Duct injury

The overall incidence of bile duct injury after CCX is about 0.3–0.6% [84]. This may become more of an issue with the increased use of the single-incision laparoscopic approach [85]. Recent data suggests that IOC does not reduce the risk for bile duct injury [86, 87]. Overall, less than one-third of bile duct injuries are recognized intraoperatively; but an IOC would increase the chance of recognizing an injury so that it can be corrected immediately as long as appropriate surgical expertise is available [88].

Most operative bile duct injuries are not recognized at the time of surgery. The possibility of injury (or a retained stone) should be considered when there are signs and symptoms of biliary obstruction postoperatively. MRCP is a good diagnostic tool, and can identify problems (such as inadvertent ligation of an aberrant right hepatic duct) that are not visible at ERCP.

There are several classifications of bile duct injuries and leaks [84, 89]. The Amsterdam version categorizes bile leaks and/or ductal injuries according to a continuum of severity and the likelihood for successful therapy with ERCP [90]. Type A injuries are minor bile leaks from the cystic duct (A1) or duct of Luschka (A2). Type B injuries are major duct leaks without injury, and endoscopic therapy is still mostly successful. A Type C injury is a major bile duct stricture; when the injury does not involve the bifurcation, it can often but not always be treated successfully with ERCP [91–93]. It is not yet clear whether treatment of postoperative major duct strictures are best treated with multiple plastic stents or fully covered metal stents [94]. Type D lesions involve a complete duct obstruction usually due to clips. This will almost always require operative correction. If there is evidence of ductal integrity without a complete transection, then it may be possible to remove the clips at surgery and then treat the injury postoperatively with ERCP using conventional methods [95]. Management of ductal injuries is discussed further in Chapter 7.

Summary

Despite an abundance of collective experience, data, and analyses, there are many reasons why there are no definitive answers regarding the best approach for evaluation and treatment of CDL in the peri-CCX setting. First, there are

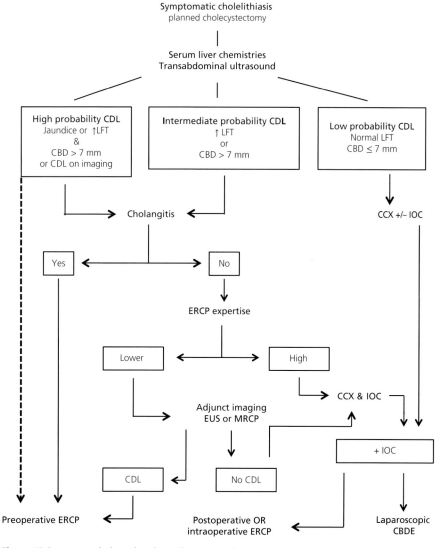

Figure 15.6 Suggested algorithm for utilization and timing of ERCP related to management of choledocholithiasis in the peri-cholecystectomy setting.

variables regarding patients including clinical presentation, comorbidities, numbers of common bile stones, sizes of stones, and bile duct diameter. Second, there are variables regarding the methods and success for detection and prediction of CDL. Third, there are variables regarding the timing of endoscopic evaluation and treatment with ERCP. Fourth, there are variables regarding laparoscopic confirmation of CDL and various treatment options. Perhaps the most important variable is the available expertise and teamwork of the endoscopic and surgical teams.

Figure 15.6 provides guidance as to a reasonable approach, one that places ERCP expertise central to the decision process. Preoperative ERCP is not indicated when the likelihood for CDL is low, but should be performed when there is cholangitis and may also be reasonable when the likelihood for CDL is high. When there is an intermediate likelihood for CDL, ERCP expertise becomes an important variable. If ERCP expertise is limited, ancillary imaging may be helpful to confirm a diagnosis of CDL before ERCP. If ERCP expertise is available, it may be reasonable to proceed with CCX and utilize IOC to clarify whether CDL is present, and, if so, treatment options would include laparoscopic CBDE, intraoperative ERCP, or postoperative ERCP.

References

1 Attasaranya S, Fogel EL, Lehman GA. Choledocholithiasis, ascending cholangitis, and gallstone pancreatitis. Medical Clin North Am. 2008;92(4):925–60.

2 Kimura Y, Takada T, Kawarada Y, *et al*. Definitions, pathophysiology, and epidemiology of acute cholangitis and cholecystitis: Tokyo Guidelines. J Hepato-biliary-pancreatic Surg. 2007;14(1):15–26.

3 Tenner S, Dubner H, Steinberg W. Predicting gallstone pancreatitis with laboratory parameters: a meta-analysis. Am J Gastroenterol. 1994;89(10):1863–6.

4 Tenner S, Baillie J, Dewitt J, Vege SS. American college of gastroenterology guideline: management of acute pancreatitis. Am J Gastroenterol. 2013;108(9):1400–15.

5 Kuo VC, Tarnasky PR. Endoscopic management of acute biliary pancreatitis. Gastrointest Endosc Clin North Am. 2013;23(4):749–68.

6 Liu CL, Fan ST, Lo CM, *et al*. Comparison of early endoscopic ultrasonography and endoscopic retrograde cholangiopancreatography in the management of acute biliary pancreatitis: a prospective randomized study. Clin Gastroenterol Hepatol. 2005;3(12):1238–44.

7 Tranter SE, Thompson MH. Spontaneous passage of bile duct stones: frequency of occurrence and relation to clinical presentation. Ann R Coll Surg Engl. 2003;85(3):174–7.

8 Roston AD, Jacobson IM. Evaluation of the pattern of liver tests and yield of cholangiography in symptomatic choledocholithiasis: a prospective study. Gastrointest Endosc. 1997;45(5):394–9.

9 Arguedas MR, Dupont AW, Wilcox CM. Where do ERCP, endoscopic ultrasound, magnetic resonance cholangiopancreatography, and intraoperative cholangiography fit in the management of acute biliary pancreatitis? A decision analysis model. Am J Gastroenterol. 2001;96(10):2892–9.

10 Tabone LE, Conlon M, Fernando E, *et al*. A practical cost-effective management strategy for gallstone pancreatitis. Am J Surg. 2013;206(4):472–7.

11 Romagnuolo J, Currie G. Noninvasive vs. selective invasive biliary imaging for acute biliary pancreatitis: an economic evaluation by using decision tree analysis. Gastrointest Endosc. 2005;61(1):86–97.

12 Shaffer EA. Gallstone disease: Epidemiology of gallbladder stone disease. Best Pract Res Clin Gastroenterol. 2006;20(6):981–96.

13 Ko CW, Lee SP. Epidemiology and natural history of common bile duct stones and prediction of disease. Gastrointest Endosc. 2002;56(6 Suppl):S165–9.

14 Dasari BV, Tan CJ, Gurusamy KS, et al. Surgical versus endoscopic treatment of bile duct stones. Cochrane Database Syst Rev. 2013;9:CD003327.

15 National Center for Health Statistics. Heath, United States, 2009: In Brief—Medical Technology. Hyattsville, MD: National Center for Health Statistics; 2010:1–17.

16 Caddy GR, Tham TC. Gallstone disease: Symptoms, diagnosis and endoscopic management of common bile duct stones. Best Pract Res Clin Gastroenterol. 2006;20(6):1085–101.

17 Collins C, Maguire D, Ireland A, et al. A prospective study of common bile duct calculi in patients undergoing laparoscopic cholecystectomy: natural history of choledocholithiasis revisited. Ann Surg. 2004;239(1):28–33.

18 Frossard JL, Hadengue A, Amouyal G, et al. Choledocholithiasis: a prospective study of spontaneous common bile duct stone migration. Gastrointest Endosc. 2000;51(2):175–9.

19 Venneman NG, Renooij W, Rehfeld JF, et al. Small gallstones, preserved gallbladder motility, and fast crystallization are associated with pancreatitis. 2005;41:738–46.

20 Shemesh E, Czerniak A, Bar-El J, et al. Choledocholithiasis: a comparison between the clinical presentations of multiple and solitary stones in the common bile duct. Am J Gastroenterol. 1989;84(9):1055–9.

21 Paul A, Millat B, Holthausen U, et al. Diagnosis and treatment of bile duct stones: results of a consensus development conference. Surg Endosc. 1998;12:856–64.

22 Cotton PB, Baillie J, Pappas TN, Meyers WS. Laparoscopic cholecystectomy and the biliary endoscopist. Gastrointest Endosc. 1991;37(1):94–7.

23 Changchien CS, Chuah SK, Chiu KW. Is ERCP necessary for symptomatic gallbladder stone patients before laparoscopic cholecystectomy? Am J Gastroenterol. 1995;90(12):2124–7.

24 Houdart R, Perniceni T, Darne B, et al. Predicting common bile duct lithiasis: determination and prospective validation of a model predicting low risk. Am J Surg. 1995;170(1):38–43.

25 Abboud PA, Malet PF, Berlin JA, et al. Predictors of common bile duct stones prior to cholecystectomy: a meta-analysis. Gastrointest Endosc. 1996;44(4):450–5.

26 van der Hul RL, Plaisier PW, Hamming JF, et al. Detection and management of common bile duct stones in the era of laparoscopic cholecystectomy. Scand J Gastroenterol. 1993;28(11):929–33.

27 Hunt DR. Common bile duct stones in non-dilated bile ducts? An ultrasound study. Australas Radiol. 1996;40(3):221–2.

28 Andrews S. Gallstone size related to incidence of post cholecystectomy retained common bile duct stones. Int J Surg. 2013;11(4):319–21.

29 Anciaux ML, Pelletier G, Attali P, et al. Prospective study of clinical and biochemical features of symptomatic choledocholithiasis. Dig Dis Sci. 1986;31(5):449–53.

30 Peng WK, Sheikh Z, Paterson-Brown S, Nixon SJ. Role of liver function tests in predicting common bile duct stones in acute calculous cholecystitis. Br J Surg. 2005;92(10):1241–7.

31 Sheen AJ, Asthana S, Al-Mukhtar A, et al. Preoperative determinants of common bile duct stones during laparoscopic cholecystectomy. Int J Clin Pract. 2008;62(11):1715–9.

32 Barr LL, Frame BC, Coulanjon A. Proposed criteria for preoperative endoscopic retrograde cholangiography in candidates for laparoscopic cholecystectomy. Surg Endosc. 1999;13(8):778–81.

33 Bergamaschi R, Tuech JJ, Braconier L, *et al*. Selective endoscopic retrograde cholangiography prior to laparoscopic cholecystectomy for gallstones. Am J Surg. 1999;178(1):46–9.

34 Prat F, Meduri B, Ducot B, *et al*. Prediction of common bile duct stones by noninvasive tests. Ann Surg. 1999;229(3):362–8.

35 Onken JE, Brazer SR, Eisen GM, *et al*. Predicting the presence of choledocholithiasis in patients with symptomatic cholelithiasis. Am J Gastroenterol. 1996;91(4):762–7.

36 Maple JT, Ben-Menachem T, Anderson MA, *et al*. The role of endoscopy in the evaluation of suspected choledocholithiasis. Gastrointest Endosc. 2010;71(1):1–9.

37 Buscarini E, Tansini P, Vallisa D, *et al*. EUS for suspected choledocholithiasis: do benefits outweigh costs? A prospective, controlled study. Gastrointest Endosc. 2003;57(4):510–8.

38 Petrov MS, Savides TJ. Systematic review of endoscopic ultrasonography versus endoscopic retrograde cholangiopancreatography for suspected choledocholithiasis. Br J Surg. 2009;96(9):967–74.

39 Sahai AV, Mauldin PD, Marsi V, *et al*. Bile duct stones and laparoscopic cholecystectomy: a decision analysis to assess the roles of intraoperative cholangiography, EUS, and ERCP. Gastrointest Endosc. 1999;49(3 Pt 1):334–43.

40 Scheiman JM, Carlos RC, Barnett JL, *et al*. Can endoscopic ultrasound or magnetic resonance cholangiopancreatography replace ERCP in patients with suspected biliary disease? A prospective trial and cost analysis. Am J Gastroenterol. 2001;96(10):2900–4.

41 Tse F, Barkun JS, Barkun AN. The elective evaluation of patients with suspected choledocholithiasis undergoing laparoscopic cholecystectomy. Gastrointest Endosc. 2004;60(3):437–48.

42 Epelboym I, Winner M, Allendorf JD. MRCP is not a cost-effective strategy in the management of silent common bile duct stones. J Gastrointest Surg. 2013;17(5):863–71.

43 Richard F, Boustany M, Britt LD. Accuracy of magnetic resonance cholangiopancreatography for diagnosing stones in the common bile duct in patients with abnormal intraoperative cholangiograms. Am J Surg. 2013;205(4):371–3.

44 Massarweh NN, Devlin A, Elrod JA, Symons RG, Flum DR. Surgeon knowledge, behavior, and opinions regarding intraoperative cholangiography. J Am Coll Surg. 2008;207(6):821–30.

45 Videhult P, Sandblom G, Rasmussen IC. How reliable is intraoperative cholangiography as a method for detecting common bile duct stones? A prospective population-based study on 1171 patients. Surg Endosc. 2009;23(2):304–12.

46 Horwood J, Akbar F, Davis K, Morgan R. Prospective evaluation of a selective approach to cholangiography for suspected common bile duct stones. Ann R Coll Surg Engl. 2010; 92(3):206–10.

47 Coppola R, Riccioni ME, Ciletti S, *et al*. Selective use of endoscopic retrograde cholangiopancreatography to facilitate laparoscopic cholecystectomy without cholangiography. A review of 1139 consecutive cases. Surg Endosc. 2001;15(10):1213–6.

48 Ueno K, Ajiki T, Sawa H, *et al*. Role of intraoperative cholangiography in patients whose biliary tree was evaluated preoperatively by magnetic resonance cholangiopancreatography. World J Surg. 2012;36(11):2661–5.

49 Pierce RA, Jonnalagadda S, Spitler JA, *et al*. Incidence of residual choledocholithiasis detected by intraoperative cholangiography at the time of laparoscopic cholecystectomy in patients having undergone preoperative ERCP. Surg Endosc. 2008;22(11):2365–72.

50 Livingston EH, Rege RV. Technical complications are rising as common duct exploration is becoming rare. J Am Coll Surg. 2005;201(3):426–33.

51 Grubnik VV, Tkachenko AI, Ilyashenko VV, Vorotyntseva KO. Laparoscopic common bile duct exploration versus open surgery: comparative prospective randomized trial. Surg Endosc. 2012;26(8):2165–71.

52 Buxbaum J. Modern management of common bile duct stones. Gastrointest Endosc Clin N Am. 2013;23(2):251–75.

53 Barkun AN, Barkun JS, Fried GM, *et al*. Useful predictors of bile duct stones in patients undergoing laparoscopic cholecystectomy. McGill Gallstone Treatment Group. Ann Surg. 1994;220(1):32–9.

54 Alkhaffaf B, Parkin E, Flook D. Endoscopic retrograde cholangiopancreatography prior to laparoscopic cholecystectomy: a common and potentially hazardous technique that can be avoided. Arch Surg. 2011;146(3):329–33.

55 Clair DG, Carr-Locke DL, Becker JM, Brooks DC. Routine cholangiography is not warranted during laparoscopic cholecystectomy. Arch Surg. 1993;128(5):551–4; discussion 4–5.

56 O'Neill CJ, Gillies DM, Gani JS. Choledocholithiasis: overdiagnosed endoscopically and undertreated laparoscopically. ANZ J Surg. 2008;78(6):487–91.

57 Boerma D, Schwartz MP. Gallstone disease. Management of common bile-duct stones and associated gallbladder stones: Surgical aspects. Best Pract Res Clin Gastroenterol. 2006; 20(6):1103–16.

58 Boerma D, Rauws EA, Keulemans YC, *et al*. Wait-and-see policy or laparoscopic cholecys-tectomy after endoscopic sphincterotomy for bile-duct stones: a randomised trial. Lancet. 2002;360(9335):761–5.

59 Urbach DR, Khajanchee YS, Jobe BA, *et al*. Cost-effective management of common bile duct stones: a decision analysis of the use of endoscopic retrograde cholangiopancreatography (ERCP), intraoperative cholangiography, and laparoscopic bile duct exploration. Surg Endosc. 2001;15(1):4–13.

60 Brown LM, Rogers SJ, Cello JP, *et al*. Cost-effective treatment of patients with symptomatic cholelithiasis and possible common bile duct stones. J Am Coll Surg. 2011;212(6):1049–60, e1–7.

61 Rhodes M, Sussman L, Cohen L, Lewis MP. Randomised trial of laparoscopic exploration of common bile duct versus postoperative endoscopic retrograde cholangiography for common bile duct stones. Lancet. 1998;351(9097):159–61.

62 Cuschieri A, Lezoche E, Morino M, *et al*. E.A.E.S. multicenter prospective randomized trial comparing two-stage vs single-stage management of patients with gallstone disease and ductal calculi. Surg Endosc. 1999;13(10):952–7.

63 Koc B, Karahan S, Adas G, *et al*. Comparison of laparoscopic common bile duct explora-tion and endoscopic retrograde cholangiopancreatography plus laparoscopic cholecystec-tomy for choledocholithiasis: a prospective randomized study. Am J Surg. 2013;206(4): 457–63.

64 Petelin JB. Surgical management of common bile duct stones. Gastrointest Endosc. 2002;56(6 Suppl):S183–9.

65 Bansal VK, Misra MC, Garg P, Prabhu M. A prospective randomized trial comparing two-stage versus single-stage management of patients with gallstone disease and common bile duct stones. Surg Endosc. 2010;24(8):1986–9.

66 Thompson MH, Tranter SE. All-comers policy for laparoscopic exploration of the common bile duct. Br J Surg. 2002;89(12):1608–12.

67 Taylor CJ, Kong J, Ghusn M, *et al*. Laparoscopic bile duct exploration: results of 160 consec-utive cases with 2-year follow up. ANZ J Surg. 2007;77(6):440–5.

68 Fanelli RD, Gersin KS. Laparoscopic endobiliary stenting: a simplified approach to the management of occult common bile duct stones. J Gastrointest Surg. 2001;5(1):74–80.

69 Bingener J, Schwesinger WH. Management of common bile duct stones in a rural area of the United States: results of a survey. Surg Endosc. 2006;20(4):577–9.

70 Petelin JB. Laparoscopic common bile duct exploration. Surg Endosc. 2003;17(11): 1705–15.

71 Sato N, Shibao K, Akiyama Y, *et al.* Routine intraoperative cholangiography during single-incision laparoscopic cholecystectomy: a review of 196 consecutive patients. J Gastrointest Surg. 2013;17(4):668–74.

72 Spinoglio G, Priora F, Bianchi PP, *et al.* Real-time near-infrared (NIR) fluorescent cholangiography in single-site robotic cholecystectomy (SSRC): a single-institutional prospective study. Surg Endosc. 2013;27(6):2156–62.

73 Deslandres E, Gagner M, Pomp A, *et al.* Intraoperative endoscopic sphincterotomy for common bile duct stones during laparoscopic cholecystectomy. Gastrointest Endosc. 1993; 39(1):54–8.

74 Cavina E, Franceschi M, Sidoti F, *et al.* Laparo-endoscopic "rendezvous": a new technique in the choledocholithiasis treatment. Hepatogastroenterology. 1998;45(23):1430–5.

75 Enochsson L, Lindberg B, Swahn F, Arnelo U. Intraoperative endoscopic retrograde cholangiopancreatography (ERCP) to remove common bile duct stones during routine laparoscopic cholecystectomy does not prolong hospitalization: a 2-year experience. Surg Endosc. 2004;18(3):367–71.

76 Noel R, Enochsson L, Swahn F, *et al.* A 10-year study of rendezvous intraoperative endoscopic retrograde cholangiography during cholecystectomy and the risk of post-ERCP pancreatitis. Surg Endosc. 2013;27(7):2498–503.

77 Lella F, Bagnolo F, Rebuffat C, *et al.* Use of the laparoscopic-endoscopic approach, the so-called "rendezvous" technique, in cholecystocholedocholithiasis: a valid method in cases with patient-related risk factors for post-ERCP pancreatitis. Surg Endosc. 2006;20(3):419–23.

78 Wang B, Guo Z, Liu Z, *et al.* Preoperative versus intraoperative endoscopic sphincterotomy in patients with gallbladder and suspected common bile duct stones: system review and meta-analysis. Surg Endosc. 2013;27(7):2454–65.

79 Sarli L, Sabadini G, Pietra N, *et al.* Laparoscopic cholecystectomy and endoscopic sphincterotomy under a single anesthetic: a case report. Surg Laparosc Endosc. 1995;5(1): 68–71.

80 Richardson JF, Lee JG, Smith BR, *et al.* Laparoscopic transgastric endoscopy after Roux-en-Y gastric bypass: case series and review of the literature. Am Surg. 2012;78(10):1182–6.

81 Sandha GS, Bourke MJ, Haber GB, Kortan PP. Endoscopic therapy for bile leak based on a new classification: results in 207 patients. Gastrointest Endosc. 2004;60(4):567–74.

82 Pioche M, Ponchon T. Management of bile duct leaks. J Visc Surg. 2013;150(3 Suppl):S33–8.

83 Tewani SK, Turner BG, Chuttani R, *et al.* Location of bile leak predicts the success of ERCP performed for postoperative bile leaks. Gastrointest Endosc. 2013;77(4):601–8.

84 Baillie J. Endoscopic approach to the patient with bile duct injury. Gastrointest Endosc Clin N Am. 2013;23(2):461–72.

85 Joseph M, Phillips MR, Farrell TM, Rupp CC. Single incision laparoscopic cholecystectomy is associated with a higher bile duct injury rate: a review and a word of caution. Ann Surg. 2012;256(1):1–6.

86 Nuzzo G, Giuliante F, Giovannini I, *et al.* Bile duct injury during laparoscopic cholecystectomy: results of an Italian national survey on 56591 cholecystectomies. Arch Surg 2005;140(10):986–92.

87 Sheffield KM, Riall TS, Han Y, *et al.* Association between cholecystectomy with vs without intraoperative cholangiography and risk of common duct injury. JAMA. 2013;310(8): 812–20.

88 Pekolj J, Alvarez FA, Palavecino M, *et al.* Intraoperative management and repair of bile duct injuries sustained during 10,123 laparoscopic cholecystectomies in a high-volume referral center. J Am Coll Surg. 2013;216(5):894–901.

89 Lau WY, Lai EC. Classification of iatrogenic bile duct injury. Hepatobiliary Pancreatic Diseases Int. 2007;6(5):459–63.

90 Bergman JJGHM, van den Brink GR, Rauws EAJ, *et al.* Treatment of bile duct lesions after laparoscopic cholecystectomy. Gut. 1996;38:141–7.

91 Csendes A, Navarrete C, Burdiles P, Yarmuch J. Treatment of common bile duct injuries during laparoscopic cholecystecotmy: endoscopic and surgical management. World J Surg 2001;25(10):1346–51.

92 Draganov P, Hoffman B, March W, *et al.* Long-term outcome in patients with benign biliary strictures treated endoscopically with multiple stents. Gastrointest Endosc 2002;55(6):680–6.

93 Costamagna G, Tringali A, Mutignani M, *et al.* Endotherapy of postoperative biliary strictures with multiple stents: results after more than 10 years of follow-up. Gastrointest Endosc 2010;72(3):551–7.

94 Garcia-Cano J. Endoscopic management of benign biliary strictures. Curr Gastroenterol Rep. 2013;15(8):336.

95 Tarnasky PR, Linder JD, Mejia A, *et al.* Bile duct obstruction after cholecystectomy caused by clips: undo what has been undone, then do what you normally do. Gastrointest Endosc. 2009;69(4):e19–21.

CHAPTER 16

Large bile duct stones

Julia McNabb-Baltar[1] & Alan Barkun[2]

[1] Division of Gastroenterology, Hepatology and Endoscopy, Brigham and Women's Hospital, Harvard Medical School, Boston, USA

[2] Division of Gastroenterology, Montreal General Hospital, McGill University, and the McGill University Health Centre, Montreal, Canada

---

KEY POINTS

- Large choledocholithiasis is defined as a stone with a diameter greater than 1–1.2 cm.

- They are challenging and associated with higher complication rates.

- Management often includes a combination of techniques to increase the size of the bile duct opening in the duodenum and decrease the size of the stones.

- Endoscopists must also assess the characteristics of a clinical setting, bile duct, and CBD stones that make these difficult to extract endoscopically and choose appropriate method(s) of removal.

- Biliary management is best performed adopting a collaborative multidisciplinary approach while remaining both evidence-based and weighing the risks and benefits for a given patient.

Case

An 84-year-old female post remote cholecystectomy, having had a myocardial infarction 2 years ago, and now on aspirin, presents to the local emergency department with a 2-day history of abdominal pain. She denies fever or jaundice. Her initial physical examination is unremarkable except for right upper quadrant tenderness. Initial investigations reveal elevated alanine aminotransferase , aspartate aminotransferase, and total bilirubin. Abdominal ultrasound demonstrates an 18-mm common bile duct (CBD) stone. What is the best management approach?

Introduction

More than 90% of all CBD stones are extracted endoscopically using standard techniques [1, 2]. Large choledocholithiasis (Figure 16.1) is defined as a stone with a diameter greater than 1–1.2 cm. This clinical entity is relevant, because it is associated with higher rates of failed extraction and complications, and poses

---

ERCP: The Fundamentals, Second Edition. Edited by Peter B. Cotton and Joseph Leung.
Companion Website: www.wiley.com\go\cotton\ercp

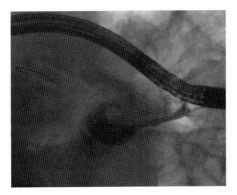

Figure 16.1 Large common bile duct stone.

Table 16.1 Possible approaches to treat large bile duct stones.

Techniques that increase the sphincterotomy opening diameter
   Endoscopic sphincnterotomy (ES)
   Balloon sphincteroplasty
   Post-ES endoscopic papillary balloon dilation
Techniques that will decrease stone size: lithotripsy
   Mechanical lithotripsy
   Extracorporal (shock wave) lithotripsy
   Intracorporeal (intraductal) lithotripsy via choledochoscopy
   (electrohydraulic, smart laser)
Role of biliary stenting
   Biliary (plastic/metal) stents
   Stents with ursodeoxycholic acid
   Naso-biliary drain
Backup methods
   Percutaneous transhepatic cholangiography (PTC)
   Surgical

specific management issues. Other stones may be considered difficult to extract including piston-shaped stones, impacted stones, or stones in the presence of biliary stricture or acute angulation of the distal CBD or short segment. Distorted anatomy after surgical reconstruction may represent another challenge for successful CBD stone removal. In this chapter, we performed a systematic review summarizing the clinical results of specific contemporary management options for the removal of large choledocholithiasis. Different techniques may be required, and even a combination thereof, to achieve favorable results. General conceptual approaches include techniques aimed at increasing the opening diameter of the bile duct into the duodenum, and methods to decrease the size of the stone (Table 16.1). We will also briefly discuss the specific role of biliary stenting, and alternatives to endoscopic methods, as well as specific issues related to patients exhibiting reconstructed anatomy, Mirizzi's syndrome, impacted stones, and intrahepatic stones.

Methods of the narrative review

We performed a literature search of Embase, MEDLINE, and Cochrane Library databases (1988 to July 2013). We used a combination of MeSH subjects headings and text words, including Gallstone OR (common AND bile AND duct AND stone*) OR (Mirizzi AND syndrome) OR Choledocholithiase OR (intrahepatic AND stone*) OR (bil* AND lithiasis) AND stent* OR Lithotripsy OR litholapaxy OR lithotrypsy OR Electrohydraulic OR (endoscopic AND sphincterotomy) OR sphincteroplasty OR (balloon AND dilation) OR (naso-biliary AND drain) OR (smart AND laser). Reference lists from selected articles were reviewed manually to identify additional citations. All data were abstracted and recorded in dedicated forms and reviewed by two independent individuals (J.M.B., A.N.B.). Resolution of any discrepancies in data abstraction was achieved through consensus. We included randomized controlled trials (RCTs) as highest-level evidence, whenever possible, and assessed stone clearance, as the main outcome, and complications as the secondary outcome.

Techniques that increase the bile duct opening in the duodenum

Endoscopic balloon dilation
The standard technique to increase the bile duct opening in the duodenum is that of endoscopic sphincterotomy (ES). Although effective, it is associated with immediate and delayed complications [3, 4]; theoretically, because it destroys the biliary sphincter permanently, it may lead to long-term complications such as pancreatico-biliary reflux, and chronic inflammation of the biliary system, although the actual clinical impact of these remains poorly documented and subject to controversy.

As a result, endoscopic balloon dilation (EBD) (Figure 16.2) has been studied because of its theoretical benefit of maintaining sphincter function, although

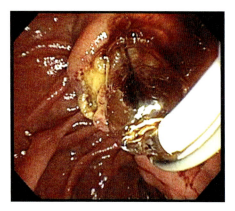

Figure 16.2 Endoscopic sphincterotomy followed by endoscopic balloon dilation.

studies assessing sphincter function after EBD and ES show conflicting results [5, 6]. We identified 9 trials, including a total of 1390 patients randomized to ES versus EBD. In 1997, Bergman and colleagues studied randomized patients without previous sphincterotomy to ES or EBD. One hundred one patients received EBD using an 8-mm balloon inflated for 45–60 s, and the same number received ES. Stones were similar in size in both groups (median size 10 versus 9 mm). Successful stone extraction rates were similar after the initial endoscopic retrograde cholangiopancreatography (ERCP) (89% in EBD versus 91% in ES, $P=0.81$). Mechanical lithotripsy (ML) was used more often in the EBD group (31 versus 13, $P<0.005$). There were no differences in overall complications rates. One patient died of retroperitoneal perforation after EBD. More acute cholecystitis was observed in the ES group (7 versus 1 in EBD, $P<0.05$). Acute pancreatitis occurred at the same frequency in both groups (7% in each group).

Using a similar technique, and randomizing 30 patients per group, Arnold and colleagues found that EBD caused more complications and longer procedure times and led to lower stone removal rates than ES (77% versus 100%) [7]. Since then, several other RCTs were conducted using various balloon diameters, ranging from 8 to 18 mm, and various inflation times, ranging from 30 s to 5 min. Most trials have showed similar results using ES or EBD [8–12]. One additional trial showed higher rates of complications in the EBD group [13]. Watanabe and colleagues randomized 180 patients to receive ES or EBD with an 8-mm-diameter balloon inflated for 2 min. Overall, the rate of complete stone extraction was greater in the ES group than in the EBD group, as was the pancreatitis rate in the EBD group (16.7% versus 6.7%, $P<0.05$). In the only US multicenter RCT, DiSario and colleagues found that although the stone extraction rate was similar using ES or EBD, EBD was associated with increased short-term morbidity when compared to ES including higher rates of pancreatitis (15.4% versus 0.8%, $P<0.001$), with two reported cases of death [14]. Their protocol used 8-mm-diameter balloons inflated for 60 s. Although they initially planned to exclude all patients with stones larger than 1 cm, 3 patients with such stone sizes were included, in a total population of 237 patients. Based on this multicenter trial with the two case fatalities from pancreatitis, this approach has fallen out of favor, at least in North America.

The ideal dilation time has also been assessed prospectively. Two trials were conducted comparing EBD time, including a total of 240 patients, that presented conflicting results. In 70 patients with a mean stone size of 8 mm, using 15-mm-diameter balloons, Bang and colleagues compared a dilation time of 20 versus 60 sec [15]. They found similar complete duct clearance in both groups, as well as rates of need forML. The use of 60-sec dilation was associated with more cases of mild pancreatitis, although this finding was not statistically significant (11.4% versus 5.7%). Longer duration of dilation, 1 versus 5 min, was assessed by a separate group [16]. The 5-min dilation group was associated with less failed stone extraction and pancreatitis (4.8% versus 15.1%, RR=0.32, $P=0.038$). This study included stones up to 2 cm. Based on these studies, the ideal dilation time is unclear.

Short-term complications of EBD versus ES remain controversial; a report described no difference in the rate of pancreatitis, but an increased rate of hyper-amylasemia in a trial of 180 patients [17]. Others, such as DiSario and colleagues, report increased pancreatitis with EBD, as discussed earlier [14]. Long-term complications of EBD versus ES have also been specifically assessed in two trials, including 314 patients. Compared to EBD, ES is a risk factor for stone recurrence and biliary sphincter dysfunction in studies with follow-up periods of up to 7 years [18, 19].

Combination endoscopic sphincterotomy and balloon dilation

Because EBD appears most beneficial in the management of small stones and less so with large stones, a combination of ES and EBD (ESBD) has been assessed specifically in the context of large CBD stones. We identified four trials accounting for 411 patients. Hoe and colleagues randomized 200 consecutive patients with stones to receive ES versus ESBD, performing a limited sphincter-otomy of maximum 50% of the sphincter followed by large balloon dilation with a diameter of up to 20 mm to match the size of the duct and stones [20]. Overall, duct clearance of large stones (>15 mm) was similar in both groups (ES versus ESBD: 96.7% versus 94.4%, not significant (NS)), as were complica-tions, including a 4% pancreatitis rate. Similar results were observed in the trial conducted by Kim et al. [21]. In 2013, Teoh and colleagues compared the two approaches and evaluated end points of duct clearance, the use of ML, and hospitalization costs [22]. Randomizing 156 patients, they found no difference in the stone clearance rate (ES versus ESBD: 88.5 versus 89.0%, NS), more use of ML in the ES group (46.2% versus 28.8%, $P=0.028$), and lower costs with ESBD ($P=0.034$).

A meta-analysis including three trials, one of which was published as an abstract form, and six retrospective studies showed no differences in the rates of stone removal in the first session (OR=1.01, 95% CI 0.92–1.11), or in the need for ML (OR=0.78, 95% CI 0.49–1.23, $P=0.29$). Results also showed equivalent complication rates (OR=0.61, 95% CI 0.17–2.25, $P=0.46$), including pancrea-titis (OR=1.11, 95% CI 0.37–3.35, $P=0.86$), but with less bleeding in the ESBD group (OR=0.10, 95% CI 0.03–0.30, $P\leq0.001$) [23].

A trial was also conducted to compare balloon dilation to ESBD. Hwang et al. randomized 131 patients with CBD stones larger than 12 mm to receive EBD or ESBD [24]. They showed similar outcomes of bile duct clearance, stone removal without need for ML, as well as comparable complication rates including pan-creatitis (6.5% versus 4.3%, $P=0.593$), impaction of stone or basket (0% versus 1.6%, $P=0.341$), and perforation (0% versus 1.4%, $P=0.341$).

Duration of balloon dilation has also been assessed for ESBD. In a RCT of 124 patients with large CBD stones, Paspatis and colleagues evaluated the efficacy of ES followed by 30 versus 60 s dilation using a maximum balloon diameter of 20 mm, and found similar rates of successful bile duct clearance and complications [25].

Other combination therapies have been assessed head to head. Stefanidis and colleagues compared ESBD with ES followed by ML in a trial involving 90 patients [26]. Specifically focusing on large stones (12–20 mm), they found similar efficacy but less complications including perforation (0% versus 2.2%, NS) and cholangitis (0 versus 13.3%, $P=0.026$) in the ESBD group compared to ES with ML [26].

Based on these considerations, multiple modalities are available to aid the endoscopist perform successful extraction of large bile duct stones. ESBD appears as effective as ES but may decrease cost of hospitalization and require less ML, which may be associated with more complications.

Techniques to decrease the size of the stones

Mechanical and pharmacological methods have been described to decrease the size of bile duct stones. Pharmacological approaches using methyl *tert*-butyl ether or ursodeoxycholic acid (UDCA) alone are of mostly historical interest because of their low success rate, especially in large stones, and complication rates, although UDCA has been used as adjuvant therapy in combination with lithotripsy and/or stents as described later.

Methods to decrease the size of stones

Lithotripsy can be performed mechanically using specialized baskets to crush the stones, or through shock wave fragmentation of bile duct stones, either extracorporeally using external generators or intracorporeally through placement of a shock wave–delivering catheter positioned under fluoroscopic guidance or direct visualization at cholangioscopy. The source of shock wave creation uses either electrohydraulic lithotripsy (EHL) generators or pulsed dye lasers (with or without safety features to minimize bile duct injury, such as with smart lasers).

ML (Figure 16.3) was studied in a cohort of 346 patients and was associated with a successful duct clearance rate of 85–90%. Complications were infrequent (3.6% overall), and included trapped or broken baskets, wire fractures, broken handles, and perforation or bile duct injury in three patients [27].Using additional methods, 94% achieved duct clearance using ES extension, EHL, stent, ESWL, laser, and surgery in one patient.

Overall, we identified four RCTs assessing lithotripsy and totaling 169 patients. Adamek and colleagues compared extracorporeal piezoelectric lithotripsy (EPL) to intracorporeal EHL in patients with failed duct clearance using

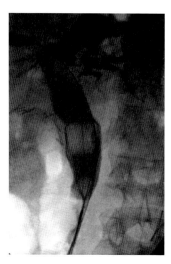

Figure 16.3 Mechanical lithotripsy.

standard approaches, in which 13 patients had large stones [28]. Assessing
35 patients that met the inclusion criteria, they found that EHL was associated
with less lithotripsy sessions than EPL (1.4 versus 2.3); both techniques
required additional endoscopy, with almost half the patients requiring three.
The duct clearance was similar in both groups. Yasuda and colleagues studied
combination therapy: EBD with extracorporeal shock wave lithotripsy (ESWL)
versus EBD and ML (29). They randomized 40 patients with large CBD stones
(>12 mm). Duct clearance was complete in all patients in both groups; ML was
associated with a rise in amylase in multivariable analysis ($P<0.05$), while
ESWL was protective.

Two groups studied intracorporeal laser lithotripsy (ILL) versus ESWL using
the smart laser (Lithognost) technology. Jakobs and colleagues randomized 34
patients to receive one of the two treatments for patients with retained stones
[30]. Initial fragmentation of stone was achieved in 52.4% of patients treated
with ESWL and 82.4% of patients treated with ILL. Overall, ILL required less
sessions and was associated with a significant reduction in cost. No major
complications were observed in either group. Neuhaus and colleagues also
assessed these two modalities [31], randomizing 60 patients with difficult stones
or anatomy nonamenable to an endoscopic approach, including 27 patients
that received treatment or stone fragment extraction through percutaneous
transhepatic cholangiographic drainage (PTCD). ILL achieved more duct
clearance (97% versus 73%, $P<0.05$) and required less treatment sessions than
ESWL (1.2 versus 3.0, $P<0.001$). The authors concluded that ILL was more
effective than ESWL in the treatment of difficult bile duct stones [31].It thus
appears that ILL may be more effective than ESWL in the management of CBD
stones, requiring fewer sessions to achieve duct clearance.

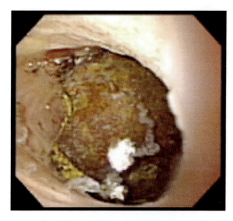

Figure 16.4 CBD stone seen using cholangioscopy. Source: Reproduced with permission of Peter Cotton.

Different methods of cholangioscopy (Figure 16.4) exist, including using the Spyglass TM technology, the mother–daughter scope, or other forms of direct cholangioscopy. These are detailed in Chapter 9. A prospective RCT by Pohl and colleagues compared the two cholangioscopy techniques of short-access mother–baby cholangioscopy (SAMBA) versus direct cholangioscopy using ultraslim gastroscopes. They randomized 30 patients in each arm, including a total of 8 with complex bile duct stones. Focusing on patients with stones, 4 ILL were performed using SAMBA and direct cholangioscopy (DC); 1 patient received successful stone extraction using SAMBA, compared to 4 using DC [32].

Role of biliary stents

Biliary stents (Figure 16.5) may be used as a temporizing measure to maintain biliary drainage between endoscopic sessions or prior to surgical assessment, or to assist in stone fragmentation. Temporary stents using plastic, pigtail, multiple, or metallic stents have all been assessed. Alternately, a naso-biliary drain may be useful in providing irrigation, or helping with stone localization for ESWL, but may cause discomfort to patients.

The role of a stent alone or in combination with UDCA has been studied. We identified 4 RCTs, including 165 patients, of which 144 were considered high-risk. Chopra and colleagues randomized 43 high-risk patients to ES with double pigtail stent versus a conventional approach using ES and ML [33]. Biliary drainage was achieved after 1 session in 98% in the former group versus 56% in the latter. Stent placement was associated with fewer complications after 3 days compared to the conventional group (7% versus 16%), but more complications at 20 months (36% versus 14%). Another trial focused on long-term stent placement in high-risk patients [34]. The authors compared two types of biliary

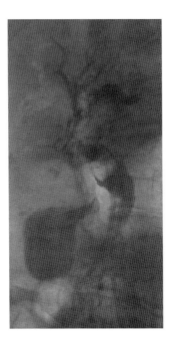

Figure 16.5 Biliary stent.

endoprostheses: polyethylene or hydrophilic hydromer-coated polyurethane. During a median follow-up of 38 months, stent patency was similar in both groups; two patients died of biliary-related causes.

Katsinelos and colleagues studied 41 subjects with stones difficult to extract [35]. They randomized the subjects to receive 10 French straight plastic stents and UDCA or placebo for 6 months. Repeat ERCP achieved a total CBD clearance in 77 and 75% of cases, respectively. Stone fragmentation and stone size reduction were not statistically significantly different between the two groups (38 and 33% in the group treatment with UDCA versus 50 and 25% in the placebo group, both NS). Lee and colleagues randomized patients with difficult stone extraction to multiple 7 French pigtail stents with or without UDCA and terpene. Stone size decreased significantly during the follow-up period of 6 months from 19 to 13 mm and 21 to 14 mm, but there were no differences in successful stone removal rates between the two treatment arms (73.7% in the stent group and 86.4% in the stent and choleretic agents group, $P = 0.826$) [36].

There exist no high-quality comparative trials assessing the use of metal stents for difficult CBD stones.

Therefore, in a selected population with high-risk, long-term stent placement can be considered. The addition of UDCA or terpene to endoprosthesis does not appear to help decrease the size of the stones with a clinically meaningful impact on management.

Backup methods

When endoscopic therapy is unsuccessful, other alternatives must be considered.

Surgery

When endoscopic treatment is not successful, surgical management may be considered. A laparoendoscopic rendezvous approach has also been assessed and described in two trials, which included a total of 191 patients. The rendezvous technique is described as follows: the sphincterotome is driven across the papilla into the CBD by a Dormia basket passed in the duodenum through the cystic duct during laparoscopic cholecystectomy (LC) [37]. In a trial from 2006 by Morino and colleagues, 91 patients with cholelithiasis and CBD stones were randomized to receive ERCP with ES followed by LC or LC with intraoperative ERCP using a rendezvous approach [38]. They recorded that the rate of CBD clearance was 80% in the ERCP with ES followed by LC versus 96% in the laparoendoscopic rendezvous approach ($P=0.06$). Hospital stay was shorter by 4 days in the latter group ($P \leq 0.00001$), with associated reduced total costs ($P < 0.05$). The interim analysis of another controlled trial supported the previous findings and noted less post-ERCP hyperamylasemia in the laparoendoscopic rendezvous approach group ($P=0.02$), but without differences in complications [39].

Percutaneous transhepatic cholangiography

When surgery is not an option, or biliary cannulation is unsuccessful, percutaneous transhepatic cholangiography (PTC) can be used to facilitate access to the biliary system through a rendezvous approach. After this, intracorporeal lithotripsy techniques can be undertaken [40].

Special circumstances

Other clinical contexts such as modified anatomy or stone location and bile duct anatomy may render CBD stone extraction difficult.

Impacted stones

Impacted stones (Figure 16.6) also represent a technical challenge for the endoscopist. Indeed, these may lead to difficult biliary cannulation when impacted in the ampulla, in which case a precut sphincterotomy may be of use. There are no RCT data addressing this situation.

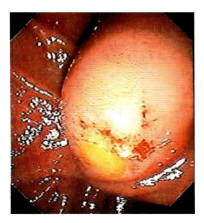

Figure 16.6 Impacted stone.

Mirizzi's syndrome

Mirizzi's syndrome (Figure 16.7) occurs in approximately 0.5% of patients with cholelithiasis, usually in presence of an anatomical variant in which the cystic duct at the gallbladder neck runs parallel to the common hepatic duct (CHD). If so, CBD or CHD obstruction may result from impaction of a stone in the cystic duct or neck of the gallbladder because of the stone itself, or due to secondary inflammation [41]. When present, it may be difficult to diagnose at ERCP, and may require surgical intervention. Pre-ERCP imaging is very helpful in raising the possibility of such a diagnosis. Historically, the role of ERCP has been limited to diagnosis and stent insertion to temporize prior to surgical intervention. In recent years, case reports have described successful stone removal using lithotripsy in elderly patients [42, 43].

Surgically altered anatomy

Surgically altered anatomy with Billroth II or Roux-en-Y reconstruction represents specific challenges to the endoscopist. Indeed, it may be difficult to identify the afferent loop; the distance between the mouth and the biliary intestinal anastomosis is usually greater than in nonsurgically altered anatomy, such that the biliary system needs to be accessed from an intestinal retrograde approach leading to an inverted biliary anatomy.

Based on these considerations, a trial assessing altered anatomy due to Billroth II gastrectomy compared ES with EBD in 34 patients. Successful biliary clearance, use of ML, and early complications were not different between the two groups. In the ES group, 3 (17%) patients had bleeding, while 1 (6%) patient in the EBD group had mild pancreatitis. EBD or ES thus appear to be safe approaches in patients with Billroth II anatomy [44].

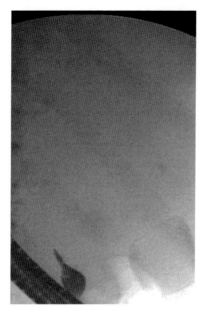

Figure 16.7 Mirizzi's syndrome. Source: Reproduced with permission of L Stein.

Surgically altered anatomy has also been assessed retrospectively in patients with a Roux-en-Y surgical hook-up. Kawasura and colleagues assessed a cohort of 204 patients, demonstrating intubation of the blind loop in 91% of patients using single-balloon enteroscopy, compared to 33% before its advent ($P=0.015$) [45].

Intrahepatic stones
Intrahepatic stones (Figure 16.8) are often located high in the biliary system and may be difficult to extract. A piston maneuver using the suction effect of an inflated extraction balloon distal to the stone may help dislodge these, bringing the stones down into the CBD where removal can more readily be achieved. Intrahepatic stones may result from localized strictures with associated bile stasis, further complicating endoscopic treatment. Endoscopy may also play a role in assessing the malignancy potential of the strictures. A percutaneous approach is commonly used in this setting [40]. Surgical management will often be the definitive treatment option. There is a paucity of high-quality comparative data addressing this difficult issue.

Long-term considerations

Cholecystectomy after endoscopic clearance of the bile duct has been assessed. McAlister and colleagues performed a Cochrane systematic review and meta-analysis of RCTs [46]. They compared cholecystectomy deferral versus elective

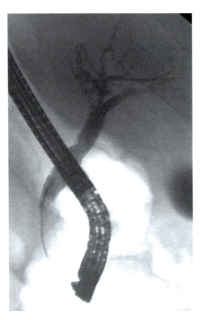

Figure 16.8 Intrahepatic stone. Source: Reproduced with permission of L Stein.

cholecystectomy, including 5 RCTs with 662 patients. The relative risk of mortality in the wait-and-see group was 1.78 compared to the elective cholecystectomy group ($P=0.010$). A subgroup analysis including only high-risk patients showed a similar mortality benefit. Patients in the cholecystectomy deferral group exhibited higher rates of recurrent biliary pain (RR 14.56, $P<00001$), jaundice or cholangitis (RR 2.53, $P=0.03$), and need for repeat cholangiography (RR 2.36, $P=0.005$). Cholecystectomy was eventually required in 35% of the wait-and-see group. Therefore, patients (including both elderly and high-risk individuals) with biliary stones appear to benefit from prophylactic cholecystectomy in this setting.

Existing guidelines and consensus recommendations

Important society guidelines related to the topic have been published by the American Society for Gastrointestinal Endoscopy (ASGE) [47], the Society of American Gastrointestinal and Endoscopic Surgeons (SAGES) [48], the American Gastroenterological Association (AGA) [49] and the American College of Gastroenterology (ACG) [50].

Back to our case

A standard sphincterotomy was performed, followed by controlled-radial expansion of a balloon to 15 mm for 3 min. Oozing bleeding was noted after deflation and stopped spontaneously. ML was then performed and the bile duct was cleared successfully.

Conclusion

In conclusion, large and difficult CBD stones represent specific challenges to the endoscopist. Advanced techniques may be used and combined to achieve better outcomes. These need to be tailored to the specific situation and patient. A multidisciplinary approach involving advanced endoscopists, interventional radiologists, and surgeons will lead to optimal patient outcomes.

References

1 Classen M, Hagenmuller F. Treatment of stones in the bile duct via duodenoscopy. Endoscopy. 1989;21 Suppl 1:375–7.

2 Peng C, Nietert PJ, Cotton PB, *et al*. Predicting native papilla biliary cannulation success using a multinational Endoscopic Retrograde Cholangiopancreatography (ERCP) Quality Network. BMC Gastroenterology. 2013;13(1):147.

3 Cotton PB, Garrow DA, Gallagher J, Romagnuolo J. Risk factors for complications after ERCP: a multivariate analysis of 11,497 procedures over 12 years. Gastrointestinal Endoscopy. 2009;70(1):80–8.

4 Freeman ML, Nelson DB, Sherman S, *et al*. Complications of endoscopic biliary sphincterotomy. The New England Journal of Medicine. 1996;335(13):909–18.

5 Yasuda I, Tomita E, Enya M, *et al.*. Can endoscopic papillary balloon dilation really preserve sphincter of Oddi function? Gut. 2001;49(5):686–91.

6 Takezawa M, Kida Y, Kida M, Saigenji K. Influence of endoscopic papillary balloon dilation and endoscopic sphincterotomy on sphincter of oddi function: a randomized controlled trial. Endoscopy. 2004;36(7):631–7.

7 Arnold JC, Benz C, Martin WR, Adamek HE, Riemann JF. Endoscopic papillary balloon dilation vs. sphincterotomy for removal of common bile duct stones: a prospective randomized pilot study. Endoscopy. 2001;33(7):563–7.

8 Oh MJ, Kim TN. Prospective comparative study of endoscopic papillary large balloon dilation and endoscopic sphincterotomy for removal of large bile duct stones in patients above 45 years of age. Scandinavian Journal of Gastroenterology. 2012;47(8–9):1071–7.

9 Lin CK, Lai KH, Chan HH, *et al*. Endoscopic balloon dilatation is a safe method in the management of common bile duct stones. Digestive and Liver Disease: Official Journal of the Italian Society of Gastroenterology and the Italian Association for the Study of the Liver. 2004;36(1):68–72.

10 Fujita N, Maguchi H, Komatsu Y, *et al*. Endoscopic sphincterotomy and endoscopic papillary balloon dilatation for bile duct stones: a prospective randomized controlled multicenter trial. Gastrointestinal Endoscopy. 2003;57(2):151–5.

11 Vlavianos P, Chopra K, Mandalia S, *et al*. Endoscopic balloon dilatation versus endoscopic sphincterotomy for the removal of bile duct stones: a prospective randomised trial. Gut. 2003;52(8):1165–9.

12 Natsui M, Narisawa R, Motoyama H, *et al*. What is an appropriate indication for endoscopic papillary balloon dilation? European Journal of Gastroenterology & Hepatology. 2002;14(6): 635–40.

13 Watanabe H, Yoneda M, Tominaga K, *et al*. Comparison between endoscopic papillary balloon dilatation and endoscopic sphincterotomy for the treatment of common bile duct stones. Journal of Gastroenterology. 2007;42(1):56–62.

14 Disario JA, Freeman ML, Bjorkman DJ, *et al.* Endoscopic balloon dilation compared with sphincterotomy for extraction of bile duct stones. Gastroenterology. 2004;127(5):1291–9.

15 Bang BW, Jeong S, Lee DH, *et al.* The ballooning time in endoscopic papillary balloon dilation for the treatment of bile duct stones. The Korean Journal of Internal Medicine. 2010;25(3):239–45.

16 Liao WC, Lee CT, Chang CY, *et al.* Randomized trial of 1-minute versus 5-minute endoscopic balloon dilation for extraction of bile duct stones. Gastrointestinal Endoscopy. 2010;72(6): 1154–62.

17 Bergman JJ, van Berkel AM, Bruno MJ, *et al.* Is endoscopic balloon dilation for removal of bile duct stones associated with an increased risk for pancreatitis or a higher rate of hyper-amylasemia? Endoscopy. 2001;33(5):416–20.

18 Yasuda I, Fujita N, Maguchi H, *et al.* Long-term outcomes after endoscopic sphincterotomy versus endoscopic papillary balloon dilation for bile duct stones. Gastrointestinal Endoscopy. 2010;72(6):1185–91.

19 Tanaka S, Sawayama T, Yoshioka T. Endoscopic papillary balloon dilation and endoscopic sphincterotomy for bile duct stones: long-term outcomes in a prospective randomized controlled trial. Gastrointestinal Endoscopy. 2004;59(6):614–8.

20 Heo JH, Kang DH, Jung HJ, *et al.* Endoscopic sphincterotomy plus large-balloon dilation versus endoscopic sphincterotomy for removal of bile-duct stones. Gastrointestinal Endoscopy. 2007;66(4):720–6; quiz 68, 71.

21 Kim HG, Cheon YK, Cho YD, *et al.* Small sphincterotomy combined with endoscopic papillary large balloon dilation versus sphincterotomy. World Journal of Gastroenterology: WJG. 2009;15(34):4298–304.

22 Teoh AY, Cheung FK, Hu B, *et al.* Randomized trial of endoscopic sphincterotomy with balloon dilation versus endoscopic sphincterotomy alone for removal of bile duct stones. Gastroenterology. 2013;144(2):341–5 e1.

23 Liu Y, Su P, Lin Y, *et al.* Endoscopic sphincterotomy plus balloon dilation versus endoscopic sphincterotomy for cholcdocholithiasis: a meta-analysis. Journal of Gastroenterology and Hepatology. 2013;28(6):937–45.

24 Hwang JC, Kim JH, Lim SG, *et al.* Endoscopic large-balloon dilation alone versus endoscopic sphincterotomy plus large-balloon dilation for the treatment of large bile duct stones. BMC Gastroenterology. 2013;13:15.

25 Paspatis GA, Konstantinidis K, Tribonias G, *et al.* Sixty- versus thirty-seconds papillary balloon dilation after sphincterotomy for the treatment of large bile duct stones: a randomized controlled trial. Digestive and Liver Disease: Official Journal of the Italian Society of Gastroenterology and the Italian Association for the Study of the Liver. 2013;45(4):301–4.

26 Stefanidis G, Viazis N, Pleskow D, *et al.* Large balloon dilation vs. mechanical lithotripsy for the management of large bile duct stones: a prospective randomized study. The American Journal of Gastroenterology. 2011;106(2):278–85.

27 Thomas M, Howell DA, Carr-Locke D, *et al.* Mechanical lithotripsy of pancreatic and biliary stones: complications and available treatment options collected from expert centers. The American Journal of Gastroenterology. 2007;102(9):1896–902.

28 Adamek HE, Buttmann A, Wessbecher R, *et al.* Clinical comparison of extracorporeal piezo-electric lithotripsy (EPL) and intracorporeal electrohydraulic lithotripsy (EHL) in difficult bile duct stones. A prospective randomized trial. Digestive Diseases and Sciences. 1995;40(6): 1185–92.

29 Yasuda I, Tomita E, Moriwaki H, *et al.* Endoscopic papillary balloon dilatation for common bile duct stones: efficacy of combination with extracorporeal shockwave lithotripsy for large stones. European Journal of Gastroenterology & Hepatology. 1998;10(12):1045–50.

30 Jakobs R, Adamek HE, Maier M, *et al*. Fluoroscopically guided laser lithotripsy versus extra-corporeal shock wave lithotripsy for retained bile duct stones: a prospective randomised study. Gut. 1997;40(5):678–82.

31 Neuhaus H, Zillinger C, Born P, *et al*. Randomized study of intracorporeal laser lithotripsy versus extracorporeal shock-wave lithotripsy for difficult bile duct stones. Gastrointestinal Endoscopy. 1998;47(5):327–34.

32 Pohl J, Meves VC, Mayer G,*et al*. Prospective randomized comparison of short-access mother-baby cholangioscopy versus direct cholangioscopy with ultraslim gastroscopes. Gastrointestinal Endoscopy. 2013;78(4):609–16.

33 Chopra KB, Peters RA, O'Toole PA, *et al*. Randomised study of endoscopic biliary endoprosthesis versus duct clearance for bileduct stones in high-risk patients. Lancet. 1996;348(9030):791–3.

34 Pisello F, Geraci G, Li Volsi F, *et al*. Permanent stenting in "unextractable" common bile duct stones in high risk patients. A prospective randomized study comparing two different stents. Langenbeck's archives of surgery/Deutsche Gesellschaft fur Chirurgie. 2008; 393(6):857–63.

35 Katsinelos P, Kountouras J, Paroutoglou G, *et al*. Combination of endoprostheses and oral ursodeoxycholic acid or placebo in the treatment of difficult to extract common bile duct stones. Digestive and Liver Disease: Official Journal of the Italian Society of Gastroenterology and the Italian Association for the Study of the Liver. 2008;40(6):453–9.

36 Lee TH, Han JH, Kim HJ, *et al*. Is the addition of choleretic agents in multiple double-pigtail biliary stents effective for difficult common bile duct stones in elderly patients? A prospective, multicenter study. Gastrointestinal Endoscopy. 2011;74(1):96–102.

37 Cavina E, Franceschi M, Sidoti F, *et al*. Laparo-endoscopic "rendezvous": a new technique in the choledocholithiasis treatment. Hepato-Gastroenterology. 1998;45(23):1430–5.

38 Morino M, Baracchi F, Miglietta C, *et al*. Preoperative endoscopic sphincterotomy versus laparoendoscopic rendezvous in patients with gallbladder and bile duct stones. Annals of Surgery. 2006;244(6):889–93; discussion 93–6.

39 Tzovaras G, Baloyiannis I, Zachari E, *et al*. Laparoendoscopic rendezvous versus preoperative ERCP and laparoscopic cholecystectomy for the management of cholecysto-choledocholithiasis: interim analysis of a controlled randomized trial. Annals of Surgery. 2012;255(3):435–9.

40 Rimon U, Kleinmann N, Bensaid P, *et al*. Percutaneous transhepatic endoscopic holmium laser lithotripsy for intrahepatic and choledochal biliary stones. Cardiovascular and Interventional Radiology. 2011;34(6):1262–6.

41 Johnson LW, Sehon JK, Lee WC, *et al*. Mirizzi's syndrome: experience from a multi-institutional review. The American Surgeon. 2001;67(1):11–4.

42 Binmoeller KF, Thonke F, Soehendra N. Endoscopic treatment of Mirizzi's syndrome. Gastrointestinal Endoscopy. 1993;39(4):532–6.

43 Tsuyuguchi T, Saisho H, Ishihara T,*et al*. Long-term follow-up after treatment of Mirizzi syndrome by peroral cholangioscopy. Gastrointestinal Endoscopy. 2000;52(5):639–44.

44 Bergman JJ, van Berkel AM, Bruno MJ, *et al*. A randomized trial of endoscopic balloon dilation and endoscopic sphincterotomy for removal of bile duct stones in patients with a prior Billroth II gastrectomy. Gastrointestinal Endoscopy. 2001;53(1):19–26.

45 Kawamura T, Mandai K, Uno K, Yasuda K. Does single-balloon enteroscopy contribute to successful endoscopic retrograde cholangiopancreatography in patients with surgically altered gastrointestinal anatomy? ISRN Gastroenterology. 2013;2013:214958.

46 McAlister VC, Davenport E, Renouf E. Cholecystectomy deferral in patients with endoscopic sphincterotomy. The Cochrane Database of Systematic Reviews. 2007(4):CD006233.

47 Adler DG, Baron TH, Davila RE, *et al*. ASGE guideline: the role of ERCP in diseases of the biliary tract and the pancreas. Gastrointestinal Endoscopy. 2005;62(1):1–8.

48 Overby DW, Apelgren KN, Richardson W, Fanelli R. Society of American G, Endoscopic S. SAGES guidelines for the clinical application of laparoscopic biliary tract surgery. Surgical Endoscopy. 2010;24(10):2368–86.

49 American Gastroenterological Association (AGA) Institute on "Management of Acute Pancreatits" Clinical Practice and Economics Committee, AGA Institute Governing Board. AGA Institute medical position statement on acute pancreatitis. Gastroenterology. 2007;132(5):2019–21.

50 Tenner S, Baillie J, DeWitt J, Vege SS. American College of G. American College of Gastroenterology guideline: management of acute pancreatitis. The American Journal of Gastroenterology. 2013;108(9):1400–15; 16.

CHAPTER 17

The patient with pain; suspected gallbladder and sphincter dysfunction

Peter B. Cotton

Digestive Disease Center, Medical University of South Carolina, Charleston, USA

Before the days of sophisticated imaging techniques, ERCP was frequently and effectively used to investigate patients with biliary/pancreatic pain and to diagnose and exclude common diseases such as bile duct stones and chronic pancreatitis. The situation is quite different now.

Nowadays, most patients with upper abdominal pain **have basic laboratory tests taken** and undergo upper endoscopy (after careful clinical enquiry and physical examination). If this is negative, abdominal scanning is indicated, by ultrasound in some countries, more likely by computed tomography (CT) in the United States. If that is negative and suspicion persists, MRCP is recommended. These scans provide excellent information about the biliary tree and pancreas, and should also detect problems in surrounding organs, such as aortic aneurysm and renal tumors. This review concerns patients in whom all of these tests are unrevealing.

The appropriate next steps are influenced by clinical features, such as age and the type of pain, and any associated complaints, such as weight loss.

Epigastric pain, especially if persistent, is suggestive of a pancreatic origin. The best next step is EUS, which can detect small tumors and less severe cases of pancreatitis. EUS is also valuable in looking for small stones in the gallbladder or bile ducts. If EUS is negative, there is no role for ERCP. The chances of finding anything are less than the risk of causing pancreatitis.

Intermittent pain in the right upper quadrant (and/or epigastrium) suggests biliary disease, specifically dysfunction of the gallbladder or sphincter of Oddi, and suspicion is enhanced if the liver tests bump with attacks of pain. This is where the algorithm of investigation gets more controversial, since hard data are scarce [1].

Gallbladder dysfunction. It is presumed that incoordination of gallbladder emptying can cause pain. Cholescintigraphy (hepatobiliaryiminodiacetic acid,

---

ERCP: The Fundamentals, Second Edition. Edited by Peter B. Cotton and Joseph Leung.
© 2015 John Wiley & Sons, Ltd. Published 2015 by John Wiley & Sons, Ltd.
Companion Website: www.wiley.com\go\cotton\ercp

DISIDA scanning after stimulation with cholecystokinin) is commonly used to detect gallbladder function. However, the value of this test in predicting the outcome of cholecystectomy is controversial, despite numerous studies [2], and there is increasing skepticism about the whole concept of a functional gall bladder disorder [3]. ERCP has no role in this context. An important point is that patients with typical biliary pain and a reduced ejection fraction are far more likely to respond than those with atypical symptoms. Since some patients with typical pain and normal ejection fractions may also respond to surgery, some experienced clinicians rely more on the symptoms than the scans. ERCP has no role in this scenario.

Sphincter of Oddi dysfunction (SOD). This is also controversial [1, 4, 5]. The concept is that inappropriate sphincter activity can cause pain by increasing the pressure in the biliary and pancreatic ducts. ERCP has been used to measure the sphincter pressure by manometry, and to perform sphincterotomy when pressures appear to be elevated. Whilst the sphincters could presumably malfunction in patients with intact gallbladders, most experts explore SOD only in patients with pains after cholecystectomy.

More than 20 years ago, Hogan and Geenen introduced a classification system for patients with suspected sphincter dysfunction [6]. It appears logical, but the evidence underlying it is thin and perhaps disappearing [7]. The definitions, as updated later, are as follows.

Type I: patients with pain, abnormal liver tests on two occasions, and a dilated bile duct (>10 mm).

Type II: abnormal liver tests or a dilated duct, but not both.

Type III: no abnormal findings.

Multiple studies suggest that Type I patients have a structural problem (stenosis or small stones) and are well treated by biliary sphincterotomy, without manometry (indeed manometry was often negative in early studies of these patients) [8].

There have been three (small) controlled studies in Type II patients, with similar results. All performed biliary sphincterotomy or sham irrespective of the results of manometry [8–13]. While the results were significantly better for the patients with elevated biliary pressures and treated by sphincterotomy, the numbers were small and the placebo responses impressive. It is surprising that biliary sphincterotomy alone was effective, when we know that many if not most patients also have elevated pancreatic sphincter pressures. Nonetheless, these reports and some cohort studies have resulted in manometry-directed sphincterotomy (of the pancreatic as well as the biliary sphincter, without further evidence) becoming standard practice in many referral centers, as sanctioned **by an National Institute of Health State of the Science conference in 2002** [14]. However, skepticism about the manometry data, and the (mistaken) early suggestion that manometry increases the risk of postprocedure pancreatitis, has led to many clinicians offering a "trial of sphincterotomy" to patients with pain and some abnormality of liver tests, or a dilated bile duct. This practice is certainly difficult to justify in patients who still have a gallbladder. Cholecystectomy may be a better (and safer) option in such cases, when symptoms are significant.

There is also room for caution in the postcholecystectomy situation, since the results of sphincterotomy are not great, and there are serious risks [8, 9, 14, 15]. More data concerning the predictors of a good (or bad) outcome, and further validation of manometry (or other tests, such as choledochoscintigraphy) would be welcome.

Management of the Type III postcholecystectomy patient with "pain only" has been even more controversial [9]. Post-ERCP pancreatitis has been reported in up to 40% of such patients [15], and still in at least 15% even with stent/non-steroidal anti-inflammatory drugs prophylaxis [16]. Perforations occur after sphincterotomy, and patients who do not respond often end up on a slippery slope with more ERCPs and eventual fruitless surgical interventions. It has been stated that "ERCP is most dangerous for those who need it least" [17], and adverse events in this context have been a common reason for medico-legal action [18].

Because of poor results and significant risks, the NIH conference cautioned against the use of ERCP in this context and recommended referral to tertiary "expert" centers capable of performing sphincter manometry. That happened progressively, despite the fact that manometry had not been shown to be valuable in that context, and several US centers were seeing literally hundreds of such patients each year. This gave the "experts" some pause, and also the opportunity to study the problem carefully.

The result was a multicenter randomized sham-controlled study called EPISOD (Evaluating Predictors and Interventions in Sphincter of Oddi Dysfunction), funded by NIH. Results reported recently showed that biliary sphincterotomy and combined biliary and pancreatic sphincterotomy were no better than sham treatment in these patients [19]. Many patients in the treatment and sham arms improved substantially, but this was attributed to a strong placebo effect. Furthermore, the authors could not find any clinical features that made success any more or less likely, and manometry was unhelpful. Not surprisingly, this report had a big impact on clinical practice, and should stimulate further research into the mechanism of pain in these patients, and better methods for treatment.

Conclusion

ERCP nowadays has very little role in the management of patients with biliary/pancreatic pain in the absence of impressive laboratory or imaging findings. There are few benefits and substantial risks. Patients and doctors should use great caution when approaching this minefield.

References

1 Behar J, Corazziari E, Guelrud M, *et al*. Functional Gallbladder and Sphincter of Oddi Disorders. Gastroenterology 2006; 130:1498–509.

2 DiBaise J, Oleynikov D. Does gallbladder ejection fraction predict outcome after cholecystectomy for suspected chronic acalculous gallbladder dysfunction? A systematic review. Am J Gastroenterol 2003;98:2605–11.

3 Bielefeldt K, Saligram S, Zickmund SL, Dudekula A, Olyaee M, Yadav D. Cholecystectomy for Biliary Dyskinesia: How Did We Get There? Dig Dis Sci. 2014 Sep 6. [Epub ahead of print]

4 Sherman S, Lehman GA. Sphincter of Oddi dysfunction: diagnosis and treatment. J Pancreas 2001;2:382–400.

5 Varadarajulu S, Hawes RH. Key issues in sphincter of Oddi dysfunction. Gastrointest Endosc Clin North Am 2003;13:671–94.

6 Hogan WJ, Geenen JE. Biliary dyskinesia. Endoscopy 1988;20 (Suppl 1):179–83.

7 Freeman ML, Gill M, Overby C, Cen YY. Predictors of outcomes after biliary and pancreatic sphincterotomy for sphincter of oddi dysfunction. J ClinGastroenterol. 2007 Jan;41(1):94–102.

8 Petersen BT. An evidence-based review of sphincter of Oddi dysfunction: part 1, presentations with "objective" biliary findings (types I and II). Gastrointest Endosc 2004;59:525–34.

9 Petersen BT. Sphincter of Oddi dysfunction, part 2: evidence-based review of the presentations, with "objective" pancreatic findings (types I and II) and of presumptive type III. Gastrointest Endosc 2004;59:670–87.

10 Sgouros SN, Periera SP. Systematic Review: sphincter of Oddi dysfunction—non-invasive diagnostic methods and long-term outcome after endoscopic sphincterotomy. Aliment Pharmacol Ther 2006;24:237–46.

11 Geenen JE, Hogan WJ, Dodds WJ, *et al*. The efficacy of endoscopic sphincterotomy after cholecystectomy in patients with sphincter of Oddi dysfunction. N Engl J Med 1989;320:82–7.

12 Toouli J, Roberts-Thomson IC, Kellow J, *et al*. Manometry based randomized trial of endoscopic sphincterotomy for sphincter of Oddi dysfunction. Gut 2000;46:98–102.

13 Sherman S, Lehman G, Jamidar P, *et al*. Efficacy of endoscopic sphincterotomy and surgical sphincteroplasty for patients with sphincter of Oddi dysfunction (SOD); randomized controlled study. Gastrointest Endosc 1994;40:P125.

14 Cohen S, Bacon BR, Berlin JA, *et al*. National Institutes of Health State-of-the-Science Conference statement: ERCP for diagnosis and therapy, January 14–16, 2002. Gastrointest Endosc 2002;56:803–9.

15 Freeman ML, Guda NM. Prevention of post-ERCP pancreatitis: a comprehensive review. Gastrointest Endosc 2004;59:845–64.

16 Elmunzer BJ, Scheiman JM, Lehman G, *et al*. A randomized trial of rectal indomethacinto prevent post-ERCP pancreatitis. N Engl J Med 2012;366:1414–22.

17 Cotton PB. ERCP is most dangerous for people who need it least. Gastrointest Endosc 2001;54(4):535–6.

18 Cotton PB. Analysis of 59 ERCP lawsuits; mainly about indications. GIE 2006;68:378–82.

19 Cotton PB, Durkalski V, Romagnuolo J, Pauls Q, Fogel E, Tarnasky P, et al. Effect of endoscopic sphincterotomy for suspected sphincter of Oddi dysfunction on pain-related disability following cholecystectomy: the EPISOD randomized clinical trial. JAMA. 2014 May;311(20):2101–9.

CHAPTER 18

Benign Biliary Strictures

John T. Cunningham

Section of Gastroenterology and Hepatology, University of Arizona Health Sciences Center, Tucson, USA

KEY POINTS

- The common causes of benign biliary strictures are postoperative (postcholecystectomy and liver transplant), chronic pancreatitis (CP), and primary sclerosing cholangitis (PSC).

- Magnetic resonance cholangiopancreatography (MRCP) now allows accurate diagnoses without risk, and the opportunity to consider the best approaches.

- A multidisciplinary approach is necessary to be able to advise patients optimally.

- Endoscopic retrograde cholangiopancreatography (ERCP) treatment with stenting (multiple plastic stents or expandable metal stents) is usually effective in postoperative strictures, less so in patients with CP, and unproven in PSC.

Introduction

The first plastic stents were introduced by Soehendra for relief of malignant obstructive jaundice [1]. Realization that small stents tend to block quickly led to the development of instruments and devices to allow placement of larger stents with longer patency [2]. The techniques rapidly became popular because they could be carried out with less morbidity than surgical bypass [3]. The situation in patients with benign biliary strictures is different because of the potential for extended survival. The challenge is to maintain duct patency long term to prevent cholangitis and resulting cirrhosis [4]. This can be achieved in most but not all cases endoscopically with multiple plastic stents or self-expanding metals stents (SEMS). Surgical bypass is an option that should be considered in every case [5].

Chronic pancreatitis (CP)

Temporary cholestasis due to biliary obstruction in acute pancreatitis can respond favorably to placement of a single 10 Fr plastic stent pending resolution of the acute process. Severe biliary strictures secondary to advanced CP occur in

ERCP: The Fundamentals, Second Edition. Edited by Peter B. Cotton and Joseph Leung.
© 2015 John Wiley & Sons, Ltd. Published 2015 by John Wiley & Sons, Ltd.
Companion Website: www.wiley.com\go\cotton\ercp

up to 11% of patients [4], and the response to treatment with repeated single plastic stents is poor [6]. Multiple plastic 10 Fr stents have been associated with a higher long-term success, but the presence of calcific pancreatitis is associated with more failures [7–11]. One study reported success of single-stent insertion in 24% of 34 patients, and only 7% in the presence of calcification. That group changed to a protocol with the insertion of a 10 Fr stent at first, followed by additional 10 Fr stents sequentially with eight patients receiving four stents and four having five stents [10]. The total duration of treatment was at least 12 months. There was one episode of inward stent migration, managed by ERCP. Overall success at a mean of 3.6 years was 92%, including five of the six patients with pancreatic calcifications. Other series with multiple stents claimed success in less than half of the patients with CP [8, 9]. Interestingly, there were no episodes of clinical cholangitis during the phase of multiple stenting. This finding is supported by another center that reported only one episode in 22 patients with stents in place for more than 6 months [12].

Self-expanding metal stents (SEMS) were introduced for use in malignant biliary obstruction, but have gradually also been employed in benign biliary strictures due to CP [13–15]. One study showed initial enthusiasm in 20 patients with no early complications and mean 3.3-year follow-up, with only two stent occlusions secondary to intimal hyperplasia [9]. A report with 50-month follow-up in 8 patients showed many needing repeat procedures, repeat SEMS (three cases), plastic stent inside SEMS (three cases), stent migration and one instance of recurrent stone formation in 13 patients, with 30 Fr × 10 cm Wallstent (Schneider, Switzerland) [15]. Two further studies with longer follow-up (5 or more years) revealed significant complications, including symptomatic occlusions in 63%, due to stone formation and intimal hyperplasia [13] and one stent-related death due to cholangitis, and two further occlusions in the five patients surviving 5 years [14].

The problem that uncovered SEMS are not readily removable [16, 17] has led to development of covered SEMS. Covered stents are less likely to become occluded by intimal hyperplasia, and are potentially removable. The first-generation stents were partially covered with a variable rim of bare metal on the proximal and distal ends. A pilot study with the partially covered 30 Fr Wallstent (Boston Scientific, Natik, MA) in 14 patients with CP reported spontaneous migration in two patients and intimal overgrowth in five patients which began at 18 months post insertion, with no plan for elective removal [18]. The second study placed the same device in 20 patients, 75% with calcific CP, with successful drainage in 95%, but the duration of stent placement was "at the discretion of the clinician," and placement was for a median of 5 months (range 1–31) [19]. All of the stents could be removed at the second session, and failure of treatment occurred in 10%, who went on to surgical correction. The drawback of that study is that the follow-up interval was only 6 months. An interim report on the 10-mm fully covered Viabil® stent in 19 patients with CP demonstrated stricture resolution in 65%, with stent

migration in one patient whose stricture had resolved [20]. To have an apprecia-
tion for what multiple plastic stents accomplish relative to metal stents, consider
that the circumference achieved by five 10 Fr stents is 31 mm, which is equivalent
to a single 10-mm-diameter metal stent. An 8-mm-diameter metal stent has a
circumference diameter of 25.3 mm, and that of four 10 Fr stents is 27 mm.

With the significant failure rate of endoscopic treatment in these patients, even
with multiple stents and SEMS, operative bypass remains a viable alternative,
especially if they are also candidates for surgery on the pancreas itself at the
same operation (e.g., pancreaticojejunostomy). The Amsterdam group reported on
42 patients who responded initially to stent placement, but were assessed for surgery due to the need for repeated stenting or complications of pancreatitis. Twenty-
six patients were poor operative candidates or refused surgery, and continued with
plastic stents or SEMS. Sixteen patients underwent some form of surgical biliary
diversion with significant postoperative morbidity in 6 (38%) but with jaundice
resolution in 15/16 and no long-term complications [21]. Late complications
occurred in 64% of the patients who were treated with stents alone.

Postoperative strictures

Benign strictures resulting from cholecystectomy or orthotopic liver transplant
(OLTX) are different from those due to CP. They are typically higher in the duct and
may extend into the bifurcation in the case of hepatic artery occlusion in patients
post OLTX or at the surgical anastomosis (Figure 18.1). The results with endoscopic
stenting for strictures below the bifurcation are similar for posttransplant and

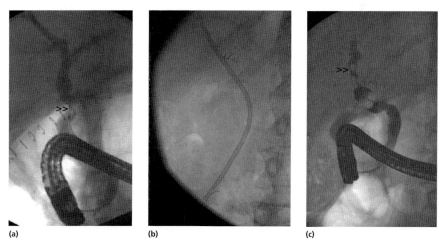

(a)   (b)   (c)

Figure 18.1 (a) Patient 1 month post liver transplant with high bilirubin, ERCP with tight
anastomotic stricture (arrow). (b) Stricture dilated with a 10 Fr dilation and a single 10 Fr
biliary stent. (c) First follow-up ERCP after stent removal with persistent stricture.

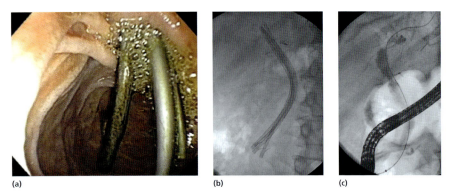

(a)   (b)   (c)

Figure 18.2 (a) End of multiple-stent trial, endoscopic view with four stents. (b) Fluoroscopic view with four stents in place. (c) Stents removed with patent anastomosis.

postcholecystectomy strictures, and are clearly better with multiple as opposed to single plastic stents (Figure 18.2) [22–25]. Long-term success rates of 80–90% have been reported with multiple plastic stents [24–27].

The concern for multiple procedures and the attendant cost resulted in the use of partially covered metal stents (pcSEMS) (Wallstent®, Boston Scientific, Natik, MA). In one study, stent migration resulted in initial failure in 13.6%, and with stricture recurrence of 47% [28]. A second study with the same device reported a high initial success rate for short-term stenting for postoperative strictures (100%) and OLTX strictures (94%); however, some of the extractions were difficult due to proximal migration, and one patient had a duct rupture during stent extraction with a dilation balloon, which resolved with plastic stents [29]. The concerns for problems with the proximal uncovered portion of the stent resulted in the development and use of fully covered SEMS (fcSEMS) [20, 30–32]. The first two studies used either the Nit-S ComVi® (Taewoong Medical Seoul, Korea) in 16 patients [30] or the Wallflex® (Boston Scientific, Natik, MA) in 11 patients, all of whom had failed prior therapy with dilation or plastic stent placement. Outward stent migration occurred in 11/27 (41%), but the stricture had resolved in most of those cases. Four of the patients ultimately underwent surgical bypass for failure or stricture recurrence. Another study in benign biliary strictures involved 62 patients treated with the Niti-S ComVi® stent, 51 patients after prior treatment and 11 patients as the first endoscopic intervention. There was a 24% migration rate but only a 9.6% failure rate and 7.1% stricture recurrences. The results were no different between initial and secondary treatments [31].

There are considerable differences in the mechanical forces exerted by the various metal stent designs, and a device that has high axial force may want to straighten after deployment, rather than conform to the shape of the biliary tree, and has the potential to imbed into the wall of the bile duct [33]. The issue of stent migration and complications during attempted stent extraction has been addressed by two studies [34, 35] using stents with anchoring fins to decrease the incidence of stent migration. A prototype stent with proximal anchoring fins (M.I. Tech, Seoul, Korea) was placed in 22 patients, versus the same device with a flared proximal end in 22 patients, all with benign biliary strictures [34]; there was no outward migration of the stents with flaps versus 33% with the flared end. All of the stents were removed without difficulty and the stricture improvement was equal with both stents. Another study reported removing all of 37 stents without difficulty, but three patients with benign strictures developed secondary biliary strictures, two in whom the stent was placed intraductally rather than transpapillary, and the stricture was at the area of the distal stent margin [35].

Technical issues that have not been fully addressed are the fact that plastic stents come in a variety of calibers and lengths, whereas the metal stents come only in 8- and 10-mm diameters, and up to 10 cm in length. For some of the highest benign lesions, the 2-cm cuff above the stenosis would only allow intraductal deployment, and the safety and success of extraction is a major issue. An unresolved issue is what constitutes adequate stricture resolution. One series with "maximal stent" placement had a goal of no discernible residual stricture [26], but there is no data to support this conclusion. Adequate stricture resolution is achieved is an inflated balloon is able to pass through the stricture, especially if the balloon is passed upstream, where there may be less tendency for deformity than if pulling downstream.

The results of expert surgery for postcholecystectomy strictures are also good. An early nonrandomized study comparing surgery versus one or two 10 Fr or 11.5 Fr stents reported similar long-term outcomes, with higher early complications in the surgical group and more delayed complications after stenting [6]. The Mayo Clinic reported a 92% 5-year stricture-free survival in 47 patients [36]. Surgical repair is more problematic in patients with strictures after liver transplantation, where an initial endoscopic approach may be preferred [22, 26, 37, 38]. Percutaneous transhepatic drainage and stenting may be valuable in some cases.

Primary sclerosing cholangitis

The diagnostic role of ERCP in PSC has diminished significantly in recent years, since MRCP now has similar sensitivity and specificity, and, in the demonstration of the presence of dominant strictures, is either intrahepatic (Figure 18.3) or extrahepatic (Figure 18.4a and b). It is also less costly than ERCP and without hazard [39]. A recent meta-analysis involving 456 subjects compared MRCP to ERCP in four centers and to ERCP or PTC in another two [40]. The overall sensitivity was 86% and the specificity 91%.

Endoscopic treatment of dominant strictures seems logical and can improve cholestasis, but the long-term value is unproven, and stenting carries a significant risk of cholangitis [41, 42]. The Amsterdam group proposed stenting for only

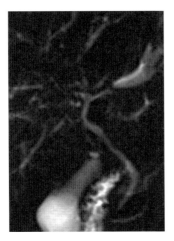

Figure 18.3 MR cholangiogram with dominant stricture of left hepatic duct and normal common duct.

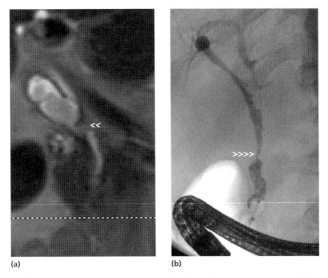

(a)   (b)

Figure 18.4 (a) MR cholangiogram showing a tight CBD stricture (arrows), and (b) ERCP showing the stricture as well as biliary pseudo-diverticulosis, classic for PSC.

1 to 2 weeks, and reported symptomatic improvement in 83% and normalization of bilirubin levels in 12/14 patients at 2 months. Additionally, there was no reintervention in 80% at 1 year and 60% at 3 years [43]. The Mayo Clinic demonstrated fewer complications after balloon dilation without stenting [44].

One report covered a 20-year prospective evaluation of 171 PSC patients treated by ERCP [45]. If alkaline phosphatase was at least 2× the upper limit of normal and treatment with balloon dilation of dominant strictures that were 1.5 mm diameter or less in the common bile duct (CBD) and 1.0 mm in the

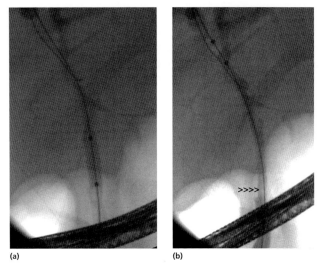

(a)   (b)

Figure 18.5 (a) ERCP with 6-mm balloon dilation of stricture and (b) stricture post dilation (arrows).

intrahepatic ducts if they were within 2 cm of the bifurcation. A small sphinc-terotomy was performed, followed by sequential dilation in up to 24 Fr in the CBD (Figure 18.5a and b) and 18 Fr to 24 Fr in the intrahepatics. Dilation was repeated at 4-week intervals until "success, as assessed by opening of the stenosis on repeat cholangiography" was achieved. A total of 97 patients underwent a total of 500 dilations; 5 additional patients had stents placed for 1–2 weeks after dilation for severe cholestasis with active clinical cholangitis. The procedural related complications were pancreatitis 2.2%, bacterial cholangitis 1.4% and a single CBD perforation (0.2%) [45].

The goal of endoscopic therapy in PSC is to relieve symptomatic cholestasis, and to delay the need for transplantation, but this is unproven, and treatment carries risks, Although balloon dilation may be safer than stent placement, the real question is when to intervene and whether that alters the course of the disease. This will be answered only with randomized prospective trials. The current recommendation is that endoscopic therapy should be primarily by balloon dilation for dominant strictures (with antibiotics for a minimum of 5-days post procedure), and that stenting (albeit short term) be limited to cases where dilation cannot maintain duct patency [46].

Conclusions

The use of therapeutic ERCP in the management of benign biliary strictures is now established practice, with a gradual transition from single to multiple stents, and to various types of self-expanding metal stents. Results are best in patients with postoperative biliary strictures (including posttransplant), less so in patients with CP (especially with calcification), and essentially unproven in PSC. Despite extensive experience and multiple cohort studies, there have been no head-to-head comparisons of different stenting approaches, or comparisons of endoscopy with surgery. Randomized trials would be ideal, but patient's lesions and associated problems vary enormously.

The lack of definitive trials makes deciding the best approach difficult. Prolonged plastic stenting with multiple stents has the drawback of requiring multiple procedures but the complications of the presence of the stents, once placed, is actually very low, and the stents are easily removed. The advantage of SEMS is the diminished number of procedures, with similar efficacy, but with some potential for complications from the stent itself.

For the time being the most prudent approach in patients with postoperative strictures seems to be to place a single plastic stent, since many benign strictures will resolve quickly. The issue is what to do if the stricture persists when ERCP is repeated at about 3 months? Place multiple plastic stents, or consider metal stent insertion, and which one? A recent review concluded that "further study of the cost analysis of fcSEMS in benign bile duct strictures is clearly required" [47]. In PSC, until controlled data are available, it is perhaps best to minimize invasion.

In deciding whether to offer endoscopic or surgical management in a particular case, there are other considerations. Some patients (especially those with CP) are not compliant with prolonged treatments with stents (resulting in a significant risk of cholangitis), and the costs of repeated stenting are not insubstantial.

There remain many questions and the field is continuing to evolve. The widespread availability of MRCP means that the patient's problem can be identified easily and safely, and should be discussed carefully in a multidisciplinary context before any invasive (and potentially hazardous) intervention is initiated. This should allow consultation with other relevant specialists and also detailed explanation to patients about their options. In some cases this should involve referral to a tertiary center, since results of all the possible treatments in complex cases are operator-dependent.

References

1 Soehendra N, Reynders-Frederix V. Palliative bile duct drainage-a new endoscopic method of introducing a transpapillary drain. Endoscopy 1980;8:8–11.
2 Speer AG, Cotton PD, MacRae KD. Endoscopic management of malignant biliary obstruction: stents of 10 French gauge are preferable to stents of 8 French gauge. Gastrointest Endosc 1988;34:412–7.
3 Smith AC, Dowsett JF, Russell RCG, *et al*. Randomised trial of endoscopic stenting versus surgical bypass in malignant low bile duct obstruction. Lancet 1994;344:1655–60.

4 Warshaw AL, Schapiro RH, Ferrucci JT Jr, Galdabini JJ. Persistent obstructive jaundice, cholangitis and biliary cirrhosis due to common bile duct stenosis in chronic pancreatitis. Gastroenterology 1976;70:562–7.

5 Deviere J, Devaere S, Baize M, *et al.* Endoscopic biliary drainage in chronic pancreatitis. Gastrointest Endsoc 1990;36:96–100.

6 Davids PHP, Tanka AKF, Rauws EAJ, *et al.* Benign biliary strictures: surgery or endoscopy? Ann Surg 1993;207:237–43.

7 Catalano MF, Linder JD, George S, *et al.* Treatment of symptomatic distal common bile duct stenosis secondary to chronic pancreatitis: comparison of single vs. multiple simultaneous stents. Gastrointest Endosc 2004;60:945–52.

8 Cahen DL, van Berkel AMM, Oskam D, *et al.* Long-term results of endoscopic drainage of common bile duct strictures in chronic pancreatitis. Eur J Gastro Hepatol 2005;17:103–8.

9 Draganov P, HoffmanB, Marsh W, *et al.* Long term outcome in patients with benign biliary strictures treated endoscopically with multiple stents. Gastrointest Endosc 2002;55:680–6.

10 Pozsar J, Sahin P, Laszlo F, *et al.* Medium-term results of endoscopic treatment of common bile duct strictures in chronic calcifying pancreatitis with increasing numbers of stents. J Clin Gastroenterol 2004;38:118–23.

11 Kahl S, Zimmermann S, Genz I, *et al.* Risk factors for failure of endoscopic stenting of chronic pancreatitis: a prospective follow-up study. Am J Gastroent 2003;98:2448–53.

12 Lawrence C, Romagnuolo J, Payne M, *et al.* Low symptomatic premature stent occlusion of multiple plastic stents for benign biliary strictures: comparing standard and prolonged stent change intervals. Gastrointest Endosc 2010;72:558–63.

13 Deviere J, Cremer M, Baize M, *et al.* Management of common bile duct stricture caused by chronic pancreatitis with metal mesh self expandable stents. Gut 1994;35:122–6.

14 Yamaguchi T, Ishihara T, Seza K, *et al.* Long-term outcome of endoscopic metallic stenting for benign biliary stenosis associated with chronic pancreatitis. World J Gastroent 2006;12: 426–30.

15 van Berkel, Cahen DL, van Westerloo DJ, *et al.* Self-expanding metal stents in benign biliary strictures due to chronic pancreatitis. Endoscopy 2004;36:381–4.

16 Kahaleh M, Toka J, Le T, *et al.* Removal of self-expanding metallic Wallstents. Gastrointest Endosc 2004;60:640–4.

17 Familiari P, Bulajic M, Mutignani M, *et al.* Endoscopic removal of malfunctioning biliary self-expandable metallic stents. Gastrointest Endosc 2005;62:903–10.

18 Cantu P, Hookey LC, Morales A, *et al.* The treatment of patients with symptomatic common bile duct stenosis secondary to chronic pancreatitis using partially covered metal stents: a pilot study. Endoscopy 2005;37:735–9.

19 Behm B, Brock A, Clarke BW, *et al.* Partially covered self-expandable metallic stents for benign biliary strictures due to chronic pancreatitis. Endoscopy 2009;41:547–51.

20 Mahajan A, Ho H, Sauer B, *et al.* Temporary placement of fully covered self-expandable metal stents in benign biliary strictures: midterm evaluation. Gastrointest Endosc 2009; 70:303–9.

21 Smits ME, Rauws EAJ, van Gulik TM, *et al.* Long-term results of endoscopic stenting and surgical drainage for biliary stricture due to chronic pancreatitis. Br J Surg 1996;83:764–8.

22 Pfau P, Kochman ML, Lewis J, *et al.* Endoscopic management of postoperative biliary complications in orthotopic liver transplantation. Gastrointest Endosc 2000;52:55–63.

23 Morelli J, Mulcahy HE, Willner IR, *et al.* Long-term outcomes for patients with post-liver transplant anastomotic biliary strictures treated by endoscopic stent placement. Gastrointest Endosc 2003;58:374–9.

24 Tuvignon N, Liguory C, Ponchon T, *et al.* Long-term follow-up after biliary stent placement for postcholecystectomy bile duct strictures: a multicenter study. Endoscopy 2011;43:208–16.

25 Costamagna G, Tringali A, Mutignani M, *et al.* Endotherapy of postoperative biliary stricture with multiple stents: results after more than 10 years follow-up. Gastrointest Endosc 2010; 72:551–7.

26 Tabibian JH, Asham EH, Han S, *et al.* Endoscopic treatment of postorthotopic liver transplantation anastomotic biliary strictures with maximal stent therapy. Gastrointest Endosc 2010;71:505–12.

27 Costamagna G, Pandolfi M, Mutignani M, *et al.* Long-term results of endoscopic management of postoperative bile duct strictures with increasing numbers of stents. Gastrointest Endosc 2001;54:162–8.

28 Chaput U, Scatton O, Bichard P, *et al.* Temporary placement of partially covered self-expandable metal stents for anastomotic biliary strictures after liver transplantation: a prospective, multicenter study. Gastointest Endosc 2010;72:1167–74.

29 Kahaleh M. Behn B, Clarke BW, *et al.* Temporary placement of covered self-expandable metal stents in benign biliary strictures: a new paradigm? Gastrointest Endosc 2008;67: 446–54.

30 Triana M, Tarantino I, Barresi L, *et al.* Efficacy and safety of fully covered self-expanding metallic stents in biliary complications after liver transplantation: a preliminary study. Liver Transplant 2009;15:1493–8.

31 Marin-Gomez LM, Sobrino-Rodriguez S, Alamo-Martinez JM, *et al.* Use of fully covered self-expandable stent in biliary complications after liver transplantation: a case series. Transplant Proceed 2010;42:2975–7.

32 Tarantino I, Mangiavilliano B, Di Mitri R, *et al.* Fully covered self-expandable metallic stents in benign biliary strictures: a multicenter study on efficacy and safety. Endoscopy 2012;44:923–7.

33 Isayama H, Nakai Y, Toyokawa Y, *et al.* Measurement of radial and axial forces of biliary self-expandable metallic stents. Gastrointest Endosc 2009;70:37–44.

34 Park DH, Lee SS, Lee TH, *et al.* Anchoring flap versus flared end, fully covered self-expandable metal stents to prevent migration in patients with benign biliary strictures: a multicenter, prospective comparative pilot study. Gastrointest Endosc 2011;73:64–70.

35 Kasher JA, Corasanti JG, Tarnasky PR, *et al.* A multicenter analysis of safety and outcome of removal of a fully covered self-expandable metal stent during ERCP. Gastrointest Endosc 2011;73:1292–7.

36 Fatima J, Barton JG, Grotz TE, *et al.* Is there a role for endoscopic therapy as a definitive treatment for post-laparoscopic bile duct injuries? J Am Coll Surg 2010;211:495–502.

37 Shah JN, Ahmad NA, Shetty K, *et al.* Endoscopic management of biliary complications after adult living donor transplantation. Am J Gastroent 2004;99:1291–5.

38 Rerknimitr R, Sherman S, Fogel EL, *et al.* Biliary tract complication after orthotopic liver transplantation with choledochocholedochostomy anastomosis: endoscopic findings and results of therapy. Gastrointest Endosc 2002;55:224–31.

39 Talwalkar JA, Angulo P, Johnson CD, *et al.* Cost-minimization analysis of MRC versus ERCP for the diagnosis of primary sclerosing cholangitis. Hepatology 2004;40:39–45.

40 Dave M, Elmunzer BJ, Dwamena BA, *et al.* Primary sclerosing cholangitis: meta-analysis of diagnostic performance of MR cholangiography. Radiology 2010;256:387–96.

41 Lee JG, Schutz SM, England RE, *et al.* Endoscopic therapy of sclerosing cholangitis. Hepatology 1995;21:661–7.

42 van Milligen AWM, van Bracht J, Rauws EA, *et al.* Endoscopic stent therapy for dominant extrahepatic bile duct strictures in primary sclerosing cholangitis. Gastrointest Endosc 1996;44:293–9.

43 Ponsioen CY, Lam K, van Milligen AWM, *et al.* Four years experience with short term stenting in primary sclerosing cholangitis. Am J Gastroenterol 1999;94:2403–7.

44 Kaya M, Peterson BT, Angulo P, *et al.* Balloon dilation compared to stenting of dominant strictures in primary sclerosing cholangitis. Am J Gastroenterol 2001;96:1059–66.

45 Gotthardt DN, Rudolph G, Kloters-Plachky P, *et al.* Endoscopic dilation of dominant stenosis in primary sclerosing cholangitis: outcome after long-term treatment. Gastrointest Endosc 2010;71:527–34.

46 Eaton JE, Talwalkar JA, Lazaridis KN, *et al.* Pathogenesis of primary sclerosing cholangitis and advances in diagnosis and management. Gastroenterology 2013;145:521–36.

47 Kaffres AJ, Liu K. Fully covered self-expandable metal stents for treatment of benign biliary strictures. Gastrointest Endosc 2013;78:13–20.

CHAPTER 19

The Role of ERCP in Pancreatico-Biliary Malignancies

John G. Lee

UC Irvine Health, H. H. Chao Comprehensive Digestive Disease Center, Orange, USA

KEY POINTS

- Endoscopic retrograde cholangiopancreatography (ERCP) and stenting is indicated in most patients with malignant obstructive jaundice due to pancreatic cancer except for select patients with resectable disease who can undergo surgery within a week of the diagnosis.

- ERCP and stenting is indicated in most patients with hilar obstruction regardless of resectability.

- The number and location of stents placed for hilar obstruction should be based on magnetic resonance cholangiopancreatography (MRCP) and computed tomography (CT) findings with the goal being to drain at least 50% of the liver.

- Available metal stents appear to work about the same.

- The published data do not show a clear advantage for the endoscopically placed covered SEM over the uncovered SEM.

- SEM is cost-effective for patients with unresectable cancer and expected survival of more than 4 months.

ERCP in diagnosis of pancreatico-biliary malignancies

Radiological diagnosis

Significance of "double-duct stricture" sign

The radiographic features of ERCP cannot reliably distinguish between benign and malignant diseases. Although the double-duct sign with simultaneous narrowing of the common bile duct and the pancreatic duct has been regarded traditionally as predictive of pancreatic cancer, its specificity is low [1, 2]. The cholangiographic appearance was nonspecific as benign-appearing strictures

ERCP: The Fundamentals, Second Edition. Edited by Peter B. Cotton and Joseph Leung.

© 2015 John Wiley & Sons, Ltd. Published 2015 by John Wiley & Sons, Ltd.

Companion Website: www.wiley.com\go\cotton\ercp

were usually found to be malignant on follow-up [3]. Autoimmune pancreatitis (AIP) can present similar to pancreatic cancer with jaundice, weight loss, pancreatic mass on CT scan, and bile and pancreatic duct strictures. Pancreatogram showing stricture greater than 1/3 of the length of the main duct, lack of dilation greater than 5 mm, multiple strictures, and side branches arising from structured segment may help distinguish AIP from cancer [4].

Tissue diagnosis

Brush cytology, biopsy, and fine-needle aspiration

Endoscopic wire-guided brush cytology and endoscopic needle aspiration or forceps biopsy can be successfully performed during ERCP for cytological diagnosis. Studies of brush cytology (usually from the bile duct) showed a sensitivity of approximately 40% and a specificity of 100% for the diagnosis of malignancy [5, 6], with sampling of both ducts and dilating increasing sensitivity to 50–70% [7, 8]. Combining the results of brush cytology, fine-needle aspiration (FNA), and/or forceps biopsy was reported to increase the overall sensitivity to 70–85% [9–11]. Although it would seem that direct cholangioscopic biopsies should be more accurate than conventional biopsies [12], another study actually showed opposite results [13] so I only perform cholangioscopic biopsies as last resort. Regardless, I recommend performing at least two different types of tissue sampling to improve the yield. Finally, endoscopic biopsies of the ampulla with IgG IV staining should be done in patients with suspected AIP as it is highly specific and in agreement with the more invasive pancreatic biopsy results [14].

Biomarkers in bile or pancreatic juice

I do not recommend using these tests in clinical practice until they have been validated in robust clinical trials especially since endoscopic ultrasound (EUS) is nearly 100% accurate in diagnosing pancreatic cancer.

Direct endoscopic examination of pancreatico-biliary malignancies

Per oral choledochoscopy and pancreatoscopy

Choledochoscopy using the mother and baby scope system can be used to visualize the bile duct, to obtain specimens, and to treat the tumor. However fiberoptic scopes including single-operator SpyGlass (Boston Scientific, Natick, MA) provide inferior image and smaller field of view compared to video cholangioscopes and are time-consuming and challenging to use at best. Unfortunately, video cholangioscopes are still very fragile and not yet commercially available in the United States. In addition, identification of an abnormality still requires tissue biopsy (which is often not easy) for definitive diagnosis. In my opinion, most patients referred for cholangioscopic examination of the distal duct or pancreatoscopy can be evaluated by EUS far more easily and accurately. Thus the main indication for diagnostic cholangioscopy is for examination of proximal bile duct lesions and for tumor ablation, for example, using photodynamic therapy (PDT) [15].

An alternative method of directly examining the biliary and pancreatic ducts is using an ultraslim or even an adult video gastroscope [16]. This is quite difficult to do without an anchoring balloon, which is not available in the United States, but can be done in some cases using the J maneuver in which the endoscope is retroflexed in the duodenum and withdrawn to engage and cannulate the duct [17].

An interesting new development in diagnostic imaging is the use of probe-based confocal laser endomicroscopy (Cellvizio CholangioFlex, Mauna Kea Technologies, Paris France). The CholangioFlex probe is 0.94 mm in diameter so it can be used with an ERCP catheter or through a cholangioscope. The tip of the catheter is radio-opaque. Endomicroscopic findings of thick white bands (>20 μm), thick dark bands (>40 μm), or dark clumps or epithelial structure have been described in cancer [18]. This group also reported that endomicroscopy had comparable accuracy to index tissue sampling (81% versus 75%, respectively) [19]. While promising, it remains to be seen whether these unblinded results can be replicated in a clinically meaningful way. Finally, until oncologists and surgeons accept an endomicroscopic diagnosis of cancer, we will still need tissue for diagnosis of cancer.

Palliation of pancreatico-biliary malignancies

ERCP is the preferred method of palliating patients with malignant obstructive jaundice. Endoscopic biliary drainage is successful in greater than 90% of patients with low morbidity and mortality [20, 21]. Although only surgery offers potential for a cure, endoscopic palliation continues to remain the therapeutic goal in most patients, because 85–90% of patients have unresectable cancer due to advanced stage and/or poor condition of the patient. Randomized trials comparing surgical bypass to endoscopic stenting found similar success rates for biliary decompression and overall survival, but lower morbidity and 30-day mortality in the stent group [20–22]. ERCP also reduced the cost and the length of the hospital stay ($P<0.001$) [23] and improved the quality of life [24]. Another study showed this improvement to be durable even after 180 days [25]. Although percutaneous biliary drainage is an alternative to ERCP, it is less successful and causes more complications compared to ERCP [26]. Patients with failed stenting or unapproachable biliary anatomy (e.g., duodenal obstruction) can also be effectively treated using EUS rendezvous or choledochoduodenostomy [27]. In conclusion, endoscopic palliation is highly successful, has a lower morbidity and mortality, and costs less compared to other palliative approaches to pancreatico-biliary malignancies.

Peroperative stenting in patients with resectable pancreatic cancer

Biliary decompression may be needed in patients with resectable disease undergoing neoadjuvant chemotherapy [28], for example, gemcitabine usually requires the bilirubin to be<2–2.5 mg/dl. Neoadjuvant therapy is being used more often because it can (i) downstage, (ii) select out unfavorable tumors that progress on therapy since surgery would not be curative anyway, (iii) allow more patients to receive chemotherapy as many are too ill after surgery. Surgery may be also delayed due to cholangitis, comorbidities, and financial or personal reasons. However, for the patient who can undergo surgery within a week of the diagnosis, a recent randomized controlled study showed that ERCP and stenting was associated with significantly higher overall complication rate (74% versus 39%) compared to early surgery without stenting in patients with preoperative bilirubin levels between 2.3 and 14.6 mg/dl [29]. This resulted from complications of stenting (46%) including pancreatitis (7%), cholangitis (26%), perforation (2%), and bleeding (2%). Fifteen percent had stent occlusion and 30% required stent exchange within the mean 5.2-week preoperative stenting period. Although no information was provided about the stent type and size, I wonder whether some patients had 7 Fr stents placed due to the very high rate of cholangitis and stent exchange. The initial stenting succeed in only 75%. Interestingly, further analyses of the data by the same group found that early surgery produced a trend toward higher mortality (78% versus 66%), shorter median survival after surgery (17.8 versus 21.6 months), and overall survival (12.2 versus 12.7 months) [30]. Stenting was associated with a significant reduction in mortality after surgery on multivariable analysis (hazard ratio=0.85, per increment of 1 week 95% CI, 0.75–0.96). Naturally, most surgical authors concluded that early surgery without stenting was better.

In summary, endoscopic stenting could be avoided in patients with resectable pancreatic cancer with serum bilirubin levels of 2.3–14.6 mg/dl who can undergo early surgery in 1 week, especially if the success rate of stenting is not higher than 75% and complication rate is not lower than 46%. In reality, the diagnosis of pancreatic cancer, its resectability, the need for neoadjuvant therapy, or the wishes of the patient may not be immediately obvious at the time of ERCP. These factors challenge the notion of early surgery even if it can be done in a week, which (while not impossible) is highly unusual in most practices in the United States. In my opinion, stenting should be considered in all other patients or for all practical purposes, with most patients presenting with obstructive jaundice from suspected pancreatic cancer.

Endoscopic stenting for malignant jaundice

Types of stent

The different types of self-expanding metal stents (SEMs) appear to work about the same for a comparable diameter with the only published randomized comparative study showing significantly more stent occlusion (39.1%) with a 6-mm uncovered Zilver stent (Cook Medical, Bloomington, IN) compared to a 10-mm Zilver stent (23.9%) or a 10-mm Wallstent (Boston Scientific, Natick, MA) (21.4%) while the patency of the two 10-mm stents were comparable [31]. When SEMs eventually occlude, cleaning or ablation of ingrowth tissue only provides temporary benefit and thus most should get another SEM or plastic stent, as published studies to not show a clear benefit of one over the other [32].

Metal versus plastic stents

Meta-analysis of 724 patients from seven published trials comparing plastic to uncovered Wallstent showed significant relative risk reduction of stent occlusion at 4 months for SEMs (RR, 0.44, 95% CI 0.3–0.63, $P<0.01$) and lower risk of recurrent obstruction (RR, 0.52; 95% CI 0.39–0.69) [33]. They concluded that using a SEM was cost-effective if the cost of an additional ERCP per patient was > $1820. There were no differences in the technical and therapeutic success, 30-day mortality, or complications. A second study showed that a partially covered Wallstent remained patent significantly longer (419 versus 133 days) with a lower stent occlusion rate (23.6% versus 53.5%) compared to a double-layer plastic stent (Olympus, Tokyo, Japan) [34]. Although there are no specific studies comparing other types of SEMs to plastic stents, I think it's reasonable to assume that the results would be similar and therefore I recommend using a SEM for patients expected to survive for more than 4 months.

Covered and uncovered metal stents

Three randomized comparative endoscopic studies of covered SEMs have been published [35–37]. The first found no significant differences comparing uncovered to covered nitinol stents and the second found no significant differences between the uncovered and partially covered Wallstents. The third reported significantly less stent occlusion and longer patency with a partially covered Diamond stent (Boston Scientific, Natick, MA). The author custom-made a covered stent from the commercially available Diamond stent, which has been withdrawn from the market since the study. A radiology study found that a percutaneously inserted fully covered SEM (Gore Viabil, Conmed, Utica, NY) had significantly long patency compared to an uncovered SEM in pancreatic cancer (Luminexx Bard Peripheral Vascular, Tempe, AZ) [38] and an uncovered Wallstent in distal cholangiocarcinoma [39]. In summary, the endoscopic results do not clearly show the covered SEMs to be better. Although a percutaneously placed fully covered SEMs may be better, I'm unsure as to whether the results would be the same if done endoscopically.

Endoscopic stenting for hilar strictures

Peroperative biliary drainage in patients with potentially resectable cholangiocarcinoma

Many surgeons feel that preoperative biliary drainage improves the outcome of patients with hilar tumor by promoting early decompression of the future liver remnant, improving liver function, and treating/preventing cholangitis. The current trend toward portal vein embolization and extended hepatectomy for cholangiocarcinoma means that many patients do not undergo immediate surgery, as liver hypertrophy is reassessed 4 weeks after embolization—these patients need drainage of the future liver remnant during this time. Endoscopic drainage is preferable to percutaneous drainage in these patients, due to the small but real risk of tumor seeding in the catheter tract. Therefore endoscopic preoperative drainage is indicated in patients with potentially resectable cholangiocarcinoma who have cholangitis or undergo portal vein embolization. Biliary drainage is more controversial in others with about half of the published studies supporting drainage; however, there are no published randomized or controlled studies on the subject. Iacono et al. recommended drainage in the majority of patients in a recent review [40] and the Asia-Pacific Consensus recommended drainage in select patients based on level II-3 evidence [41].

Unilateral versus bilateral drainage for hilar obstruction

There is considerable debate in the literature about whether unilateral drainage is sufficient in patients with hilar strictures. However, rather than discussing the number of stents, it makes more sense to think in terms of the amount of liver drained with the goal being to drain at least 50% of the liver be it through single or multiple stents [42]. Thus a Bismuth I stricture should be adequately drained with a single stent while a Bismuth IV lesion would probably require multiple stents draining multiple liver segments. Theoretically, draining the left side should be better because it has fewer side branches near the hilum, but this has not been confirmed clinically [43]. In my opinion, the most elegant and physiological approach to stenting a hilar tumor is to first map the lesion using MRCP and assess any liver atrophy using CT to determine which duct(s) to stent without contaminating functionally useless ducts. Finally since most studies define successful drainage as reduction in the bilirubin to 30–50% of the initial value, a successfully drained patient could still be jaundiced and additional stent placement should always be considered for patients who do not improve after one or more stents (Figure 19.1).

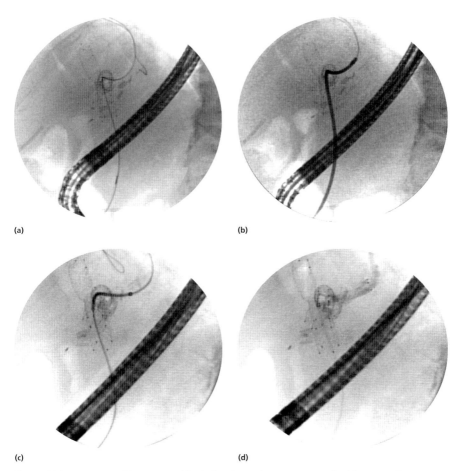

(a)

(b)

(c)

(d)

Figure 19.1 A 64-year-old woman with cholangiocarcinoma presented with worsening jaundice. She initially had metal stents placed in right and left intrahepatic ducts for Bismuth IV stricture with resolution of jaundice. She returned 4 months later with jaundice and an additional metal stent was placed in the right side with resolution of jaundice. She now returns 3 months later with worsening jaundice. (a) A guide wire was placed through the left intrahepatic stent. Contrast was not used to minimize the risk of cholangitis. (b) The side hole of the stent and the stricture was dilated using a 10 Fr Soehendra stent retriever (Cook Endoscopy, Bloomington, IN). (c) A fourth metal stent was placed through the side hole of the left intrahepatic stent. (d) Cholangiogram showed drainage of additional left-sided ducts with subsequent resolution of jaundice.

Plastic versus metal stent

The mesh design of an uncovered SEM should drain multiple ducts; not surprisingly, it resulted in higher successful drainage (70.4% versus 46.3%, $P=0.011$) and longer median patency (103 versus 35 days, $P=0.000$) compared to a plastic stent [44]. Mukai et al. performed bilateral stenting in about half of the 60 patients randomized to 7 Fr plastic stents or 10-mm

SEMs [45]. The 6-month patency rate was significantly higher for SEM (81% versus 20%, $P=0.0012$) and twice as many patients (60%) had their initial SEM at the time of death. The SEM group also had significantly lower cost, longer stent patency, and lower reintervention rate. In conclusion, I recommend metal stent for palliation of hilar stricture in patients with unresectable disease (Figure 19.2).

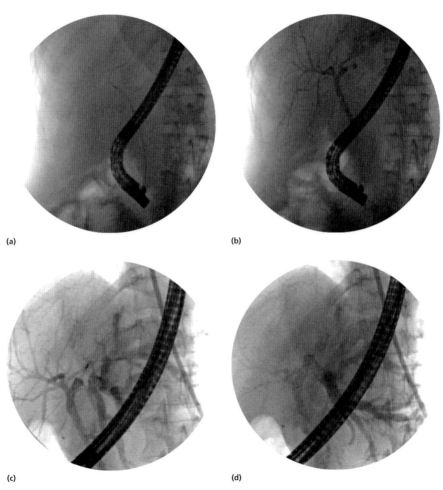

(a)   (b)

(c)   (d)

Figure 19.2 A 73-year-old woman presented with metastatic cholangiocarcinoma with left-sided intrahepatic dilation on imaging. (a) A guide wire was placed into the left system without any contrast injection. (b) Cholangiogram shows a normal-looking right system and high-grade stricture of the left system. (c) Further selective cannulation into the secondary left intrahepatic duct showed a stricture with pronounced proximal dilation. (d) A metal stent was placed with selective drainage of left-sided cholangiocarcinoma.

Other techniques of endoscopic palliation

Intraductal photodynamic therapy

Two randomized controlled studies of PDT have been published. The first compared PDT plus stenting to stenting in 39 patients and found significantly longer survival after PDT (493 versus 98 days, $P<0.0001$) [46] and the second reported significantly higher median survival after PDT compared to stenting alone (21 versus 7 months respectively, $P<0.0109$) [46]. A meta-analysis of six published trials reported a survival advantage of 265 days with PDT [47]. Nevertheless, it is not entirely clear how PDT would prolong survival in advanced cholangiocarcinoma since it doesn't even completely debulk the tumor and does not treat any extrabiliary disease; in comparison even when it completely debulks the tumor as in patients with esophageal cancer, it does not prolong survival. A systematic review of 342 patients from 20 PDT trials found cholangitis (27.5%) and phototoxicity (10.2%) as the most common complications [48].

Other treatments

Brachytherapy, radiofrequency ablation, and high-intensity intraductal ultrasound have been reported in small case reports [49–51]. All of these techniques are considered experimental at this time.

Ampullary carcinoma

Although ERCP is usually used for palliation in ampullary cancer, a potentially curative endoscopic resection and stenting may be possible in patients with all of the following: (i) protruded adenoma, (ii) papillary or well-differentiated histology, (iii) no duodenal invasion on EUS, (iv) no pancreatic duct invasion, and v) pancreatic duct diameter <3 mm if the patient is unfit or unwilling to undergo surgery [52]. The ampulla must be resected and retrieved in en bloc to assess lateral and deep margins and to document a "R0" resection.

Outstanding issues and future trends

The management of pancreatico-biliary malignancies involves a multidisciplinary approach combining the expertise of gastroenterologists, radiologists, oncologist, and surgeons. ERCP is an important diagnostic and therapeutic modality and plays a crucial role in the management of these patients. Emerging newer diagnostic modalities are helpful in defining the role of ERCP in the management of pancreatico-biliary malignancies. ERCP in combination with EUS and FNA offers an effective means of tissue sampling.

At the present time ERCP offers effective, safe, and cost-efficient palliation of these tumors. Although endoscopic stenting is an established palliation for malignant obstructive jaundice, major complications, including blockage of plastic stents by bacterial biofilm and biliary sludge, still limit its clinical benefits. Prolonged palliation of jaundice is achieved by the use of SEMSs but they too are limited by tissue and tumor ingrowth. Better innovations in technology and future studies will further widen the scope of this technique in the management of pancreatico-biliary malignancies.

References

1 Menges M, Lerch MM, Zeitz M. The double duct in patients with malignant and benign pancreatic lesions. *Gastrointest Endosc* 2000; 52: 74–7.

2 Ralls PW, Halls J, Renner I, Juttner H. Endoscopic retrograde cholangiopancreatography (ERCP) in pancreatic disease: a reassessment of the specificity of ductal abnormalities in differentiating benign from malignant disease. *Radiology* 1980; 134: 347–52.

3 Bain VG, Abraham N, Jhangri GS, *et al.* Prospective study of biliary strictures to determine the predictors of malignancy. *Can J Gastroenterol* 2000; 14: 397–402.

4 Sugumar A, Levy MJ, Kamisawa T, *et al.* Endoscopic retrograde pancreatography criteria to diagnose autoimmune pancreatitis: an international multicentre study. *Gut* 2011; 60: 666–70.

5 Shah SA, Movson J, Ransil BJ, Waxman I. pancreatic duct stricture length at ERCP predicts tumor size and pathological stage of pancreatic cancer. *Am J Gastroenterol* 1997; 92 (6): 964–7.

6 Scudera PL, Koizumi J, Jacobson IM. Brush cytology evaluation of lesions encountered during ERCP. *Gastrointest Endosc* 1990; 36: 281–4.

7 Ryan ME. Cytologic brushings of ductal lesions during ERCP. *Gastrointest Endosc* 1991; 37: 139–42.

8 McGuire DE, Venu RP, Brown RD, *et al.* Brush cytology for pancreatic carcinoma: an analysis of factors influencing results. *Gastrointest Endosc* 1996; 44: 300–4.

9 Vandervoort J, Soetikno RM, Montes H, *et al.* Accuracy and complication rate of brush cytology from bile duct versus pancreatic duct. *Gastrointest Endosc* 1999; 49: 322–7.

10 Jailwala J, Fogel EL, Sherman S, *et al.* Triple-tissue sampling at ERCP in malignant biliary obstruction. *Gastrointest Endosc* 2000; 51: 283–90.

11 Farrell RJ, Jain AK, Brandwein SL, *et al.* The combination of stricture dilation, endoscopic needle aspiration and biliary brushings significantly improves diagnostic yield from malignant bile duct strictures. *Gastrointest Endosc* 2001; 54: 587–94.

12 Hartman DJ, Slivka A, Giusto DA, Krasinskas AM. Tissue yield and diagnostic efficacy of fluoroscopic and cholangioscopic techniques to assess indeterminate biliary strictures. *Clin Gastroenterol Hepatol* 2012; 10: 1042–6.

13 Draganov PV, Chauhan S, Wagh MS, *et al.* Diagnostic accuracy of conventional and cholangioscopy-guided sampling of indeterminate biliary lesions at the time of ERCP: a prospective, long-term follow-up study. *Gastrointest Endosc* 2012; 75: 347–53.

14 Moon SH, Kim MH, Park do H, *et al.* IgG4 immunostaining of duodenal papillary biopsy specimens may be useful for supporting a diagnosis of autoimmune pancreatitis. *Gastrointest Endosc* 2010; 71: 960–6.

15 Choi HJ, Moon JH, Ko BM, *et al.* Clinical feasibility of direct peroralcholangioscopy-guided photodynamic therapy for inoperable cholangiocarcinoma performed by using an ultra-slim upper endoscope (with videos). *Gastrointest Endosc* 2011; 73: 808–13.

16 Itoi T, Moon JH, Waxman I. Current status of direct peroralcholangioscopy. *Dig Endosc* 2011; 23 Suppl 1: 154–7.

17 Brauer BC, Chen YK, Shah RJ. Single-step direct cholangioscopy by freehand intubation using standard endoscopes for diagnosis and therapy of biliary diseases. *Am J Gastroenterol* 2012; 107: 1030–5.

18 Meining A, Shah RJ, Slivka A, *et al*. Classification of probe-based confocal laser endomicroscopy findings in pancreaticobiliary strictures. *Endoscopy* 2012;44:251–7.

19 Meining A, Chen YK, Pleskow D, *et al*. Direct visualization of indeterminate pancreaticobiliary strictures with probe-based confocal laser endomicroscopy: a multicenter experience. *Gastrointest Endosc* 2011; 74: 961–8.

20 Andersen JR, Sorensen SM, Kruse A, *et al*. Randomized trial of endoprosthesis versus operative bypass and malignant obstructive jaundice. *Gut* 1989; 30: 1132–5.

21 Shepherd HA, Diba A, Ross AP, *et al*. Endoscopic biliary prosthesis and the palliation of malignant biliary obstruction: a randomized trial. *Br J Surg* 1988; 75: 1166–8.

22 Smith AC, Dowset JF, Russell RCG, *et al*. Randomized trial of endoscopic stenting versus surgical bypass in malignant low bile duct obstruction. *Lancet* 1994; 344: 1655–60.

23 Raikar G, Melin M, Ress A, *et al*. Cost-effective analysis of surgical palliation versus endoscopic stenting in the management of unresectable pancreatic cancer. *Ann Surg Oncol* 1996; 3: 470–5.

24 Luman W, Cull A, Palmer K. Quality of life in patient's stented malignant biliary obstruction. *Eur J Gastroenterol Hepatol* 1997; 9: 481–4.

25 Barkay O, Mosler P, Schmitt CM, *et al*. Effect of endoscopic stenting of malignant bile duct obstruction on quality of life. *J Clin Gastroenterol* 2013; 47: 526–31.

26 Speer AG, Cotton PB, Russell RCG, *et al*. Randomized trial of endoscopic versus percutaneous stent insertion in malignant obstructive jaundice. *Lancet* 1987; 2: 57–62.

27 Iwashita T, Lee JG, Shinoura S, *et al*. Endoscopic ultrasound-guided rendezvous for biliary access after failed cannulation. *Endoscopy* 2012; 44: 60–5.

28 Lim KH, Chung E, Khan A, *et al*. Neoadjuvant therapy of pancreatic cancer: the emerging paradigm? *Oncologist* 2012; 17: 192–200.

29 van der Gaag NA, Rauws EA, van Eijck CH, *et al*. Preoperative bilairy drainage for cancer of the head of the pancreas. *N Engl J Med* 2010; 362: 129–37.

30 Eshuis WJ, van der Gaag NA, Rauws EA, *et al*. Therapeutic delay and survival after surgery for cancer of the pancreatic head with or without preoperative biliary drainage. *Ann Surg* 2010; 252: 840–8.

31 Loew BJ, Howell DA, Sanders MK, *et al*. Comparative performance of uncoated, self-expanding metal biliary stents of different designs in 2 diameters: final results of an international multicenter, randomized, controlled trial. *Gastrointest Endosc* 2009; 70: 445–53.

32 Shah T, Desai S, Haque M, *et al*. Management of occluded metal stents in malignant biliary obstruction: similar outcomes with second metal stents compared to plastic stents. *Dig Dis Sci* 2012; 57: 2765–73.

33 Moss AC, Morris E, Leyden J, MacMathuna P. Do the benefits of metal stents justify the costs? A systematic review and meta-analysis of trials comparing endoscopic stents for malignant biliary obstruction. *Eur J Gastroenterol Hepatol* 2007; 19: 1119–24.

34 Isayama H, Yasuda I, Ryozawa S, *et al*. Results of a Japanese multicenter, randomized trial of endoscopic stenting for non-resectable pancreatic head cancer: covered Wallstent versus DoubleLayer stent. *Dig Endosc* 2011; 23: 310–5.

35 Kullman E, Frozanpor F, Soderlund C, *et al*. Covered versus uncovered self-expandable nitinol stents in the palliative treatment of malignant distal biliary obstruction: results from a randomized, multicenter study. *Gastrointest Endosc* 2010; 72: 915–23.

36 Telford JJ, Carr-Locke DL, Baron TH, *et al*. A randomized controlled trial comparing uncovered and partially covered self-expandable metal stents in the palliation of distal malignant biliary obstruction. *Gastrointest Endosc* 2010; 72: 907–14.

37 Isayama H, Komatsu Y, Tsujino T, *et al*. A prospective randomised study of "covered" versus "uncovered" diamond stents for the management of distal malignant biliary obstruction. *Gut* 2004; 53: 729–34.

38 Krokidis M, Fanelli F, Orgera G, *et al*. Percutaneous palliation of pancreatic head cancer: randomized comparison of ePTFE/FEP-covered versus uncovered nitinol biliary stents. *Cardiovasc Intervent Radiol* 2011; 34: 352–61.

39 Krokidis M, Fanelli F, Orgera G, *et al*. Percutaneous treatment of malignant jaundice due to extrahepaticcholangiocarcinoma: covered Viabil stent versus uncovered Wallstents. *Cardiovasc Intervent Radiol* 2010; 33: 97–106.

40 Iacono C, Ruzzenente A, Campagnaro T, *et al*. Role of preoperative biliary drainage in jaundiced patients who are candidates for pancreatoduodenectomy or hepatic resection: highlights and drawbacks. *Ann Surg* 2013; 257: 191–204.

41 Rerknimitr R, Angsuwatcharakon P, Ratanachu-ek T, *et al*. Asia-Pacific consensus recommendations for endoscopic and interventional management of hilar cholangiocarcinoma. *J Gastroenterol Hepatol* 2013; 28: 593–607.

42 Vienne A, Hobeika E, Gouya H, *et al*. Prediction of drainage effectiveness during endoscopic stenting of malignant hilar strictures: the role of liver volume assessment. *Gastrointest Endosc* 2010; 72: 728–35.

43 Polydorou AA, Chisholm EM, Romanos AA, *et al*. A comparison of right versus left hepatic duct endoprosthesis insertion in malignant hilar biliary obstruction. *Endoscopy* 1989; 21: 266–71.

44 Sangchan A, Kongkasame W, Pugkhem A, *et al*. Efficacy of metal and plastic stents in unresectable complex hilar cholangiocarcinoma: a randomized controlled trial. *Gastrointest Endosc* 2012: 76: 93–9.

45 Mukai T, Yasuda I, Nakashima M, *et al*. Metallic stents are more efficacious than plastic stents in unresectable malignant hilar biliary strictures: a randomized controlled trial. *J Hepatobiliary Pancreat Sci* 2013; 20: 214–22.

46 Ortner ME, Caca K, Berr F, *et al*. Successful photodynamic therapy for nonresectable cholangiocarcinoma: a randomized prospective study. *Gastroenterology* 2003; 125: 1355–63.

47 Zoepf T, Jakobs R, Arnold JC,*et al*. Palliation of nonresectable bile duct cancer: improved survival after photodynamic therapy. *Am J Gastroenterol* 2005; 100: 2426–30.

48 Leggett CL, Gorospe EC, Murad MH, *et al*. Photodynamic therapy for unresectable cholangiocarcinoma: a comparative effectiveness systematic review and meta-analyses. *Photodiagnosis Photodyn Ther* 2012; 9: 189–95.

49 49.Válek V, Kysela P, Kala Z,*et al*. Brachytherapy and percutaneous stenting in the treatment of cholangiocarcinoma: a prospective randomised study. *Eur J Radiol* 2007; 62: 175–9.

50 Steel AW, Postgate AJ, Khorsandi S,*et al*. Endoscopically applied radiofrequency ablation appears to be safe in the treatment of malignant biliary obstruction. *Gastrointest Endosc* 2011; 73: 149–53.

51 Prat F, Lafon C, De Lima DM, *et al*. Endoscopic treatment of cholangiocarcinoma and carcinoma of the duodenal papilla by intraductal high-intensity US: results of a pilot study. *Gastrointest Endosc* 2002; 56: 909–15.

52 Aiura K, Hibi T, Fujisaki H, *et al*. Proposed indications for limited resection of early ampulla of Vater carcinoma: clinico-histopathological criteria to confirm cure. *J Hepatobiliary Pancreat Sci* 2012: 19: 707–16.

CHAPTER 20

ERCP in acute and recurrent acute pancreatitis

Gregory A. Coté

Medical University of South Carolina, Charleston, USA

KEY POINTS

- Up to 20% of individuals who endure one episode of acute pancreatitis (AP) will have two or more recurrent events (recurrent acute pancreatitis (RAP)).

- Individuals with RAP have a substantial risk of progression to chronic pancreatitis.

- First-tier diagnostic testing for a patient with AP should include a thorough history (alcohol, smoking, family, medications, trauma/surgery), laboratories (calcium, triglycerides), and cross-sectional imaging (transabdominal ultrasound (US) with or without computed tomography (CT) scan).

- Gallstone pancreatitis is most likely in patients with an intact gallbladder, extrahepatic biliary dilation, and/or transient elevation in liver chemistries at the time of presentation.

- Early (<72 h after presentation) endoscopic retrograde cholangiopancreatography (ERCP) is indicated for patients with AP *and* one of the following: (i) concomitant acute cholangitis; (ii) severe AP with biliary obstruction.

- Empiric biliary sphincterotomy is reasonable for patients with gallstone pancreatitis who are poor candidates for cholecystectomy or those post-cholecystectomy who have a high probability of occult choledocholithiasis/sludge as the underlying cause.

- Given its risk profile, ERCP as an imaging test for individuals with RAP should be preceded by second-tier diagnostic imaging (magnetic resonance imaging (MRI)/ magnetic resonance cholangiopancreatography (MRCP) or EUS) to evaluate for chronic pancreatitis, congenital abnormalities, and obstructive etiologies.

- RAP is appropriately classified as idiopathic after negative first- and second-tier diagnostic imaging, and an evaluation for autoimmune pancreatitis or genetic abnormalities in some populations.

- If ERCP is performed for idiopathic, RAP, the endoscopist should be prepared to perform sphincter of Oddi manometry (SOM) during the same session.

- Among patients with idiopathic, RAP, pancreatic sphincter of Oddi dysfunction is associated with a greater likelihood of recurrent episodes following ERCP, irrespective of endoscopic therapy.

ERCP: The Fundamentals, Second Edition. Edited by Peter B. Cotton and Joseph Leung.
© 2015 John Wiley & Sons, Ltd. Published 2015 by John Wiley & Sons, Ltd.
Companion Website: www.wiley.com\go\cotton\ercp

Introduction

AP is an acute inflammatory process of the pancreas often caused by gallstones, alcohol, smoking, or some combination. Up to 20% of cases are idiopathic, and these individuals are at risk of suffering two or more AP episodes and progressing to chronic pancreatitis. The short- and long-term morbidity of AP is highly variable, and has a mortality rate of at least 1% [1–5]. In conjunction with chronic pancreatitis, AP is the most common inpatient gastrointestinal indication for hospitalization, accounting for more than 250 000 admissions in the United States annually [1, 6, 7].

With improvements in cross-sectional imaging, the diagnostic and therapeutic roles of ERCP in the management of patients with AP and RAP are evolving. In its nascence, ERCP was unparalleled in its ability to delineate pancreatic and biliary ductal anatomy, facilitating the diagnosis of choledocholithiasis, pancreas divisum, intraductal papillary mucinous neoplasm (IPMN), chronic pancreatitis, and others. Now, MRCP and endoscopic ultrasound (EUS) have largely replaced ERCP as an imaging modality. Is ERCP being relegated to a purely therapeutic procedure? This chapter will discuss the established and potential applications of ERCP in the diagnosis and treatment of patients with AP and RAP.

Acute biliary pancreatitis

Gallstones represent the single most common cause of AP in the Western world [8]. Its course is highly variable, with a mortality rate of approximately 5% while some patients are able to manage their disease in the ambulatory setting [9, 10]. The pathophysiology of gallstone pancreatitis is debated, but probably results from partial or complete occlusion of pancreatic outflow, reflux of bile acids into the pancreatic duct, or both [11]. Numerous clinical trials and meta-analyses have identified patients who benefit from early ERCP in the management of gallstone pancreatitis (Figure 20.1).

Gallstone pancreatitis should be suspected in the setting of an intact gallbladder or when there is elevation in alanine aminotransferase (ALT) > 3× upper limit of normal, the latter having a positive predictive value of 95% [12]. However, AP of any etiology may extrinsically compress the extrahepatic biliary tree, causing a mild elevation in liver chemistries or even common bile duct (CBD) dilation; therefore, mild elevation in liver chemistries is not pathognomonic for gallstone pancreatitis. Supporting evidence includes the presence of a dilated CBD or gallstones documented by transabdominal US, CT, or other imaging.

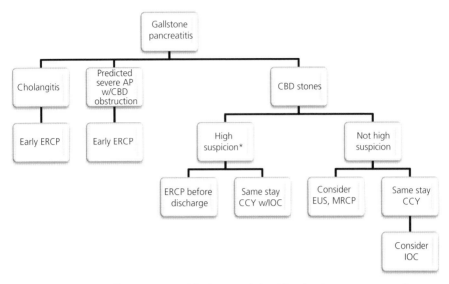

Figure 20.1 ERCP in gallstone pancreatitis. Suggested algorithm for the management of patients with gallstone AP. Early (within 72 h of presentation) ERCP is clearly beneficial for patients with concomitant cholangitis or predicted severe AP and bile duct obstruction. Otherwise, there are no subgroups that clearly benefit from early ERCP. Same-stay ERCP or cholecystectomy will reduce the likelihood of readmission or recurrent episodes. *The use of CCY with IOC and ERCP depends on local expertise in surgical exploration of the bile duct and ERCP. AP, acute pancreatitis; CBD, common bile duct; CCY, cholecystectomy; EUS, endoscopic ultrasound; IOC, intraoperative cholangiogram; MRCP, magnetic resonance cholangiopancreatography.

Early ERCP for the treatment of gallstone pancreatitis

There are two scenarios in which early ERCP, typically defined as within 72 h of presentation or symptom onset, is clearly beneficial. First, some patients with gallstone pancreatitis may present with concomitant acute cholangitis, a topic elaborated elsewhere in this textbook. These individuals are often jaundiced and demonstrating signs of systemic infection such as high fever, rigors, and sepsis-like physiology. Early ERCP significantly reduces mortality (relative risk (RR) 0.20, 95% confidence interval 0.06, 0.68) and local (RR 0.45, [0.20, 0.99]) and systemic complications (RR 0.37, [0.18, 0.78]) compared to conservative therapy [13].

Individuals predicted to have severe gallstone AP with concurrent biliary obstruction also benefit from early ERCP. Objective measures of severe AP include systemic inflammatory response syndrome (SIRS), Ranson's criteria, the Apache II score, the Balthazar CT severity index, and the BISAP score [14–18].

SIRS, high levels of blood urea nitrogen and hematocrit at the time of admission, and failure for these laboratories to decline during the first 24–48 h are probably the easiest bedside tools for clinicians.

Gallstone pancreatitis before cholecystectomy

Early ERCP should be applied selectively since these procedures may be more complex, particularly in the setting of substantial periampullary edema (Figure 20.2). In the absence of biliary obstruction or cholangitis, routine ERCP is rarely indicated for cases of mild or moderate AP in patients with an intact gallbladder. In the majority of these cases, patients will spontaneously pass CBD stones before cholangiography. Unless a CBD stone is definitively identified on preoperative imaging, these patients should undergo cholecystectomy during the initial hospitalization whenever possible [19, 20]. Same-stay chole-cystectomy reduces the likelihood of readmission for smoldering or RAP. An intraoperative cholangiogram should be performed in patients who have not previously undergone MRCP, EUS, or ERCP, to exclude retained CBD stones. The management of CBD stones identified intraoperatively depends on local expertise in CBD exploration and ERCP [21–24]. A single-stage operative approach combining cholecystectomy with CBD exploration and stone extrac-tion may be slightly less expensive and reduces length of stay compared to a two-stage approach. Intraoperative cholangiography and laparoscopic CBD exploration are performed infrequently, largely due to variable comfort and expertise [25]. As a result, ERCP is often performed before or after cholecystec-tomy to clear retained CBD stones if necessary.

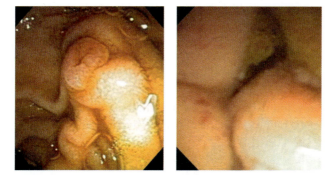

Figure 20.2 The major papilla in the setting of acute pancreatitis. Normally, the major papilla is easily visualized at a distance from the duodenoscope (left image). However, patients with acute pancreatitis may have substantial periampullary edema, causing compression of the duodenum and marked distortion of the major papilla (right image). As a result, early ERCP should be applied to selected populations with acute pancreatitis.

Empiric biliary sphincterotomy

ERCP with biliary sphincterotomy is a reasonable alternative to cholecystectomy for patients with gallstone pancreatitis who are poor operative candidates. In a retrospective cohort study of 1119 patients with gallstone pancreatitis and no history of cholecystectomy, the likelihood of developing recurrent pancreatitis after 1, 2, and 5 years was significantly lower for patients who underwent ERCP (5.2, 7.4, and 11.1%, respectively) compared to those who did not (11.3, 16.1, and 22.7%; hazard ratio 0.45, [0.30, 0.69]) [26]. Therefore, patients with gallstone pancreatitis and a contraindication to cholecystectomy should undergo ERCP with empiric biliary sphincterotomy. Endoscopic placement of a transpapillary, double-pigtail stent into the gallbladder may further attenuate the likelihood of symptomatic gallstones, but further studies are needed [27].

Suspected gallstone pancreatitis after cholecystectomy

In patients who have previously undergone cholecystectomy, nonbiliary etiologies for AP should be thoroughly vetted before proceeding with ERCP. Elevation in liver chemistries does not equate with biliary pancreatitis, since any cause of AP may lead to compression of the extrahepatic duct. In addition, unrelated causes for liver chemistry elevation should be considered, including alcohol, medications, fatty liver disease, and viral hepatitis. Second-tier imaging tests such as MRCP or EUS should precede ERCP, unless standard imaging such as transabdominal US or CT confirm the presence of a CBD stone. The rationale for conservatively applying ERCP is twofold: first, the risk of post-ERCP pancreatitis is highest in patients without biliary obstruction, many of who meet criteria for sphincter of Oddi dysfunction [28, 29]; second, the diagnostic yield and therapeutic benefit of ERCP and empiric biliary sphincterotomy are unknown in patients with nongallstone etiologies of AP [30].

If a CBD stone is identified on cross-sectional imaging, then ERCP with biliary sphincterotomy and stone extraction is appropriate. ERCP during the index hospitalization reduces the likelihood of readmission for gallstone pancreatitis [20].

Recurrent acute pancreatitis

Since AP occurs from a multitude of etiologies, many of which remain unrecognized after the first episode, the probability of having two or more episodes ranges from 5 to 30% [1, 8, 26]. Patients may not have their second episode until several years after the initial episode, and those having two episodes are likely to have three or more, assuming the underlying cause is untreated or unknown [31]. It is important to distinguish RAP from a single episode of AP with smoldering symptoms. Patients who develop recurrent, or have persistent symptoms related to local complications from a single episode of AP, such as a pancreatic fistula or pseudocyst, are better described as suffering from smoldering AP with local complications rather than RAP.

The highest-risk etiologies for RAP in an adult population include alcohol with recidivism, untreated gallstone disease (as summarized earlier), pancreatic duct obstruction, metabolic derangements such as hypertriglyceridemia and hypercalcemia, and genetic abnormalities (Figure 20.3). While genetic mutations were predominantly considered in a pediatric and young adult population, older adults are increasingly likely to have mutations identified with the use of complete gene sequencing [32]. Individuals with a relevant family history, personal history of chronic pancreatitis, and pancreas divisum have the highest probability of a high-risk mutation, although none of these are mandatory [33, 34]. ERCP remains in the diagnostic algorithm for patients with RAP, after a comprehensive evaluation for alternative etiologies (Figure 20.4).

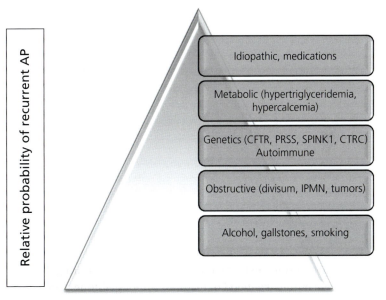

Figure 20.3 Etiologies of acute and recurrent acute pancreatitis. This figure illustrates a condensed list of potential etiologies for AP, with relative probabilities for recurrent episodes (RAP). Smoking, alcohol, and untreated gallstone disease represent the most common etiologies, whereas medication-/drug-induced pancreatitis remains a poorly recognized entity. Once the listed etiologies have been ruled out, RAP patients are typically classified as idiopathic. These individuals have a 15–30% chance of recurring episodes and progression to chronic pancreatitis. AP, acute pancreatitis; CFTR, cystic fibrosis transmembrane conductance regulator; CTRC, chymotrypsin C (CTRC); IPMN, intraductal papillary mucinous neoplasm; PRSS1, protease serine 1; RAP, recurrent acute pancreatitis; SPINK1, serine protease inhibitor, Kazal type 1.

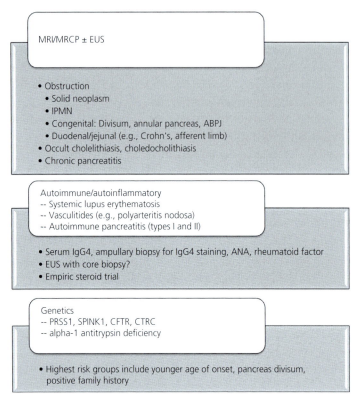

Figure 20.4 Suggested second-tier diagnostic tests for patients with unexplained acute and recurrent acute pancreatitis before ERCP. Suggested second-tier diagnostic tests for patients with unexplained AP or RAP. In appropriate populations, all of these should be applied before proceeding with ERCP. ANA, antinuclear antibody; CFTR, cystic fibrosis transmembrane conductance regulator; CTRC, chymotrypsin C (CTRC); EUS, endoscopic ultrasound; IPMN, intraductal papillary mucinous neoplasm; MRI/MRCP, magnetic resonance imaging/magnetic resonance cholangiopancreatography; PRSS1, protease serine 1; SPINK1, serine protease inhibitor, Kazal type 1.

Diagnostic yield of ERCP in RAP

If no clear etiology for RAP is identifiable after second-tier imaging (MRI/MRCP and/or EUS) and advanced diagnostics in select populations as summarized in Figure 20.4, the patient is appropriately classified as idiopathic [35]. Older studies report a diagnostic yield of ERCP between 38 and 80% [36–43]. These series are muddled by inconsistent definitions of idiopathic and variable pre-ERCP testing. Furthermore, the most common "cause" for RAP identified at ERCP is sphincter of Oddi dysfunction, a controversial entity that will be discussed later in this chapter. Nevertheless, abnormalities found at ERCP but missed on previous testing include occult choledocholithiasis, chronic

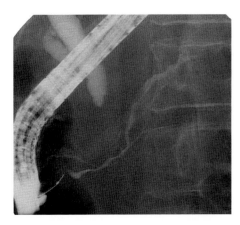

Figure 20.5 Autoimmune pancreatitis. A 58-year-old man presented with painless jaundice. ERCP demonstrates a distal common bile duct stricture and long pancreatic duct stricture without upstream dilation. He was found to have elevation in serum IgG4 levels and both strictures resolved following a 3-month course of systemic steroids. He was diagnosed with type I autoimmune pancreatitis, also known as lymphoplasmacytic sclerosing pancreatitis.

pancreatitis with or without pancreatic duct stones and strictures, complete pancreas divisum, and ampullary tumors [36, 38, 39, 41–43]. Structural abnormalities such as obstructing tumors and pancreas divisum are more likely in older (age > 60) individuals [40]. Autoimmune pancreatitis, often presenting as a malignant masquerader, is most common in older (age > 50) men and may be accompanied by obstructive jaundice with a pseudomass in the pancreas [44, 45]. Ideally, the diagnosis of autoimmune pancreatitis is made without ERCP, but given its similarities to pancreatic cancer an ERCP is often performed. Features suggestive of autoimmune pancreatitis include the presence of long strictures without upstream pancreatic duct dilation, absence of pancreatic calcifications, and presence of intrahepatic duct strictures or other extrapancreatic manifestations (Figure 20.5).

The likelihood of occult choledocholithiasis or microlithiasis (biliary crystals) is highest in patients with an intact gallbladder [38, 43]. Overall, the prevalence of microlithiasis as the underlying cause for idiopathic RAP is probably overstated, with a recent cohort attributing microlithiasis in 10 of 75 (13%) cases [46]. ERCP may be accompanied by aspiration of bile to analyze for crystals using a polarizing microscope. Critics of this approach emphasize the lack of evidence correlating bile crystals with response to therapy—cholecystectomy, biliary sphincterotomy, or ursodeoxycholic acid [47]. Most studies evaluating the role of empiric cholecystectomy for the treatment of unexplained AP were performed before the widespread utilization of EUS and MRCP. The efficacy of empiric cholecystectomy is substantially reduced when the patient has normal or near-normal liver chemistries and no evidence of gallbladder stones on transabdominal US [48]. Compared to patients with both of these abnormalities, the likelihood of recurrent pancreatitis after cholecystectomy was significantly higher (9% versus 61%) when neither was present.

Future cohort studies need to quantify the diagnostic yield of ERCP in patients with idiopathic recurrent acute pancreatitis (iRAP) who have previously undergone MRCP, EUS, and autoimmune and genetic testing. Since the yield is probably <20%, diagnostic ERCP is no longer recommended in the absence of SOM [38, 49, 50]. Secretin-enhanced MRCP and EUS and other noninvasive functional tests do not consistently correlate with the results of SOM; therefore, their role in the diagnostic algorithm for patients with idiopathic RAP requires further investigation [51–55]. That said, the implications of diagnosing an RAP patient with sphincter of Oddi dysfunction remain uncertain.

Sphincter of Oddi dysfunction: Cause or consequence of RAP?

There are several indirect pieces of evidence in animals and humans supporting the notion that obstruction of the pancreatic duct leads to AP:

1 Pancreatic duct obstruction precipitates AP in animal models, and early decompression of the duct attenuates progression to pancreatic necrosis [56, 57].

2 In an animal model, sphincter of Oddi spasm induced by application of a topical cholinergic agonist increased intraductal pressure and AP [58].

3 Use of a prophylactic pancreatic stent reduces the likelihood of post-ERCP pancreatitis [59].

4 The amount and force while infusing bile acids or other solutions into the pancreatic duct causes AP in animal models and correlates with disease severity [60, 61].

5 Multiple pancreatic duct injections, contrast opacification extending to the pancreatic tail, and acinarization increase the risk of post-ERCP pancreatitis [28].

Along these lines, sphincter of Oddi dysfunction (SOD) has been documented in 30–65% of iRAP patients undergoing ERCP with SOM. SOD is usually defined as an elevation >40 mmHg in basal biliary, pancreatic, or both sphincter pressures [36, 62–65]. Among individuals with choledocholithiasis, those having concomitant RAP were found to have significantly higher basal sphincter pressures, along with higher gradients between the common duct and duodenum [66]. This insinuates that pancreatitis, and not choledocholithiasis, causes or is the consequence of SOD.

While SOD is associated with RAP, it remains unclear whether SOD represents the underlying cause or if RAP produces a fibroinflammatory reaction in and around the papilla, leading to stenosis. In a series of 446 surgical sphincteroplasties primarily performed for SOD (22% of whom had RAP) and without prior endoscopic therapy, inflammation and fibrosis—not otherwise detailed in the manuscript—were observed in 29% and 10% of ampullary biopsies, respectively; biopsies from the transampullary septum identified inflammation in 15% and fibrosis in 27% of all cases [67]. This suggests that a fibroinflammatory process specifically occurs at the sphincter of Oddi, in the setting of RAP and chronic pancreatitis; it remains unclear if this is the inciting factor or simply a part of a systemic fibroinflammatory process that impacts the entire pancreas. The "consequence" theory is further supported by observations that SOD occurs in the setting of chronic pancreatitis [68], and that individuals with RAP and SOD have a more severe phenotype compared to those with RAP and normal sphincter manometry [30]. In a randomized trial that included 89 patients with idiopathic RAP, 69 (78%) with pancreatic SOD, the risk of having at least one episode of AP during long-term follow-up (median 78 months) was four times higher among patients with pancreatic SOD.

Biliary, pancreatic, or dual sphincterotomies for idiopathic RAP?

Empiric biliary sphincterotomy is an appropriate alternative to cholecystectomy for patients with gallstone pancreatitis (one or more episodes) who are poor operative candidates. Beyond this population, the benefit of endoscopic biliary, pancreatic, or dual sphincterotomies is unproven. Studies evaluating the efficacy of SOD treatment, via surgical sphincteroplasty or endoscopic sphincterotomy, are limited by their small samples sizes, retrospective design, and short-term follow-up [69–74]. In addition, study outcomes vary: attenuation of all recurrent episodes, number of AP episodes during follow-up, and pain, to name a few. To date, the largest idiopathic RAP trial compared biliary with biliary and pancreatic sphincterotomy in patients with pancreatic SOD ($n=69$), and biliary sphincterotomy with sham in patients with normal SOM ($n=20$) [30]. Among patients with pancreatic SOD, the frequency of RAP during follow-up was nearly identical in those randomized to biliary sphincterotomy alone (49%) and dual sphincterotomy (47%), with a trend to higher recurrence rates during the first year among those having dual sphincterotomy during the initial ERCP. Similarly, patients with normal SOM derived no benefit from empiric biliary sphincterotomy (recurrence rate 27%), compared to sham patients having a recurrence rate of 11%. Limitations of this study included its small number of normal pancreatic SOM patients, single-center design, and high frequency (>75%) of persistent/recurrent pancreatic SOD in the subgroup who underwent follow-up ERCP. The latter suggests endoscopic pancreatic sphincterotomy is an inadequate therapy for pancreatic SOD. However, surgical sphincteroplasty is equally unimpressive, having considerable morbidity, similar rates of restenosis or persistent sphincter hypertension (30%), and reduced efficacy in patients with chronic pancreatitis [67, 75, 76]. Further, optimists reading the aforementioned study would argue that 50% of pancreatic SOD patients with RAP suffered no recurrent bouts during follow-up; unfortunately, we do not know if this is better than the natural history of this mysterious disease.

At this time, endoscopic pancreatic sphincterotomy cannot be advocated as a curative intervention for RAP. However, it may confer benefits other than attenuation of AP episodes, including a potential impact on the frequency and severity of future episodes [77]. Future longitudinal studies of ERCP in RAP must include a rigorous definition of idiopathic, long-term (minimum 3–5 years) follow-up, and objective outcomes including AP incidence, frequency, and severity, development of chronic pancreatitis, and subjective measures of wellness and quality of life.

Pancreas divisum

Pancreas divisum is defined by dominant pancreatic juice outflow via the dorsal pancreatic duct through a secondary opening in the duodenum, the minor papilla (Figure 20.6). This represents the most common congenital anomaly of the pancreas, having a prevalence of 5–10% [34, 78, 79]. Pancreas divisum may be complete (no communication between the ventral and dorsal ducts) or incomplete (vestigial communication persists), but most consider these entities equivalent. In theory, divisum predisposes to AP and chronic pancreatitis by causing a relative obstruction to juice flow. However, like sphincter of Oddi dysfunction, the clinical relevance of pancreas divisum as an underlying cause or

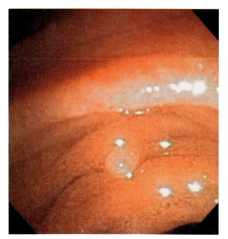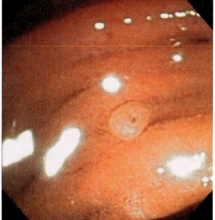

Figure 20.6 Minor papilla. Endoscopic inspection of the minor papilla can try one's patience. A patent orifice is rarely self-evident (left image). After careful and sustained inspection, sometimes for several minutes, the minor orifice becomes apparent when divisum is present (right image). Administration of secretin or cholecystokinin analogs increases pancreatic juice outflow, thereby facilitating identification and cannulation of the minor papilla.

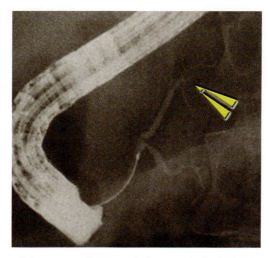

Figure 20.7 Pancreas divisum: ventral pancreatic duct terminal arborization. Inadvertent cannulation of the ventral pancreatic duct demonstrates truncation with terminal arborization (arrowhead). The presence of terminal arborization is highly suggestive of complete pancreas divisum, with failure of the ventral duct to communicate with the dorsal segment.

risk factor for AP is debated. The alternative hypothesis is that pancreas divisum is a phenotypic clue to underlying genetic mutations that predispose to pancreatitis through mechanisms other than duct obstruction [34, 80–82].

ERCP has been largely replaced by MRCP and to a lesser degree by EUS, for the diagnosis of pancreas divisum [55, 83–86]. Still, pancreas divisum may be found incidentally during ERCP; this may occur in the setting of inadvertent cannulation and injection of the ventral pancreatic duct or when ventral duct cannulation is unsuccessful. Opacification of the ventral pancreatic duct in the setting of complete pancreas divisum reveals terminal arborization (Figure 20.7), as opposed to pseudodivisum, when the ventral duct is completely obstructed by an occult tumor or chronic pancreatitis. Cannulation of the dorsal pancreatic duct is only recommended when a decision has been made to perform pancreatic duct therapy in the setting of chronic pancreatitis, or for minor papillotomy in patients with RAP. Among patients with pancreas divisum, the risk of ERCP is lower if the dorsal duct is avoided; however, once minor papilla cannulation is attempted the risk becomes comparable to high-risk ERCP with standard anatomy [87].

Minor papillotomy for the treatment of RAP in the setting of pancreas divisum

To date, there is one prospective trial of patients with pancreas divisum and RAP who were randomized to dorsal duct stenting for 1 year ($n = 10$) or control (n=9) [88]. The incidence and frequency of RAP, hospitalizations, and emergency room visits were all significantly lower in the population who underwent stent placement. Other retrospective cohort studies report mixed results [89–91]. Patients who are less likely to respond to minor papillotomy include those with nonobstructive chronic pancreatitis (i.e., without main duct obstruction) and those with chronic or recurrent abdominal pain but without evidence of RAP.

Miscellaneous obstructive etiologies for acute pancreatitis, and the role of ERCP

In addition to pancreas divisum, annular pancreas and anomalous pancreatobiliary union represent congenital anatomic abnormalities that have been associated with AP. Children with annular pancreas often present with AP, while adults are more likely to present with duodenal obstruction [92]. Anomalous pancreatobiliary union (Figure 20.8) may present with or without a choledochal cyst; this is an important consideration of unexplained pancreatitis in children. Endoscopic papillotomy may attenuate further episodes of AP, although the long-term risk of cholangiocarcinoma usually prompts cholecystectomy and bile duct resection at a young age [93, 94].

Pancreatic duct obstruction secondary to IPMN, pancreatic adenocarcinoma, or metastatic tumors to the pancreas may present with AP. In certain cases, ERCP may have a palliative role by removing mucus plugs or tumor emboli from the duct, as well as palliative stenting. There are limited data to suggest placement of

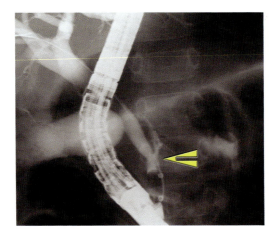

Figure 20.8 Anomalous pancreatobiliary union. A 3-year-old girl presented with acute pancreatitis and transient elevation in her liver chemistries. After an MRCP demonstrated a distal common bile duct filling defect, ERCP confirmed the presence of anomalous pancreatobiliary union, with the pancreatic duct emerging from a 1-cm common channel entering the major papilla.

larger-diameter (10 Fr) pancreatic duct stents may improve pain and exocrine insufficiency related to pancreatic cancer [95].

Future directions

Priorities in ERCP and AP research include the need for large-scale prospective cohort studies and clinical trials with long-term follow-up of individuals with idiopathic AP and RAP. The clinical significance of pancreas divisum and sphincter of Oddi dysfunction require sham-controlled trials with blinded and otherwise unbiased outcome measures. Additionally, ERCP represents a convenient vehicle for advanced imaging modalities such as contrast-enhanced and molecular intraductal US, optical coherence tomography, among others. These and other tools may identify a subgroup of individuals who may be at risk for the development of RAP and chronic pancreatitis or pancreatic cancer.

Summary

ERCP has an established therapeutic role in the management of acute gallstone pancreatitis. Early ERCP is appropriate in patients with concomitant acute cholangitis or severe AP with biliary obstruction. Same-stay cholecystectomy, ERCP, or both are appropriate for gallstone pancreatitis in an effort to reduce the likelihood of readmission and recurring episodes.

   Given its risk profile, ERCP should not be a first-tier diagnostic test to evaluate for choledocholithiasis or other etiologies of AP and RAP. Still, ERCP remains an appropriate diagnostic test for patients with idiopathic RAP, defined as two or more discrete episodes of AP without a clear explanation after a thorough evaluation. Future studies in patients with RAP will need to clarify the clinical significance of pancreatic SOD and pancreas divisum, and whether endoscopic therapies can impact the natural history of this enigmatic disease.

References

1 Yadav D, Lowenfels AB. The epidemiology of pancreatitis and pancreatic cancer. Gastroenterology. 2013 Jun;144(6):1252–61.
2 Appelros S, Borgstrom A. Incidence, aetiology and mortality rate of acute pancreatitis over 10 years in a defined urban population in Sweden. The British Journal of Surgery. 1999 Apr;86(4):465–70.
3 Goldacre MJ, Roberts SE. Hospital admission for acute pancreatitis in an English population, 1963–98: database study of incidence and mortality. BMJ. 2004 Jun 19;328(7454):1466–9.
4 Satoh K, Shimosegawa T, Masamune A, *et al.* Nationwide epidemiological survey of acute pancreatitis in Japan. Pancreas. 2011 May;40(4):503–7.

5 Shen HN, Lu CL, Li CY. Epidemiology of first-attack acute pancreatitis in Taiwan from 2000 through 2009: a nationwide population-based study. Pancreas. 2012 Jul;41(5): 696–702.

6 Whitcomb DC. Clinical practice. Acute pancreatitis. The New England Journal of Medicine. 2006 May 18;354(20):2142–50.

7 Peery AF, Dellon ES, Lund J, *et al*. Burden of gastrointestinal disease in the United States: 2012 update. Gastroenterology. 2012 Nov;143(5):1179–87.

8 Yadav D, O'Connell M, Papachristou GI. Natural history following the first attack of acute pancreatitis. The American Journal of Gastroenterology. 2012 Jul;107(7):1096–103.

9 Roberts SE, Akbari A, Thorne K, *et al*. The incidence of acute pancreatitis: impact of social deprivation, alcohol consumption, seasonal and demographic factors. Alimentary Pharmacology & Therapeutics. 2013 Sep;38(5):539–48.

10 Lankisch PG, Breuer N, Bruns A, *et al*. Natural history of acute pancreatitis: a long-term population-based study. The American Journal of Gastroenterology. 2009 Nov;104(11):2797–805; quiz 806.

11 Lerch MM, Gorelick FS. Models of acute and chronic pancreatitis. Gastroenterology. 2013 Jun;144(6):1180–93.

12 Wilcox CM, Kilgore M. Cost minimization analysis comparing diagnostic strategies in unexplained pancreatitis. Pancreas. 2009 Mar;38(2):117–21.

13 Tse F, Yuan Y. Early routine endoscopic retrograde cholangiopancreatography strategy versus early conservative management strategy in acute gallstone pancreatitis. The Cochrane Database of Systematic Reviews. 2012;5:CD009779.

14 Mounzer R, Langmead CJ, Wu BU, *et al*. Comparison of existing clinical scoring systems to predict persistent organ failure in patients with acute pancreatitis. Gastroenterology. 2012 Jun;142(7):1476–82; quiz e15–6.

15 Wu BU, Bakker OJ, Papachristou GI, *et al*. Blood urea nitrogen in the early assessment of acute pancreatitis: an international validation study. Archives of Internal Medicine. 2011 Apr 11;171(7):669–76.

16 Wu BU, Johannes RS, Sun X, *et al*. Early changes in blood urea nitrogen predict mortality in acute pancreatitis. Gastroenterology. 2009 Jul;137(1):129–35.

17 Wu BU, Johannes RS, Sun X, *et al*. The early prediction of mortality in acute pancreatitis: a large population-based study. Gut. 2008 Dec;57(12):1698–703.

18 Brown A, Orav J, Banks PA. Hemoconcentration is an early marker for organ failure and necrotizing pancreatitis. Pancreas. 2000 May;20(4):367–72.

19 Gurusamy KS, Nagendran M, Davidson BR. Early versus delayed laparoscopic cholecystectomy for acute gallstone pancreatitis. The Cochrane Database of Systematic Reviews. 2013 Sep 2;9:CD010326.

20 van Baal MC, Besselink MG, Bakker OJ, *et al*. Timing of cholecystectomy after mild biliary pancreatitis: a systematic review. Annals of Surgery. 2012 May;255(5):860–6.

21 Dasari BV, Tan CJ, Gurusamy KS, *et al*. Surgical versus endoscopic treatment of bile duct stones. The Cochrane Database of Systematic Reviews. 2013;9:CD003327.

22 Lu J, Cheng Y, Xiong XZ, *et al*. Two-stage vs single-stage management for concomitant gallstones and common bile duct stones. World Journal of Gastroenterology. 2012 Jun 28;18(24): 3156–66.

23 Brown LM, Rogers SJ, Cello JP, *et al*. Cost-effective treatment of patients with symptomatic cholelithiasis and possible common bile duct stones. Journal of the American College of Surgeons. 2011 Jun;212(6):1049–60, e1–7.

24 Rogers SJ, Cello JP, Horn JK, *et al*. Prospective randomized trial of LC+LCBDE vs ERCP/S+LC for common bile duct stone disease. Archives of Surgery. 2010 Jan;145(1): 28–33.

25 Sheffield KM, Han Y, Kuo YF, *et al*. Variation in the use of intraoperative cholangiography during cholecystectomy. Journal of the American College of Surgeons. 2012 Apr;214(4):668–79; discussion 79–81.

26 Hwang SS, Li BH, Haigh PI. Gallstone pancreatitis without cholecystectomy. JAMA Surgery. 2013 Sep 1;148(9):867–72.

27 Elmunzer BJ, Novelli PM, Taylor JR, *et al*. Percutaneous cholecystostomy as a bridge to definitive endoscopic gallbladder stent placement. Clinical Gastroenterology and Hepatology. 2011 Jan;9(1):18–20.

28 Freeman ML, DiSario JA, Nelson DB, *et al*. Risk factors for post-ERCP pancreatitis: a prospective, multicenter study. Gastrointestinal Endoscopy. 2001 Oct;54(4):425–34.

29 Freeman ML, Nelson DB, Sherman S, *et al*. Complications of endoscopic biliary sphincterotomy. The New England Journal of Medicine. 1996 Sep 26;335(13):909–18.

30 Cote GA, Imperiale TF, Schmidt SE, *et al*. Similar efficacies of biliary, with or without pancreatic, sphincterotomy in treatment of idiopathic recurrent acute pancreatitis. Gastroenterology. 2012 Dec;143(6):1502–9, e1.

31 Trapnell JE, Duncan EH. Patterns of incidence in acute pancreatitis. British Medical Journal. 1975 Apr 26;2(5964):179–83.

32 Ballard DD, Flueckiger JR, Fogel EL, *et al*. Testing adults with pancreatic disease for genetic abnormalities: Factors associated with having a positive genetic test [Abstract]. Gastroenterology. 2013;144(5(S1)):S460.

33 Montagnani M, Cazzato S, Mutignani M, *et al*. A patient with pancreas divisum, recurrent acute pancreatitis, and homozygosity for the cystic fibrosis transmembrane regulator-associated protein 5T allele. Clinical Gastroenterology and Hepatology. 2013 May;11(5):579–81.

34 Bertin C, Pelletier AL, Vullierme MP, *et al*. Pancreas divisum is not a cause of pancreatitis by itself but acts as a partner of genetic mutations. The American Journal of Gastroenterology. 2012 Feb;107(2):311–7.

35 Somogyi L, Martin SP, Venkatesan T, Ulrich CD, 2nd. Recurrent acute pancreatitis: an algorithmic approach to identification and elimination of inciting factors. Gastroenterology. 2001 Feb;120(3):708–17.

36 Coyle WJ, Pineau BC, Tarnasky PR, *et al*. Evaluation of unexplained acute and acute recurrent pancreatitis using endoscopic retrograde cholangiopancreatography, sphincter of Oddi manometry and endoscopic ultrasound. Endoscopy. 2002 Aug;34(8):617–23.

37 Hamilton I, Bradley P, Lintott DJ, *et al*. Endoscopic retrograde cholangiopancreatography in the investigation and management of patients after acute pancreatitis. The British Journal of Surgery. 1982 Sep;69(9):504–6.

38 Wilcox CM, Varadarajulu S, Eloubeidi M. Role of endoscopic evaluation in idiopathic pancreatitis: a systematic review. Gastrointestinal Endoscopy. 2006 Jun;63(7):1037–45.

39 Kaw M, Brodmerkel GJ, Jr. ERCP, biliary crystal analysis, and sphincter of Oddi manometry in idiopathic recurrent pancreatitis. Gastrointestinal Endoscopy. 2002 Feb;55(2):157–62.

40 Testoni PA, Caporuscio S, Bagnolo F, Lella F. Idiopathic recurrent pancreatitis: long-term results after ERCP, endoscopic sphincterotomy, or ursodeoxycholic acid treatment. The American Journal of Gastroenterology. 2000 Jul;95(7):1702–7.

41 Feller ER. Endoscopic retrograde cholangiopancreatography in the diagnosis of unexplained pancreatitis. Archives of Internal Medicine. 1984 Sep;144(9):1797–9.

42 Lee MJ, Choi TK, Lai EC, *et al*. Endoscopic retrograde cholangiopancreatography after acute pancreatitis. Surgery, Gynecology & Obstetrics. 1986 Oct;163(4):354–8.

43 Venu RP, Geenen JE, Hogan W, *et al*. Idiopathic recurrent pancreatitis. An approach to diagnosis and treatment. Digestive Diseases and Sciences. 1989 Jan;34(1):56–60.

44 Hart PA, Kamisawa T, Brugge WR, *et al*. Long-term outcomes of autoimmune pancreatitis: a multicentre, international analysis. Gut. 2012 Dec;62(12):1771–6.

45 Kamisawa T, Chari ST, Lerch MM, *et al*. Recent advances in autoimmune pancreatitis: type 1 and type 2. Gut. 2013 Sep;62(9):1373–80.

46 Garg PK, Tandon RK, Madan K. Is biliary microlithiasis a significant cause of idiopathic recurrent acute pancreatitis? A long-term follow-up study. Clinical Gastroenterology and Hepatology. 2007 Jan;5(1):75–9.

47 Rubin M, Pakula R, Konikoff FM. Microstructural analysis of bile: relevance to cholesterol gallstone pathogenesis. Histology and Histopathology. 2000 Jul;15(3):761–70.

48 Trna J, Vege SS, Pribramska V, *et al*. Lack of significant liver enzyme elevation and gall-stones and/or sludge on ultrasound on day 1 of acute pancreatitis is associated with recurrence after cholecystectomy: a population-based study. Surgery. 2012 Feb;151(2): 199–205.

49 Freeman ML. Adverse outcomes of ERCP. Gastrointestinal Endoscopy. 2002 Dec;56(6 Suppl):S273–82.

50 Ong TZ, Khor JL, Selamat DS, *et al*. Complications of endoscopic retrograde cholangiog-raphy in the post-MRCP era: a tertiary center experience. World Journal of Gastroenterology. 2005 Sep 7;11(33):5209–12.

51 Cicala M, Habib FI, Vavassori P, *et al*. Outcome of endoscopic sphincterotomy in post chole-cystectomy patients with sphincter of Oddi dysfunction as predicted by manometry and quantitative choledochoscintigraphy. Gut. 2002 May;50(5):665–8.

52 Young SB, Arregui M, Singh K. HIDA scan ejection fraction does not predict sphincter of Oddi hypertension or clinical outcome in patients with suspected chronic acalculous chole-cystitis. Surgical Endoscopy. 2006 Dec;20(12):1872–8.

53 Baillie J, Kimberly J. Prospective comparison of secretin-stimulated MRCP with manometry in the diagnosis of sphincter of Oddi dysfunction types II and III. Gut. 2007 Jun;56(6): 742–4.

54 Chowdhury AH, Humes DJ, Pritchard SE, *et al*. The effects of morphine-neostigmine and secretin provocation on pancreaticobiliary morphology in healthy subjects: a randomized, double-blind crossover study using serial MRCP. World Journal of Surgery. 2011 Sep;35(9): 2102–9.

55 Mariani A, Arcidiacono PG, Curioni S, *et al*. Diagnostic yield of ERCP and secretin-enhanced MRCP and EUS in patients with acute recurrent pancreatitis of unknown aetiology. Digestive and Liver Disease. 2009 Oct;41(10):753–8.

56 Lerch MM, Saluja AK, Runzi M, *et al*. Pancreatic duct obstruction triggers acute necrotizing pancreatitis in the opossum. Gastroenterology. 1993 Mar;104(3):853–61.

57 Runzi M, Saluja A, Lerch MM, *et al*. Early ductal decompression prevents the progression of biliary pancreatitis: an experimental study in the opossum. Gastroenterology. 1993 Jul;105(1):157–64.

58 Chen JW, Thomas A, Woods CM, *et al*. Sphincter of Oddi dysfunction produces acute pancreatitis in the possum. Gut. 2000 Oct;47(4):539–45.

59 Sofuni A, Maguchi H, Mukai T, *et al*. Endoscopic pancreatic duct stents reduce the incidence of post-endoscopic retrograde cholangiopancreatography pancreatitis in high-risk patients. Clinical Gastroenterology and Hepatology. 2011 Oct;9(10):851–8; quiz e110.

60 Arendt T, Hansler M, Stoffregen C, Folsch UR. Does high pancreatic duct pressure compromise the duct mucosal barrier function to pancreatic exocrine proteins? acta pathologica, microbio-logica, et immunologica Scandinavica. 1996 Sep;104(9):615–22.

61 Haciahmetoglu T, Ertekin C, Dolay K, *et al*. The effects of contrast agent and intraductal pressure changes on the development of pancreatitis in an ERCP model in rats. Langenbeck's archives of surgery/Deutsche Gesellschaft fur Chirurgie. 2008 May;393(3):367–72.

62 Fazel A, Geenen JE, MoezArdalan K, Catalano MF. Intrapancreatic ductal pressure in sphincter of Oddi dysfunction. Pancreas. 2005 May;30(4):359–62.

63 Fischer M, Hassan A, Sipe BW, *et al.* Endoscopic retrograde cholangiopancreatography and manometry findings in 1,241 idiopathic pancreatitis patients. Pancreatology. 2010;10(4): 444–52.

64 Elta GH. Sphincter of Oddi dysfunction and bile duct microlithiasis in acute idiopathic pancreatitis. World Journal of Gastroenterology. 2008 Feb 21;14(7):1023–6.

65 Toouli J, Roberts-Thomson IC, Dent J, Lee J. Sphincter of Oddi motility disorders in patients with idiopathic recurrent pancreatitis. The British Journal of Surgery. 1985 Nov;72(11): 859–63.

66 Guelrud M, Mendoza S, Vicent S, *et al.* Pressures in the sphincter of Oddi in patients with gallstones, common duct stones, and recurrent pancreatitis. Journal of Clinical Gastroenterology. 1983 Feb;5(1):37–41.

67 Madura JA, Madura JA, 2nd, Sherman S, Lehman GA. Surgical sphincteroplasty in 446 patients. Archives of Surgery. 2005 May;140(5):504–11; discussion 11–3.

68 Okazaki K, Yamamoto Y, Ito K. Endoscopic measurement of papillary sphincter zone and pancreatic main ductal pressure in patients with chronic pancreatitis. Gastroenterology. 1986 Aug;91(2):409–18.

69 Jacob L, Geenen JE, Catalano MF, Geenen DJ. Prevention of pancreatitis in patients with idiopathic recurrent pancreatitis: a prospective nonblinded randomized study using endoscopic stents. Endoscopy. 2001 Jul;33(7):559–62.

70 Jathal A, Sherman S, Fogel EL, *et al.* Long-term clinical outcome of endoscopic pancreatobiliary sphincterotomy (PBES) versus biliary sphincterotomy (BES) alone in sphincter of Oddi dysfunction associated with idiopathic recurrent pancreatitis. Gastrointestinal Endoscopy. 2001 Apr;53(5):AB93.

71 Samavedy R, Schmidt S, Fogel EL, *et al.* Long term outcomes of endoscopic therapy for idiopathic acute recurrent pancreatitis (IARP) [Abstract]. Gastrointestinal Endoscopy. 2007 Apr;65(5):AB248.

72 Guelrud M, Plaz J, Mendoza S, Beker B, *et al.* Endoscopic treatment in type-II pancreatic sphincter dysfunction [Abstract]. Gastrointestinal Endoscopy. 1995 Apr;41(4):398.

73 Catalano MF, Sivak MV, Falk GW, *et al.* Idiopathic pancreatitis (IP): Diagnostic role of sphincter of Oddi manometry (SOM) and response to endoscopic sphincterotomy (ES) [Abstract]. Gastrointestinal Endoscopy. 1993 Mar–Apr;39(2):310.

74 Wehrmann T. Long-term results (≥10 years) of endoscopic therapy for sphincter of Oddi dysfunction in patients with acute recurrent pancreatitis. Endoscopy. 2011 Mar;43(3): 202–7.

75 Tzovaras G, Rowlands BJ. Transduodenal sphincteroplasty and transampullary septectomy for sphincter of Oddi dysfunction. Annals of the Royal College of Surgeons of England. 2002 Jan;84(1):14–9.

76 Morgan KA, Romagnuolo J, Adams DB. Transduodenal sphincteroplasty in the management of sphincter of Oddi dysfunction and pancreas divisum in the modern era. Journal of the American College of Surgeons. 2008 May;206(5):908–14; discussion 14–7.

77 Toouli J. The sphincter of Oddi and acute pancreatitis—revisited. HPB. 2003;5(3):142–5.

78 Burtin P, Person B, Charneau J, Boyer J. Pancreas divisum and pancreatitis: a coincidental association? Endoscopy. 1991 Mar;23(2):55–8.

79 Gonoi W, Akai H, Hagiwara K, *et al.* Pancreas divisum as a predisposing factor for chronic and recurrent idiopathic pancreatitis: initial in vivo survey. Gut. 2011 Aug;60(8):1103–8.

80 Cohn JA, Friedman KJ, Noone PG, *et al.* Relation between mutations of the cystic fibrosis gene and idiopathic pancreatitis. The New England Journal of Medicine. 1998 Sep 3; 339(10):653–8.

81 DiMagno MJ, Dimagno EP. Pancreas divisum does not cause pancreatitis, but associates with CFTR mutations. The American Journal of Gastroenterology. 2012 Feb;107(2):318–20.

82 Fogel EL, Toth TG, Lehman GA, *et al.* Does endoscopic therapy favorably affect the outcome of patients who have recurrent acute pancreatitis and pancreas divisum? Pancreas. 2007 Jan;34(1):21–45.

83 Manfredi R, Costamagna G, Brizi MG, *et al.* Pancreas divisum and "santorinicele": diagnosis with dynamic MR cholangiopancreatography with secretin stimulation. Radiology. 2000 Nov;217(2):403–8.

84 Carnes ML, Romagnuolo J, Cotton PB. Miss rate of pancreas divisum by magnetic resonance cholangiopancreatography in clinical practice. Pancreas. 2008 Aug;37(2):151–3.

85 Mosler P, Akisik F, Sandrasegaran K, *et al.* Accuracy of magnetic resonance cholangiopancreatography in the diagnosis of pancreas divisum. Digestive Diseases and Sciences. 2012 Jan;57(1):170–4.

86 Kushnir VM, Wani SB, Fowler K, *et al.* Sensitivity of endoscopic ultrasound, multidetector computed tomography, and magnetic resonance cholangiopancreatography in the diagnosis of pancreas divisum: a tertiary center experience. Pancreas. 2013 Apr;42(3):436–41.

87 Moffatt DC, Cote GA, Avula H, *et al.* Risk factors for ERCP-related complications in patients with pancreas divisum: a retrospective study. Gastrointestinal endoscopy. 2011 May;73(5): 963–70.

88 Lans JI, Geenen JE, Johanson JF, Hogan WJ. Endoscopic therapy in patients with pancreas divisum and acute pancreatitis: a prospective, randomized, controlled clinical trial. Gastrointestinal Endoscopy. 1992 Jul–Aug;38(4):430–4.

89 Ertan A. Long-term results after endoscopic pancreatic stent placement without pancreatic papillotomy in acute recurrent pancreatitis due to pancreas divisum. Gastrointestinal Endoscopy. 2000 Jul;52(1):9–14.

90 Gerke H, Byrne MF, Stiffler HL, *et al.* Outcome of endoscopic minor papillotomy in patients with symptomatic pancreas divisum. Journal of the Pancreas. 2004 May;5(3):122–31.

91 Chacko LN, Chen YK, Shah RJ. Clinical outcomes and nonendoscopic interventions after minor papilla endotherapy in patients with symptomatic pancreas divisum. Gastrointestinal Endoscopy. 2008 Oct;68(4):667–73.

92 Zyromski NJ, Sandoval JA, Pitt HA, *et al.* Annular pancreas: dramatic differences between children and adults. Journal of the American College of Surgeons. 2008 May;206(5):1019–25; discussion 25–7.

93 Samavedy R, Sherman S, Lehman GA. Endoscopic therapy in anomalous pancreatobiliary duct junction. Gastrointestinal Endoscopy. 1999 Nov;50(5):623–7.

94 Todani T, Watanabe Y, Fujii T, *et al.* Cylindrical dilatation of the choledochus: a special type of congenital bile duct dilatation. Surgery. 1985 Nov;98(5):964–9.

95 Costamagna G, Alevras P, Palladino F, *et al.* Endoscopic pancreatic stenting in pancreatic cancer. Can J Gastroenterol. 1999 Jul–Aug;13(6):481–7.

CHAPTER 21

Chronic pancreatitis

Wiriyaporn Ridtitid[1,2], Evan L. Fogel[3], & Stuart Sherman[3]

[1] *Indiana University School of Medicine, Indianapolis, USA*
[2] *Chulalongkorn University, King Chulalongkorn Memorial Hospital, Thai Red Cross Society, Bangkok,Thailand*
[3] *Digestive and Liver Disorders, Indiana University Health, University Hospital, Indianapolis, USA*

KEY POINTS

- Malignancy should be ruled out once a PD stricture is detected.

- The best candidates for endoscopic stent placement are symptomatic patients with a single stricture of the main PD in the head with upstream dilation.

- A single plastic stent (PS) provides good short-term pain relief whereas placement of multiple simultaneous PS may have a better long-term outcome. Randomized control trials (RCTs) comparing single versus multiple PSs are required.

- Uncovered self-expanding metal stents (USEMS) should not be used for treating benign PD strictures. Data supporting the use of fully covered self-expanding metal stents (FCSEMS) for PD strictures in CP are still lacking.

Introduction

Chronic pancreatitis (CP) is a progressive inflammatory disease of the pancreas, characterized by irreversible destruction of pancreatic parenchymal and ductal structures with fibrosis. The predominant symptom of CP is chronic abdominal pain. Pain in CP is multifactorial in origin and can result from increased pressure in the main pancreatic duct (PD), leading to intraparenchymal/interstitial hypertension, and from peripancreatic/celiac neural inflammation. Intraductal hypertension occurs primarily due to obstruction of the pancreatic juice outflow from the PD strictures, intraductal stones, decreased compliance of the main PD, and major/minor papillary stenosis. Complications of CP such as pseudocysts, PD leaks/ascites, and biliary and duodenal obstruction can contribute to abdominal pain. The aims of medical, endoscopic, and surgical therapies are to alleviate symptoms, slow disease progression, and resolve complications. Endoscopic modalities, including endoscopic retrograde cholangiopancreatography (ERCP) and endoscopic ultrasound (EUS), provide both diagnosis and

---

ERCP: The Fundamentals, Second Edition. Edited by Peter B. Cotton and Joseph Leung.
© 2015 John Wiley & Sons, Ltd. Published 2015 by John Wiley & Sons, Ltd.
Companion Website: www.wiley.com\go\cotton\ercp

treatment in patients with CP. This chapter presents the role of ERCP for managing PD strictures, PD stones, and pseudocysts, which account for the majority of complications in the setting of CP.

When to do ERCP in chronic pancreatitis

For diagnosis of CP

ERCP can provide evaluation of PD abnormalities, including dilatations, strictures, stones, leaks, communicating pancreatic pseudocysts, side branch changes, and pancreatic function assessment with the intraductal secretin stimulation test (IDST). The IDST has a sensitivity of 50–95% and a specificity of 89–100% for the diagnosis of CP [1, 2]. Using the Cambridge classification system, ERCP can define the severity of CP based on features of the PD [3]. However, ERCP cannot be used to obtain information regarding the pancreatic parenchyma. While ERCP is very sensitive for detecting advanced changes of CP, it has a relatively low sensitivity (50–65%) for mild CP [2]. Because of the high risk of post-ERCP complications (higher for patients with mild CP and lower for those with advanced disease) in this setting and the availability of more sensitive tests such as EUS, ERCP is rarely used to diagnose CP [4]. ERCP should be reserved for patients with suspected pancreatic disease after noninvasive and less invasive studies have been nondiagnostic [1, 5]. In patients with known CP, ERCP should be restricted to symptomatic patients where endoscopic and/or surgical therapy is planned [6].

For treatment of CP

In patients with painful CP with ductal obstruction, both endoscopic and surgical management provide adequate drainage of pancreatic juice and relieve PD hypertension. To date, there are two randomized controlled trials (RCTs) comparing endoscopic and surgical interventions in patients with painful obstructive CP [7, 8]. Dite and colleagues reported similar pain control following surgery and endotherapy at the 1-year follow-up interval (92%) [7]. However, at 5 years, patients treated surgically had better pain relief than those undergoing endotherapy (86% versus 65%; $p = 0.009$). Cahen and colleagues found significantly better pain control following surgery compared to endoscopic treatment after 2 years (75% versus 32%; $p = 0.007$) [8]. Patients were subsequently followed for 5 years, and those treated surgically were more likely to achieve partial/complete pain relief (80% versus 38%; $p = 0.042$), with fewer procedures than those undergoing endoscopic treatment [9]. Morbidity and mortality did not differ between groups [7, 8]. However, the small sample size, different surgical procedures, and unclear disease characteristics such as the number of pancreatic stones and the location of pancreatic strictures may lead to bias. Although the evidence appears to favor surgery, most experts recommend endoscopic therapy as the first-line treatment for properly selected patients with painful CP who do not respond to medical therapy or who are poor surgical candidates, due to its lesser degree of invasiveness [10–13]. Furthermore, endotherapy for CP can predict the response to surgical treatment and may be also applied as a bridge to surgery [1, 12, 14].

Pancreatic duct strictures

When to do ERCP in PD strictures

Benign PD strictures caused by recurrent inflammation or fibrosis around the main PD are common complications of CP [15, 16]. In a retrospective study of 355 patients, the risk of malignancy in isolated PD strictures was 12% [15]. The stricture location in the pancreatic head or neck positively correlated with malignancy (odds ratio = 42), whereas the presence of irregular side branches or a history of pancreatitis negatively correlated with pancreatic cancer [15]. Once a PD stricture is identified, malignancy should be excluded with a contrast-enhanced computed tomography (CT) scan and/or EUS. Depending on the location of the stricture and other ductal features, ERCP might be indicated for possible treatment if no mass is detected. In patients with alarm symptoms and no other evidence of CP, tissue sampling should be performed during ERCP with further imaging studies if needed [17]. The endoscopic management of benign pancreatic strictures consists of stent placement with or without dilation and pancreatic sphincterotomy (Figure 21.1a–d) [17–19]. At ERCP, the best candidates for endoscopic stent placement are symptomatic patients with a single stricture of the main PD in the head with upstream dilation [16–19].

Results of ERCP in PD stricture management

Several studies have shown the efficacy of endotherapy in patients with CP and PD strictures (Table 21.1) [16, 20–29]. Early series with a single plastic stent (PS) ± stricture dilation reported good short-term pain relief (70–94%). However, multiple ERCP sessions were required for stent exchanges either on demand or at regular intervals. A subsequent study of 19 CP patients with refractory PD strictures demonstrated the feasibility and safety of placement of multiple 8.5–11.5 Fr PS, limited only by stricture "tightness" and duct diameter [26]. The median number of stents was 3 (range 2–4) placed for 6–12 months. During a median follow-up period of 38 months, 84% of patients were pain-free after stent removal. The placement of a self-expandable metal stent (SEMS) has been reported in an attempt to maintain PD patency for a long term and reduce the number of interventions required for benign stricture management [27–30]. In a study from Brussels with SEMS placement for benign PD obstruction,

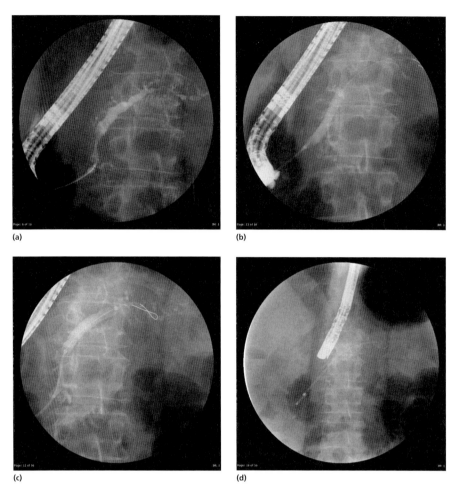

Figure 21.1 (a) Main pancreatic duct stricture in the head and body of the pancreas. (b and c) Balloon dilation of pancreatic duct stricture in the head and body of pancreas. (d) Pancreatic stent placement.

20 patients treated with uncovered SEMS (USEMS) had immediate pain relief [30]. Nevertheless, after 6 months, a high percentage of stent occlusion was noted because of epithelial hyperplasia. Since USEMS are generally not removable, this approach is not advocated as a long-term treatment. Partially covered SEMS (PCSEMS) or fully covered SEMS (FCSEMS) were placed in 16 patients with immediate pain relief [30]. However, stent migration ($n=8$) was a main complication in those with PCSEMS or FCSEMS insertion. Recent studies have reported relief of pain in 90–100% of cases while stents were in place and there was resolution of PD strictures in 67–90% of patients treated with temporary FCSEMS [27–29]. However, long-term follow-up data are lacking.

Table 21.1 Selected studies of endotherapy in patients with chronic pancreatitis and pancreatic duct strictures.

Study (year)	Number	Type of stent	Short-term pain relief (%)	Long-term pain relief (%)	Mean follow-up (months)	Complications (%)
Cremer et al. [16]	75	Single PS (10 Fr)	94	NA	37	16
Binmoeller et al. [20, 59]	93	Single PS (5, 7, 10 Fr)	74	65	58	6.5
Rosch et al. [21]	478	Single PS	NA	63	58.8	NA
Vitale et al. [22]	89	Single PS (5, 7, 10 Fr)	83	68	43	19
Eleftherladis et al. [23]	100	Single PS (8.5, 10 Fr)	70	62	69	23
Weber et al. [24]	17	Single PS (7–11.5 Fr)	89	NA	24	19
Weber et al. [25]	14	Single PS (7–11.5 Fr)	NA	57	60	NA
Costamagna et al. [26]	19	Multiple PS (8.5–11.5 Fr)	100	84	38	0
Sauer et al. [27]	6	FCSEMS (8–10 mm)	67	NA	1–8	0
Moon et al. [28]	32	Modified FCSEMS (6–10 mm)	90.6	NA	5	0
Giacino et al. [29]	10	FCSEMS (8–10 mm)	90	NA	19.8	20

Based on the available information, definitive recommendations regarding the appropriate duration of pancreatic stent placement, time to exchange stent(s), and number and size of pancreatic stents cannot be made. A previous study demonstrated fewer hospitalizations for abdominal pain in patients treated with 10 Fr PS when compared with those treated with smaller-diameter stents (8.5 Fr and smaller) [31]. In most studies, the optimal duration of PS placement before final stent removal ranged from 12 to 23 months [16, 20, 23, 24]. The occlusion rate of PD stents appears to be similar to bile duct stents of similar diameter. A recently published European Society of Gastrointestinal Endoscopy (ESGE) guideline recommends treating dominant main PD strictures with a single 10 Fr PS, with stent exchange performed at regular intervals (e.g., 3 months) for 1 year even in asymptomatic patients to prevent complications related to pancreatic stent occlusion [10].

> **KEY POINTS**
>
> - In patients with chronic calcific pancreatitis (CCP), endotherapy is most likely to be effective when the stones are small, less than three in number, not impacted, and present at the head and/or body of the pancreas without a downstream stricture.
> - If available, extracorporeal shockwave lithotripsy (ESWL) should be considered as a first-line approach in the management of large PD stones, impacted stones, and stones upstream to a stricture. PD clearance is needed following this modality in the same or different session to achieve the best outcome.
> - The role of ESWL without ERCP to clear the PD warrants further investigation.
> - Single-operator pancreatoscopy with visually directed laser and electrohydraulic lithotripsy is an evolving technique in the management of PD stones.

Pancreatic duct stones

When to do ERCP with PD stones

In patients with CCP and obstructing main PD stones, endotherapy is generally accepted as an alternative to surgery. Endoscopic management will often require lithotripsy, most commonly ESWL, to fragment the stones and facilitate their removal [32]. Simple small stones can be retrieved by endoscopic techniques alone using either stone extraction balloons or baskets (Figure 21.2a–c). Factors favoring endoscopic removal include the presence of stones in the head and/or body of the pancreas, the absence of a downstream stricture, stones measuring 10 mm or less, the presence of three stones or less, and the absence of impacted stones [33]. In contrast to bile duct stones, pancreatic stones will often require lithotripsy for successful removal. Although mechanical lithotripsy is an option, capturing an impacted stone to use this technique is rarely accomplished. Visually directed electrohydraulic and laser lithotripsy using a pancreatoscope has been more commonly utilized with the advent of single-operator pancreatoscopes [2, 17, 34–38]. Currently, ESWL is considered as a first-line approach in the treatment of large PD stones, impacted stones, and stones upstream to a stricture [10, 39] (Figure 21.3a–c). PD stones in the head area and the presence of a single stone are important factors associated with the success of ductal clearance after ESWL [40, 41]. In addition, intravenous secretin during ESWL appears to aid in ductal clearance by flushing out the stone fragments during ESWL [42].

Results of ERCP in PD stone management

Endoscopic treatment provides similar pain relief in patients with PD stones alone or in combination with a PD stricture [21, 33]. The outcome of endoscopic stone removal with or without ESWL is summarized in Table 21.2 [33, 40, 41, 43–50]. In patients who undergo ERCP with stone removal, complete stone

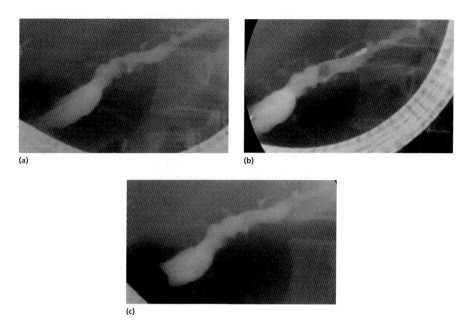

Figure 21.2 (a) Initial pancreatogram showed a filling defect in the pancreatic duct. (b) Pancreatic duct stone removal with basket extraction. (c) Final pancreatogram showed no stone remained in the pancreatic duct.

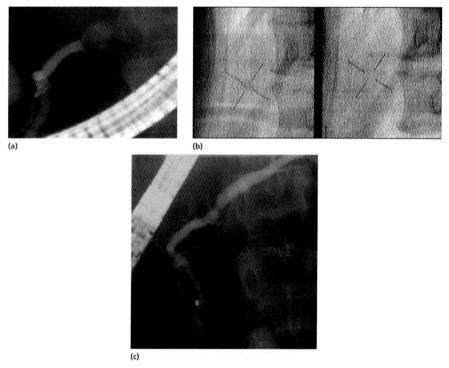

Figure 21.3 (a) Initial pancreatogram demonstrates a large stone obstructing the pancreatic duct. (b) Fluoroscopic image pre-extracorporeal shockwave lithotripsy (ESWL) identifies the stone (left); no stone is seen after successful ESWL (right). (c) No intraductal stone is identified at follow-up pancreatogram.

Table 21.2 Selected studies of endotherapy for pancreatic duct stones with or without extracorporeal shockwave lithotripsy in patients with chronic pancreatitis.

Study (year)	Number	Procedures	Follow-up (months)	Complete stone removal (%)	Pain relief (%)
Sherman et al. [33]	32	ERCP	25.2	59.4	67.7
Delhaye et al. [43]	123	ESWL+ERCP	14.4	59	45
Schneider et al. [44]	50	ESWL+ERCP	20	60	62
Dumonceau et al. [40]	41	ESWL+ERCP	24	50	54
Adamek et al. [41]	83	ESWL+ERCP	40	NA	76
Brand et al. [45]	48	ESWL+ERCP	7	44	82
Farnbacher et al. [46]	125	ESWL+ERCP	29	64	48
Tandan et al. [47]	1006	ESWL+ERCP	6	76	84
Inui et al. [49]	555	ESWL 318/ ESWL+ERCP 237	44.3	70/73	91
Dumonceau et al. [50]	55	ESWL 26/ ESWL+ERCP 29	52	NA	58/55
Seven et al. [48]	120	ESWL+ERCP	51.6	NA	50
Tandan et al. [39]	636	ESWL+ERCP	24–60 (364 patients)	77.5	68.7
			>60 (272 patients)	76	60.3

removal and clinical improvement (measured by pain, pancreatitis, or analgesic requirements) were seen in 60 and 68%, respectively [33]. In studies of patients undergoing ESWL followed by ERCP, complete stone removal was achieved in 44–76% and pain relief in 45–91% during a 6–52-month follow-up period [40, 41, 43–49]. An RCT comparing ESWL alone ($n=26$) versus ESWL combined with ERCP ($n=29$) demonstrated similar pain improvement in both groups with 2-year follow-up [50]. However, treatment costs were three times higher in patients treated with ERCP with ESWL [50]. Recently, a long-term study of 636 CP patients with large PD stones who had ESWL followed by endoscopic removal was reported [39]. Among the 364 patients followed up for 24–60 months, 77.5% had complete stone removal. Of those, 69% had complete pain relief. For the 272 patients followed up for more than 5 years, 76% had complete duct clearance. Of those, 60% had complete pain relief. The causes of CCP in this study were primarily tropical and nonalcoholic, which may have a better response to ESWL with subsequent endotherapy [39].

KEY POINTS

- Endoscopic pseudocyst drainage techniques have similar efficacy as open surgery at a lower cost and shorter hospital stay.
- The route of endoscopic pseudocyst drainage depends on the presence of a communication between the pseudocyst and PD, the distance between the lesion and gastric/duodenal wall, and the size of the collection.
- Conventional transmural drainage techniques can be performed when the pseudocyst is bulging into the gut lumen without collateral blood vessels present. EUS is necessary when these criteria are not met.

Pancreatic pseudocysts

When to do ERCP in pancreatic pseudocysts

Pancreatic pseudocysts can result as a complication of CP, occurring in 20–40% of patients during the course of CP [1, 51, 52]. An American Society for Gastrointestinal Endoscopy (ASGE) guideline recommends pseudocyst drainage in patients with symptoms (abdominal pain or early satiety), complications (such as gastric outlet/duodenal/biliary obstruction or infection), and/or a progressively enlarging collection [53]. While surgical drainage has been the traditional treatment for pancreatic pseudocysts, endotherapy provides a less invasive approach. A recent randomized trial in 40 pseudocyst patients showed equal efficacy of endoscopic and open surgical cystogastrostomy [54]. After a follow-up period of 24 months, there was no pseudocyst recurrence in patients undergoing endoscopic drainage and one in the surgically treated group. However, endoscopic treatment was associated with a shorter hospital stay, better physical and mental health of patients, and lower costs.

The route of endoscopic drainage for pseudocysts involves transpapillary, transmural, or combined transpapillary and transmural methods. The approach depends on the presence of a communication between the pseudocyst and PD, the distance between the collection and gastric/duodenal wall, and the size of the collection [17, 53]. The transpapillary approach is preferred if a relatively small pseudocyst (<5 cm) communicating with the main PD is present (Figure 21.4a–c). Currently, transmural drainage can be performed by conventional techniques using a duodenoscope or under EUS guidance. Without EUS guidance, conventional transmural drainage may be considered when the cyst causes a visible luminal bulge, collateral blood vessels are absent, and the distance between the pseudocyst and gastric/duodenal lumen is less than 1 cm using radiologic imaging

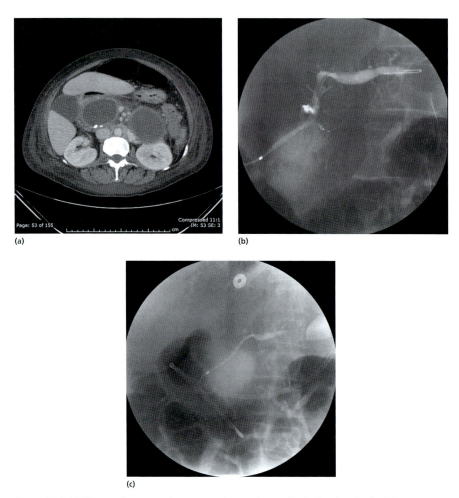

(a)   (b)

(c)

Figure 21.4 (a) CT scan demonstrating pancreatic pseudocysts in the head and tail of the pancreas. (b) Pancreatic duct leak in the pancreatic head with a complete pancreatic duct obstruction in the upstream body of the pancreas. (c) Pancreatic stent placement across the leak site in the head of the pancreas. Note: nasoduodenal tube has been placed.

techniques [17]. EUS-guided drainage is preferred when there is a nonbulging lesion or collateral vessels are present [10]. It is critical to treat associated ductal disease to achieve the best outcome from therapy.

Results of ERCP in pancreatic pseudocysts

The technical success rate of endoscopic pseudocyst drainage ranges from 73 to 100% [55–64], as shown in Table 21.3. Persistent cyst resolution was seen in 61–90% during a follow-up time of 5–37 months. Complications were seen in 5–36% of patients. In an ESGE clinical guideline [10], three studies comparing transpapillary and transmural pseudocyst drainage (173 patients) were analyzed

Table 21.3 Selected studies of endoscopic pseudocyst drainage.

References	CP* (%)	Technical success (%)	Transpapillary (n)	Transmural (n) Cysto gastrostomy	Cysto duodenostomy	Long-term success (%)	Follow-up (months)	Complications (%)
Grimm et al. [55]	100	87.5	5	1	8	NA	NA	31.2
Kozarek et al. [56]	44	85.7	12	0	0	61	16	35.7
Catalano et al. [57]	57	100	17	0	0	76	37	5
Smits et al. [58]†	100	73	12	10	7	65	32	21
Binmoeller et al. [20, 59]‡	92	94	31	6	10	70	22	9
Baron et al. [60]	46	82	NA	NA	NA	66	26	24
Kahaleh et al. [61]§	NA	94	0	74 (conventional 53 versus EUS 46)		88	14	19
Hookey et al. [64]¶	57	93	15	60 (conventional 65 versus EUS 51)		88	21	11
Varadarajulu et al. [63]**	NA	97	0	17 (conventional 15 versus EUS 15)		90	5	7
Park et al. [62]††	47	97	25	60 (conventional 29 versus EUS 31)		85	6	8

*The percentage of patients undergoing pseudocyst drainage who had chronic pancreatitis.

Of chronic pancreatitis patients undergoing pseudocyst drainage in the referred studies, 8†, 4‡, 25§, 41¶, 13**, and 25†† patients underwent combined transpapillary and transmural techniques (these patients are included in the transpapillary or transmural columns).

[59, 64, 65]. Transpapillary drainage had similar long-term success (94.6% versus 89.7%; $p=0.391$) and lower morbidity (1.8% versus 15.4%; $p=0.008$) than transmural drainage. However, the transpapillary technique was performed in patients with smaller pseudocysts than transmural drainage. In a recently published meta-analysis of four studies (two RCTs and two prospective non-randomized studies) of 229 patients comparing EUS-guided drainage to conventional drainage techniques, the technical success rate was significantly higher for EUS guidance than for conventional drainage, primarily due to the failure of conventional techniques in the setting of nonbulging lesions [66]. All 18 patients who failed conventional drainage subsequently crossed over and were successfully drained using EUS guidance. Allowing for this, using intent-to-treat analysis, EUS-guided drainage was not superior to conventional drainage in terms of short-term success (symptom resolution and at least 30% reduction in cyst size at 4–6 weeks after treatment) or long-term success (complete symptom resolution and complete radiologic resolution of the pseudocyst at a minimum of 6 months following treatment).

Conclusion

Ideally, management of symptomatic CP requires a multidisciplinary approach, involving medical, endoscopic, surgical, and radiologic therapies. To date, the evidence demonstrates a more durable outcome in terms of pain improvement for patients with obstructive CP treated surgically compared to endoscopic methods with similar morbidity and mortality during long-term follow-up. Since it is less invasive, endotherapy may still be a first-line treatment option in a properly selected group. Patients with CP should be evaluated individually to determine the appropriate management. Further comparative RCTs are required to determine the role of endotherapy versus surgery in patients with CP.

Acknowledgement

Dr. Ridtitid's ERCP fellowship was sponsored in part by an International Gastrointestinal Training Grant from the American College of Gastroenterology.

References

1 Adler DG, Lichtenstein D, Baron TH, *et al*. The role of endoscopy in patients with chronic pancreatitis. *Gastrointest Endosc* 2006;63:933–7.
2 Lehman GA. Role of ERCP and other endoscopic modalities in chronic pancreatitis. *Gastrointest Endosc* 2002;56:S237–40.

3 Sarner M, Cotton PB. Classification of pancreatitis. *Gut* 1984;25:756–9.

4 Testoni PA. Preventing post-ERCP pancreatitis: where are we? *JOP* 2003;4:22–32.

5 Schofl R. Diagnostic endoscopic retrograde cholangiopancreatography. *Endoscopy* 2001 Feb;33:147–57.

6 Cohen SA, Siegel JH. Endoscopic retrograde cholangiopancreatography and the pancreas: when and why? *Surg Clin North Am* 2001;81:321–8.

7 Dite P, Ruzicka M, Zboril V, Novotny I. A prospective, randomized trial comparing endoscopic and surgical therapy for chronic pancreatitis. *Endoscopy* 2003;35:553–8.

8 Cahen DL, Gouma DJ, Nio Y, *et al.* Endoscopic versus surgical drainage of the pancreatic duct in chronic pancreatitis. *N Engl J Med* 2007;356:676–84.

9 Cahen DL, Gouma DJ, Laramee P, *et al.* Long-term outcomes of endoscopic vs surgical drainage of the pancreatic duct in patients with chronic pancreatitis. *Gastroenterology* 2011;141:1690–5.

10 Dumonceau JM, Delhaye M, Tringali A, *et al.* Endoscopic treatment of chronic pancreatitis: European Society of Gastrointestinal Endoscopy (ESGE) Clinical Guideline. *Endoscopy* 2012;44(8):784–800.

11 Reddy DN, Ramchandani MJ, Talukdar R. Individualizing therapy for chronic pancreatitis. *Clin Gastroenterol Hepatol* 2012;10:803–4.

12 Clarke B, Slivka A, Tomizawa Y, *et al.* Endoscopic therapy is effective for patients with chronic pancreatitis. *Clin Gastroenterol Hepatol* 2012;10(7):795–802.

13 Forsmark CE. Management of chronic pancreatitis. *Gastroenterology* 2013;144:1282–91 e3.

14 Delhaye M, Arvanitakis M, Bali M, *et al.* Endoscopic therapy for chronic pancreatitis. *Scand J Surg* 2005;94:143–53.

15 Kalady MF, Peterson B, Baillie J, *et al.* Pancreatic duct strictures: identifying risk of malignancy. *Ann Surg Oncol* 2004;11:581–8.

16 Cremer M, Deviere J, Delhaye M, *et al.* Stenting in severe chronic pancreatitis: results of medium-term follow-up in seventy-six patients. *Endoscopy* 1991;23:171–6.

17 Avula H, Sherman S. What is the role of endotherapy in chronic pancreatitis? *Therap Adv Gastroenterol* 2010;3:367–82.

18 Oza VM, Kahaleh M. Endoscopic management of chronic pancreatitis. *World J Gastrointest Endosc* 2013;5:19–28.

19 Attasaranya S, Abdel Aziz AM, Lehman GA. Endoscopic management of acute and chronic pancreatitis. *Surg Clin North Am* 2007;87:1379–402.

20 Binmoeller KF, Jue P, Seifert H, *et al.* Endoscopic pancreatic stent drainage in chronic pancreatitis and a dominant stricture: long-term results. *Endoscopy* 1995;27:638–44.

21 Rosch T, Daniel S, Scholz M, *et al.* Endoscopic treatment of chronic pancreatitis: a multicenter study of 1000 patients with long-term follow-up. *Endoscopy* 2002;34:765–71.

22 Vitale GC, Cothron K, Vitale EA, *et al.* Role of pancreatic duct stenting in the treatment of chronic pancreatitis. *Surg Endosc* 2004;18:1431–4.

23 Eleftherladis N, Dinu F, Delhaye M, *et al.* Long-term outcome after pancreatic stenting in severe chronic pancreatitis. *Endoscopy* 2005 Mar;37:223–30.

24 Weber A, Schneider J, Neu B, *et al.* Endoscopic stent therapy for patients with chronic pancreatitis: results from a prospective follow-up study. *Pancreas* 2007;34:287–94.

25 25.Weber A, Schneider J, Neu B, *et al.* Endoscopic stent therapy in patients with chronic pancreatitis: a 5-year follow-up study. *World J Gastroenterol* 2013;19:715–20.

26 Costamagna G, Bulajic M, Tringali A, *et al.* Multiple stenting of refractory pancreatic duct strictures in severe chronic pancreatitis: long-term results. *Endoscopy* 2006;38:254–9.

27 Sauer B, Talreja J, Ellen K, *et al.* Temporary placement of a fully covered self-expandable metal stent in the pancreatic duct for management of symptomatic refractory chronic pancreatitis: preliminary data (with videos). *Gastrointest Endosc* 2008;68:1173–8.

28 Moon SH, Kim MH, Park do H, *et al.* Modified fully covered self-expandable metal stents with antimigration features for benign pancreatic-duct strictures in advanced chronic pancreatitis, with a focus on the safety profile and reducing migration. *Gastrointest Endosc* 2010;72:86–91.

29 Giacino C, Grandval P, Laugier R. Fully covered self-expanding metal stents for refractory pancreatic duct strictures in chronic pancreatitis. *Endoscopy* 2012;44:874–7.

30 Eisendrath P, Deviere J. Expandable metal stents for benign pancreatic duct obstruction. *Gastrointest Endosc Clin N Am* 1999;9:547–54.

31 Sauer BG, Gurka MJ, Ellen K, *et al.* Effect of pancreatic duct stent diameter on hospitalization in chronic pancreatitis: does size matter? *Pancreas* 2009;38:728–31.

32 Costamagna G, Boskoski I. Stonebreakers: the era of pancreatic stones treatment. *Expert Rev Gastroenterol Hepatol* 2012;6:521–3.

33 Sherman S, Lehman GA, Hawes RH, *et al.* Pancreatic ductal stones: frequency of successful endoscopic removal and improvement in symptoms. *Gastrointest Endosc* 1991;37:511–7.

34 Howell DA, Dy RM, Hanson BL, *et al.* Endoscopic treatment of pancreatic duct stones using a 10F pancreatoscope and electrohydraulic lithotripsy. *Gastrointest Endosc* 1999;50:829–33.

35 Hirai T, Goto H, Hirooka Y, *et al.* Pilot study of pancreatoscopic lithotripsy using a 5-fr instrument: selected patients may benefit. *Endoscopy* 2004;36:212–6.

36 Kozarek RA, Brandabur JJ, Ball TJ, *et al.* Clinical outcomes in patients who undergo extracorporeal shock wave lithotripsy for chronic calcific pancreatitis. *Gastrointest Endosc* 2002;56:496–500.

37 Maydeo A, Kwek BE, Bhandari S, *et al.* Single-operator cholangioscopy-guided laser lithotripsy in patients with difficult biliary and pancreatic ductal stones (with videos). *Gastrointest Endosc* 2011;74:1308–14.

38 Choi EK, Lehman GA. Update on endoscopic management of main pancreatic duct stones in chronic calcific pancreatitis. *Korean J Intern Med* 2012;27:20–9.

39 Tandan M, Reddy DN, Talukdar R, *et al.* Long-term clinical outcomes of extracorporeal shockwave lithotripsy in painful chronic calcific pancreatitis. *Gastrointest Endosc* 2013;78: 726–33.

40 Dumonceau JM, Deviere J, Le Moine O, *et al.* Endoscopic pancreatic drainage in chronic pancreatitis associated with ductal stones: long-term results. *Gastrointest Endosc* 1996;43: 547–55.

41 Adamek HE, Jakobs R, Buttmann A, *et al.* Long term follow up of patients with chronic pancreatitis and pancreatic stones treated with extracorporeal shock wave lithotripsy. *Gut* 1999; 45:402–5.

42 Choi EK, McHenry L, Watkins JL, *et al.* Use of intravenous secretin during extracorporeal shock wave lithotripsy to facilitate endoscopic clearance of pancreatic duct stones. *Pancreatology* 2012;12:272–5.

43 Delhaye M, Vandermeeren A, Baize M, Cremer M. Extracorporeal shock-wave lithotripsy of pancreatic calculi. *Gastroenterology* 1992;102:610–20.

44 Schneider HT, May A, Benninger J, *et al.* Piezoelectric shock wave lithotripsy of pancreatic duct stones. *Am J Gastroenterol* 1994;89:2042–8.

45 Brand B, Kahl M, Sidhu S, *et al.* Prospective evaluation of morphology, function, and quality of life after extracorporeal shockwave lithotripsy and endoscopic treatment of chronic calcific pancreatitis. *Am J Gastroenterol* 2000;95:3428–38.

46 Farnbacher MJ, Schoen C, Rabenstein T, *et al.* Pancreatic duct stones in chronic pancreatitis: criteria for treatment intensity and success. *Gastrointest Endosc* 2002;56(4):501–6.

47 Tandan M, Reddy DN, Santosh D, *et al.* Extracorporeal shock wave lithotripsy and endotherapy for pancreatic calculi—a large single center experience. *Indian J Gastroenterol* 2010;29:143–8.

48 Seven G, Schreiner MA, Ross AS, *et al.* Long-term outcomes associated with pancreatic extracorporeal shock wave lithotripsy for chronic calcific pancreatitis. *Gastrointest Endosc* 2012;75:997–1004.

49 Inui K, Tazuma S, Yamaguchi T, *et al.* Treatment of pancreatic stones with extracorporeal shock wave lithotripsy: results of a multicenter survey. *Pancreas* 2005;30:26–30.

50 Dumonceau JM, Costamagna G, Tringali A, *et al.* Treatment for painful calcified chronic pancreatitis: extracorporeal shock wave lithotripsy versus endoscopic treatment: a randomised controlled trial. *Gut* 2007;56:545–52.

51 Grace PA, Williamson RC. Modern management of pancreatic pseudocysts. *Br J Surg* 1993;80: 573–81.

52 Andren-Sandberg A, Dervenis C. Pancreatic pseudocysts in the 21st century. Part I: Classification, pathophysiology, anatomic considerations and treatment. *JOP* 2004;5:8–24.

53 Jacobson BC, Baron TH, Adler DG, *et al.* ASGE guideline: The role of endoscopy in the diagnosis and the management of cystic lesions and inflammatory fluid collections of the pancreas. *Gastrointest Endosc* 2005;61:363–70.

54 Varadarajulu S, Bang JY, Sutton BS, *et al.* Equal efficacy of endoscopic and surgical cystogastrostomy for pancreatic pseudocyst drainage in a randomized trial. *Gastroenterology* 2013;145: 583–90.

55 Grimm H, Meyer WH, Nam VC, Soehendra N. New modalities for treating chronic pancreatitis. *Endoscopy* 1989;21:70–4.

56 Kozarek RA, Ball TJ, Patterson DJ, *et al.* Endoscopic transpapillary therapy for disrupted pancreatic duct and peripancreatic fluid collections. *Gastroenterology* 1991;100:1362–70.

57 Catalano MF, Geenen JE, Schmalz MJ, *et al.* Treatment of pancreatic pseudocysts with ductal communication by transpapillary pancreatic duct endoprosthesis. *Gastrointest Endosc* 1995;42:214–8.

58 Smits ME, Rauws EA, Tytgat GN, Huibregtse K. The efficacy of endoscopic treatment of pancreatic pseudocysts. *Gastrointest Endosc* 1995;42:202–7.

59 Binmoeller KF, Seifert H, Walter A, Soehendra N. Transpapillary and transmural drainage of pancreatic pseudocysts. *Gastrointest Endosc* 1995;42:219–24.

60 Baron TH, Harewood GC, Morgan DE, Yates MR. Outcome differences after endoscopic drainage of pancreatic necrosis, acute pancreatic pseudocysts, and chronic pancreatic pseudocysts. *Gastrointest Endosc* 2002;56:7–17.

61 Kahaleh M, Shami VM, Conaway MR, *et al.* Endoscopic ultrasound drainage of pancreatic pseudocyst: a prospective comparison with conventional endoscopic drainage. *Endoscopy* 2006;38:355–9.

62 Park DH, Lee SS, Moon SH, *et al.* Endoscopic ultrasound-guided versus conventional transmural drainage for pancreatic pseudocysts: a prospective randomized trial. *Endoscopy* 2009;41: 842–8.

63 Varadarajulu S, Christein JD, Tamhane A, *et al.* Prospective randomized trial comparing EUS and EGD for transmural drainage of pancreatic pseudocysts (with videos). *Gastrointest Endosc* 2008;68:1102–11.

64 Hookey LC, Debroux S, Delhaye M, *et al.* Endoscopic drainage of pancreatic-fluid collections in 116 patients: a comparison of etiologies, drainage techniques, and outcomes. *Gastrointest Endosc* 2006;63:635–43.

65 Barthet M, Lamblin G, Gasmi M, *et al.* Clinical usefulness of a treatment algorithm for pancreatic pseudocysts. *Gastrointest Endosc* 2008;67:245–52.

66 Panamonta N, Ngamruengphong S, Kijsirichareanchai K, *et al.* Endoscopic ultrasound-guided versus conventional transmural techniques have comparable treatment outcomes in draining pancreatic pseudocysts. *Eur J Gastroenterol Hepatol* 2012;24:1355–62.

CHAPTER 22

Role of ERCP in complicated pancreatitis

Todd H. Baron

Division of Gastroenterology & Hepatology, University of North Carolina at Chapel Hill, Chapel Hill, USA

KEY POINTS

- Patients with severe, acute gallstone pancreatitis may benefit from early ERCP and stone extraction.

- ERCP can be technically challenging in the setting of early AP due to edema within the duodenum.

- Delayed local complications of AP include pancreatic pseudocysts, pancreatic abscess, and walled-off pancreatic necrosis.

- Endoscopic intervention for complicated pancreatitis is optimally performed in a tertiary care setting.

Introduction

Acute pancreatitis (AP) can take two forms: interstitial and necrotizing. Both forms can have the same etiologies but usually result in divergent clinical outcomes. Clinically severe acute pancreatitis (SAP) is almost always due to necrotizing pancreatitis and/or necrosis of surrounding peripancreatic fat [1]. The early management of SAP relies on critical care support. Some patients with acute gallstone pancreatitis may benefit from early endoscopic retrograde cholangiopancreatography (ERCP). Most patients survive the early phase of systemic inflammatory response syndrome (SIRS) and multisystem organ failure. Most have a prolonged course of sterile necrosis while others develop delayed infection. Fluid collections may form after AP and include acute peripancreatic fluid collections, pancreatic pseudocysts, acute necrotic collections, and walled-off necrosis. Endoscopy can be used to manage each of these entities [2, 3].

ERCP: The Fundamentals, Second Edition. Edited by Peter B. Cotton and Joseph Leung.

© 2015 John Wiley & Sons, Ltd. Published 2015 by John Wiley & Sons, Ltd.

Companion Website: www.wiley.com\go\cotton\ercp

Acute interstitial pancreatitis

In patients who present with interstitial acute pancreatitis (IAP), morbidity and mortality are low and care is supportive. Acute SIRS is absent and pancreatic parenchyma is preserved. The main goal is to identify the etiology. Gallstone pancreatitis is suspected based upon the presence of cholelithiasis and elevated serum transaminases in the absence of other risk factors for pancreatitis (such as heavy alcohol abuse, hypertriglyceridemia, and drugs). ERCP and biliary sphincterotomy are used when there is a high probability of bile duct stones based upon persistently elevated liver tests (particularly serum bilirubin) and a dilated biliary system. The vast majority of patients will have already passed stones and the mainstay of therapy is laparoscopic cholecystectomy. Intraoperative cholangiography is used to identify persistent bile duct stones, which can be managed laparoscopically, or with post-operative ERCP. ERCP and biliary sphincterotomy are reserved for secondary prevention of acute gallstone pancreatitis in those with prior cholecystectomy, those who are prohibitive operative candidates based upon age and/or comorbid illnesses, and as a bridge to laparoscopic cholecystectomy in selected patients.

Severe acute pancreatitis

SAP is nearly always due to necrotizing pancreatitis with loss of parenchyma of at least 30% and/or due to surrounding peripancreatic fat necrosis. Patients with SAP are recognized by acute severity of illness and SIRS. These patients are best managed in the intensive care unit (ICU) with appropriately aggressive fluid resuscitation. Early ERCP is often considered for patients with severe gallstone pancreatitis as a way of minimizing loss of pancreatic parenchyma by relieving outflow obstruction at the level of the ampulla. Despite early studies in this field showing promise, the data have not supported early ERCP in these patients. In addition, early ERCP carries risks of sedation, perforation, and introduction of infection into pancreatic necrosis if an inadvertent pancreatogram is performed in the setting of a pancreatic ductal disruption. Studies show that only patients with underlying cholangitis (evidenced by persistent or progressive jaundice) benefit from early ERCP in the setting of SAP [4]. It may be difficult to differentiate acute cholangitis in the setting of SAP as fever, leukocytosis, and abnormal liver function tests (LFTs) may be present as a result of the inflammatory process. Indeed, any cause of SAP can result in edema in the head of the pancreas as the bile duct courses through it. This can cause jaundice due to obstruction, though this type of biliary obstruction often occurs several days to a week after onset of AP rather than at initial presentation.

From a technical standpoint, ERCP in patients with SAP is often difficult due to the diffuse edema that occurs in the second part of the duodenum from the surrounding inflammation. This makes identification of the papilla and/or cannulation difficult, if not impossible. Endoscopic ultrasound (EUS) or magnetic resonance cholangiopancreatography (MRCP) may allow determination of bile duct stones and allow ERCP to be avoided. If a bile duct stone is confirmed and ERCP fails, options include percutaneous transhepatic cholangiography with or without catheter placement for subsequent ERCP, with or without rendezvous. EUS-guided approaches to the bile duct can also be considered.

Local complications of acute pancreatitis

The nomenclature of AP has recently been modified [2]. Several local complications can arise, for which ERCP can be helpful. These include acute peripancreatic fluid collections, acute pancreatic pseudocysts, pancreatic abscesses, and walled-off pancreatic necrosis (WON).

Acute peripancreatic fluid collection

These fluid collections develop in the early phase of pancreatitis (less than 4 weeks after onset of AP), do not have a well-defined wall, are homogeneous, and may be multiple. Most acute fluid collections remain sterile, usually spontaneously resolve, and rarely require intervention. Since these are composed of fluid, drainage can be performed by a transmural (transgastric or transduodenal approach) when rapidly progressive in size and/or development of infection. EUS guidance is usually undertaken to endoscopically drain these collections. While a transpapillary approach is theoretically possible, it has not been used for management of these collections.

Pancreatic pseudocyst

A pancreatic pseudocyst is a peripancreatic fluid collection surrounded by a well-defined wall and is devoid of solid material. The collection must present at least 4 weeks after onset of AP to be defined as a pseudocyst. Acute pancreatic pseudocysts arise from disruption of the pancreatic duct or side branches in the absence of parenchymal necrosis. Thus, these collections occur as a consequence of IAP or very limited, focal pancreatic necrosis. These collections can be drained by ERCP using a transpapillary approach or a transmural approach. Since these are composed of liquid, it is not imperative to use large transmural tracts for successful drainage.

Acute necrotic collection

Collections occurring within the first 4 weeks of an episode of acute necrotizing pancreatitis are referred to as acute necrotic collections. They are composed of variable amounts of liquid and solid (necrotic) material. These collections can be located within the pancreas and/or peripancreatic areas. Ability to endoscopically drain such collections is based upon whether any semblance of organization is present. Need for drainage is based primarily upon the presence of severe infection. If endoscopic therapy is undertaken and the collection is at least partially organized (walled off), initial transmural drainage of infected fluid can improve acute sepsis. However, for removal of necrotic material, large transmural drainage routes are usually required.

Walled-off necrosis (WON)

WON is an encapsulated collection of pancreatic and/or peripancreatic necrosis that has a well-defined wall (Figure 22.1). Necrosis does not usually become walled off earlier than 4 weeks after the onset of acute necrotizing pancreatitis.

Timing and indications for endoscopic intervention of necrosis

It is accepted that for patients with sterile necrosis any intervention should be delayed as long as possible from the onset of AP and for a minimum of 4 weeks. Most patients with pancreatic necrosis can be managed with medical therapy until resolution. Endoscopic management cannot be undertaken until the

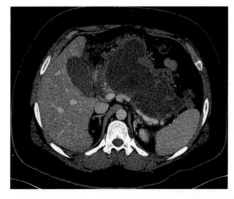

Figure 22.1 CT findings of walled-off necrosis. This image was obtained 7 weeks after the onset of SAP.

necrotic process has become walled off. This may occur as early as 2–3 weeks but often requires 4 weeks. We offer endoscopic therapy to patients with WON who have had a prolonged course of sterile necrosis, intractable pain, gastric outlet obstruction, inability to eat, or rapidly enlarging collections present at 4 or more weeks after the onset of pancreatitis. It is believed that endoscopic intervention (as described later) will return the patient to a normal health status more rapidly than "watchful waiting" (supportive care), though without clear-cut evidence. Less common indications include the inability to wean from mechanical ventilation due to increased intra-abdominal pressure and documented large, high amylase level pleural effusions or ascites.

The decision to intervene is easier in patients in whom there is a high suspicion for or known infected necrosis, and intervention has been made as early as 3 weeks after the onset of AP and in septic patients with AP and WON (as determined by computed tomography (CT)).

Necrosectomy methods

Preprocedural planning/sedation

It is imperative that a cross-sectional imaging procedure (CT or magnetic resonance imaging (MRI)) be obtained within several days prior to planned intervention to best determine the degree of organization (demarcation) and anticipated access points, and for the evaluation of major vessels either within the cavity or between the cavity and gastric or duodenal wall. In addition, one should pay attention to the degree of paracolic extension and communication between what appear to be multiple cavities. Such connections can often be appreciated on coronal CT images. One should be suspicious of a fistula between the lumen and collection when spontaneous air is present. This tract can be used for entry as described later.

A preprocedural international normalized ratio (INR) and platelet count should be obtained and corrected, as necessary.

Preprocedural antibiotics should be administered in patients not already receiving them. Extended intravenous penicillin agents (piperacillin/tazobactam), quinolone agents (levofloxacin), or a carbapenem (meropenem) are recommended agents.

Sedation using anesthesia support is recommended as these patients are often ill, procedures are prolonged, aspiration risk is high, and intraprocedural adverse events (bleeding, pneumoperitoneum) can occur.

Puncture and access

When endoscopic transmural access is performed, one or more transmural access points are targeted for drainage depending on imaging, most often CT. For WON collections located in the mid-body and tail, a transgastric route is usually undertaken. A transgastric approach is often a more direct approach to subsequently pass an endoscope directly into the cavity and into paracolic gutter extensions. A transduodenal approach is usually the only and best option for collections confined to the pancreatic head.

The initial transmural puncture can be performed in a variety of ways, with or without EUS guidance. Non-EUS-guided punctures can be performed using an ERCP scope. Advantages to using the duodenoscope are the ability to puncture at a perpendicular angle to the collection, the use of an elevator, and the ability to enter collections in the cardia or fundus in a retroflexed position. The disadvantages are a lack of dedicated large-caliber needles that allow passage of 0.035 in. guidewires and a lack of ultrasound guidance to detect underlying vessels. Using a duodenoscope the puncture is performed "blindly" using electrocautery with a biliary needle knife or cystotome (Cook Endoscopy, Winston-Salem, NC). Alternatively, a sclerotherapy needle can be used which accepts a 0.018 in. guidewire (Marcon-Haber, Cook Endoscopy). The needle, however, is short and not designed for guidewire passage; the wire often does not pass through the sheath after it is angled. Exchanges are difficult, and the small-diameter wire is not sufficiently robust to allow accessories to pass through the thicker gastric wall. In these cases, a triple-lumen needle knife or other cautery device is passed over the wire and into the cavity to allow entry and subsequent upsizing to a 0.035 in. guidewire. Unfortunately, standard EUS needles are not long enough to pass through duodenoscopes.

Standard upper endoscopes can also be used to create the puncture but a perpendicular approach to the posterior gastric wall may not be possible unless the collection is massively bulging into the gastric lumen so that an end-on view of the collection is feasible. However, a standard 19-gauge EUS needle will pass through a forward-viewing endoscope and obviates the need for changing endoscopes if direct endoscopic necrosectomy (DEN) is performed.

Most commonly, EUS-guided puncture is performed using an oblique-viewing endoscope. The advantages to EUS guidance are the ability to target the lesion, to potentially avoid blood vessels, and the possibility to assess the degree of underlying necrosis [5]. The disadvantages are the relative inflexibility, the need to have a straight access due to stiffness of the needle, the tangential nature of the puncture, and the tendency of the punctures to be more proximal both because of the access angle and due to the proximal location of the exit site relative to the transducer. Finally, echoendoscope mechanics and optics tend to be less favorable than ERCP endoscopes.

Once the cavity has been successfully accessed (Figure 22.2), the transmural tract is balloon-dilated to allow passage of a forward-viewing endoscope into the cavity. A minimum diameter of 15 mm is required (Figure 22.3). In some cases, 20 mm dilation is performed at the time of initial puncture, though this may be associated with higher risks of bleeding and perforation due to tearing of vessels and separation of the wall of the collection.

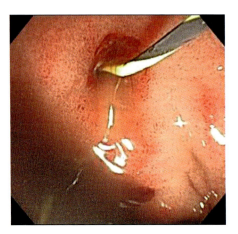

Figure 22.2 Guidewire passage through the medial wall of the duodenum (same patient as Figure 22.1).

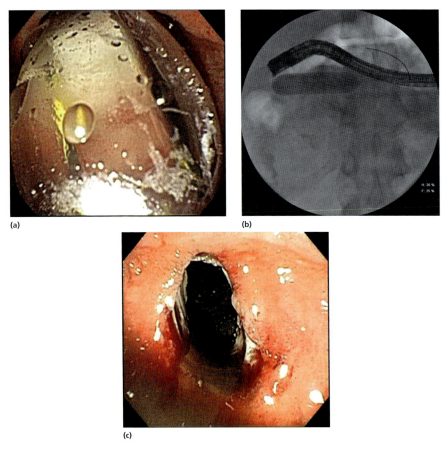

(a)

(b)

(c)

Figure 22.3 Large-balloon dilation of tract. (a) 18 mm balloon dilation seen endoscopically and (b) fluoroscopically. (c) Resultant endoscopic view of tract in duodenal wall.

Another approach is to dilate the transmural site to a small diameter followed by the placement of large-bore (16–23 mm mid-body diameter) self-expandable metal stents (SEMS) across the gastric or duodenal wall for maintaining access for DEN [6–10]. In the United States, the only large-diameter fully covered SEMS are esophageal, with the shortest lengths being 6–7 cm. This is still relatively long compared to the distance between the luminal site and the inside of the cavity and results in an excessive stent length inside the lumen or the cavity. Shorter-length devices (2 cm) with larger flanges are available outside of the United States, and at least one is expected to receive Food and Drug Administration (FDA) approval in the near future.

Necrosectomy

Once the access site is secured, a forward-viewing endoscope is driven into the cavity (Figure 22.4) and DEN is performed. Diagnostic channel scopes have the advantage of flexibility but the small working channel makes suctioning thick secretions difficult and also fills up with debris, making it difficult to pass accessories for debridement. A therapeutic channel endoscope also has water jet capabilities to aid in loosening adherent necrosis. A jumbo channel endoscope with a 6 mm channel and dual suction designed for removal of clots during gastrointestinal bleeding can be used. This endoscope is rather inflexible but large fragments of necrotic debris can be suction once loosened into smaller fragments.

The endoscope is passed into the cavity and necrotic material is removed using mechanical measures. Accessories used include standard polypectomy snares, polyp retrieval nets, and grasping forceps. The most effective forceps

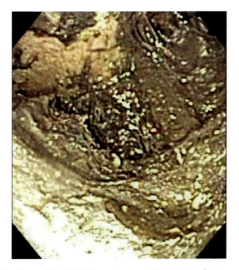

Figure 22.4 Endoscopic view with WON showing necrotic material.

have large, long prongs (pelican–alligator forceps) rather than shorter, traditional rat-toothed forceps, which tear small pieces of tissue. It is preferable to use spiral snares (Olympus Corporation, Center Valley, PA) to grasp and remove tissue. Unfortunately, these snares deform after many uses and it is not uncommon to use several during the course of one procedure. Once the tissue is grasped, it is withdrawn from the cavity and deposited in the lumen.

DEN can be time-consuming and labor-intensive. Many passages of the endoscope into and out of the WON are necessary. Complete necrosectomy in one session is usually not possible, particularly when there is a large necrotic burden.

If stents were not placed prior to DEN, they are placed at the end of the procedure. Commonly, two or more 7–10 Fr double pigtail stents are placed. A nasocystic irrigation tube is sometimes placed between necrosectomy sessions, though its use is not clear [11].

Subsequent direct necrosectomy procedures

The timing of subsequent direct necrosectomy procedures is not standardized. One approach is to perform scheduled, repeat procedures [12]. The duration between procedures can be as short as 24 h or as long as several weeks.

Postprocedural care

Outpatients who undergo necrosectomy can be kept as outpatients as long as the procedure is performed uneventfully and the patient meets discharge criteria. Antibiotics are continued per orally for at least several weeks and in most cases until the necrosis completely resolves. The patient may resume (or initiate) oral intake the day of the procedure, assuming no adverse events occur and there is no nausea, vomiting, or pain. Acid-secretory agents should be withheld, if possible (absence of severe reflux esophagitis), as the presence of acid may reduce infection due to bacteriostatic properties and acid entry into the necrotic cavity could break down necrotic debris.

Repeat cross-sectional imaging is done on a case-by-case basis. Antithrombotic medications can be reinitiated approximately 24–48 h later, based upon the risk of bleeding and thrombosis.

Management of paracolic gutter extensions

Paracolic gutter extensions can be difficult to treat, particularly when extending well into the pelvis. The central areas of necrosis in the pancreatic bed are accessible and communicate with the paracolic extensions and are thus potentially amenable to percutaneous approaches.

Adverse events

Adverse events can occur intraprocedurally or postprocedurally. Intraprocedural events include sedation, bleeding, and perforation.

Bleeding most often occurs at the entry site. Fortunately, it is usually self-limited and ceases by the end of the procedure. Uncontrolled or persistent bleeding can be managed by dilute epinephrine injection, balloon tamponade, clips, and electrocautery. Refractory or massive bleeding can be managed by placement of a large-diameter fully covered esophageal SEMS [13, 14]. Intracavitary bleeding is also usually self-limited. Severe intracavitary bleeding can be the most life-threatening and angst-producing for the physician. Hemostatic measures are similar to those for other bleeding including cautery and clip placement. If the bleeding is arterial, emergent embolization can be undertaken. Venous bleeding cannot be treated with interventional embolization techniques and may require surgery.

Perforation can also be at the entry site or in the cavity. Intraprocedural perforation can result in tension pneumoperitoneum, a life-threatening emergency that requires prompt needle catheter decompression [15]. Similar to bleeding, perforation may occur at the entry site and be managed with clips, diversion (in addition to internal pigtail stent placement), and placement of a large-caliber SEMS [16]. Large intracavity perforations often require surgical or percutaneous management.

Air embolism can be silent or result in procedure-related death [17]. It is believed to be preventable by the use of carbon dioxide for insufflation rather than air.

Introduction of organisms (bacteria and fungi) inevitably occurs during endoscopic intervention and may result in infectious complications. Thus, the need for removal of fluid and solid debris and administration of antibiotics are essential.

Outcomes

There are now many series demonstrating the efficacy of DEN [18, 19]. However, one must be careful in interpreting the literature. Successful resolution can be defined as complete nonsurgical resolution, including the use of adjuvant percutaneous therapy, or successful when only flexible endoscopic measures are used. Patients with WON are a heterogeneous group based upon size of collection, total necrotic burden, paracolic gutter extension, nutritional status, comorbid medical illnesses, and time from onset of necrosis to intervention. This makes it difficult to compare outcomes between centers and between disciplines.

In a systematic review of more than 1100 endoscopic necrosectomies in 260 patients, the overall mortality was 5% with a procedure-related morbidity of 27% [20]. Complete resolution of pancreatic necrosis using endoscopy alone was achieved in 76%. However, these studies include all types of endoscopic interventions.

Table 22.1 Types of pancreatic fluid collections complicating acute pancreatitis (AP).

Term	Definition
Acute peripancreatic fluid collection	A collection of enzyme-rich pancreatic juice occurring early in the course of AP, located in or near the pancreas, and always lacking a well-defined wall of granulation tissue or fibrous tissue.
Acute pseudocyst	A collection of pancreatic juice enclosed by a wall of nonepithelialized granulation tissue, requires at least 4 weeks to form, and is devoid of significant solid debris.
Acute necrotic collection	An intrapancreatic collection containing a variable amount of liquid and solid, typically associated with peripancreatic fat necrosis. Occurs less than 4 weeks after the onset of AP.
Walled-off pancreatic necrosis	Evolution of early necrosis to a partially encapsulated collection of pancreatic juice and necrotic debris. Well-defined inflammatory wall. Requires at least 4 weeks to form.

Table 22.2 Endoscopic approaches to walled-off pancreatic necrosis.

Endoscopic approach	Advantages	Disadvantages
Single or multiple transmural entry with nasocystic irrigation	Technically easy	Discomfort of nasal tube
Single-entry transmural with percutaneous endoscopic gastrostomy/jejunostomy (PEG-PEJ) for irrigation	Avoids nasal tube	Technically more difficult than nasocystic irrigation External tube
Transmural entry with direct endoscopic necrosectomy	Avoids external drains	Technically difficult Time-consuming Labor-intensive
Hybrid percutaneous irrigation endoscopic transmural approach	Minimal endoscopic procedures	Requires both interventional radiologist and gastroenterologist External tube
Hybrid percutaneous–endoscopic direct necrosectomy using external/internal large-diameter stents	Allows endoscopic access to areas not accessible translumenally	Requires both interventional radiologist and gastroenterologist External stent Abdominal wall pain Stent cost

Conclusions

In patients with AP, a variety of complications may occur. Early ERCP for gall-stone pancreatitis does not appear to alter outcome, except in those patients with coexistent acute cholangitis. Endoscopic interventions for local complications can be technically difficult and associated with severe adverse events.

References

1 Bakker OJ, van Santvoort H, Besselink MG, *et al*. Extrapancreatic necrosis without pancreatic parenchymal necrosis: a separate entity in necrotising pancreatitis? Gut. 2013 Oct;62(10): 1475–80.

2 Banks PA, Bollen TL, Dervenis C, *et al*. Classification of acute pancreatitis—2012: revision of the Atlanta classification and definitions by international consensus. Gut. 2013 Jan;62(1): 102–11.

3 Freeman ML, Werner J, van Santvoort HC, *et al*. Interventions for necrotizing pancreatitis: summary of a multidisciplinary consensus conference. Pancreas. 2012 Nov;41(8):1176–94.

4 de C Ferreira LE, Baron TH. Acute biliary conditions. Best Pract Res Clin Gastroenterol. 2013 Oct;27(5):745–56.

5 Jürgensen C, Arlt A, Neser F, *et al*. Endoscopic ultrasound criteria to predict the need for intervention in pancreatic necrosis. BMC Gastroenterol. 2012 May 14;12:48.

6 Belle S, Collet P, Post S, Kaehler G. Temporary cystogastrostomy with self-expanding metallic stents for pancreatic necrosis. Endoscopy. 2010;42:493–5.

7 Antillon MR, Bechtold ML, Bartalos CR, Marshall JB. Transgastric endoscopic necrosectomy with temporary metallic esophageal stent placement for the treatment of infected pancreatic necrosis (with video). Gastrointest Endosc. 2009 Jan;69(1):178–80.

8 Sarkaria S, Sethi A, Rondon C, *et al*. Pancreatic necrosectomy using covered esophageal stents: a novel approach. J Clin Gastroenterol. 2014 14 Feb;48(2):145–52.

9 Itoi T, Nageshwar Reddy D, Yasuda I. New fully-covered self-expandable metal stent for endoscopic ultrasonography-guided intervention in infectious walled-off pancreatic necrosis (with video). J Hepatobiliary Pancreat Sci. 2013 Mar;20(3):403–6.

10 Krishnan A, Ramakrishnan R. EUS-guided endoscopic necrosectomy and temporary cysto-gastrostomy for infected pancreatic necrosis with self-expanding metallic stents. Surg Laparosc Endosc Percutan Tech. 2012 Oct;22(5):e319–21.

11 Jürgensen C, Neser F, Boese-Landgraf J, *et al*. Endoscopic ultrasound-guided endoscopic necrosectomy of the pancreas: is irrigation necessary? Surg Endosc. 2012 May;26(5): 1359–63.

12 Coelho D, Ardengh JC, Eulálio JM, *et al*. Management of infected and sterile pancreatic necrosis by programmed endoscopic necrosectomy. Dign Dis. 2008;26(4):364–9.

13 Iwashita T, Lee JG, Nakai Y, *et al*. Successful management of arterial bleeding complicating endoscopic ultrasound-guided cystogastrostomy using a covered metallic stent. Endoscopy. 2012;44 Suppl 2 UCTN:E370–1.

14 Akbar A, Reddy DN, Baron TH. Placement of fully covered self-expandable metal stents to control entry-related bleeding during transmural drainage of pancreatic fluid collections (with video). Gastrointest Endosc. 2012 Nov;76(5):1060–3.

15 Baron TH, Wong Kee Song LM, *et al*. A comprehensive approach to the management of acute endoscopic perforations (with videos). Gastrointest Endosc. 2012 Oct;76(4):838–59.

16 Iwashita T, Lee JG, Nakai Y, *et al*. Successful management of perforation during cystogastrostomy with an esophageal fully covered metallic stent placement. Gastrointest Endosc. 2012 Jul;76(1):214–5.

17 Seifert H, Biermer M, Schmitt W, *et al*. Transluminal endoscopic necrosectomy after acute pancreatitis: a multicentre study with long-term follow-up (the GEPARD Study). Gut. 2009 Sep;58(9):1260–6.

18 Voermans RP, Veldkamp MC, Rauws EA, *et al*. Endoscopic transmural debridement of symptomatic organized pancreatic necrosis (with videos). Gastrointest Endosc. 2007 Nov;66(5):909–16.

19 Charnley RM, Lochan R, Gray H, *et al*. Endoscopic necrosectomy as primary therapy in the management of infected pancreatic necrosis. Endoscopy. 2006 Sep;38(9):925–8.

20 Haghshenasskashani A, Laurence JM, Kwan V, *et al*. Endoscopic necrosectomy of pancreatic necrosis: a systematic review. Surg Endosc. 2011 Dec;25(12):3724–30.

Guidelines

Working Group IAP/APA Acute Pancreatitis Guidelines. IAP/APA evidence-based guidelines for the management of acute pancreatitis. Pancreatology. 2013 Jul–Aug;13(4 Suppl 2):e1–15.

Tenner S, Baillie J, DeWitt J, Vege SS; American College of Gastroenterology. American College of Gastroenterology guideline: management of acute pancreatitis. Am J Gastroenterol. 2013 Sep;108(9):1400–15; 1416.

van Geenen EJ, van Santvoort HC, Besselink MG, van der Peet DL, van Erpecum KJ, Fockens P, Mulder CJ, Bruno MJ. Lack of consensus on the role of endoscopic retrograde cholangiography in acute biliary pancreatitis in published meta-analyses and guidelines: a systematic review. Pancreas. 2013 Jul;42(5):774–80.

Freeman ML, Werner J, van Santvoort HC, Baron TH, Besselink MG, Windsor JA, Horvath KD, vanSonnenberg E, Bollen TL, Vege SS; International Multidisciplinary Panel of Speakers and Moderators. Interventions for necrotizing pancreatitis: summary of a multidisciplinary consensus conference. Pancreas. 2012 Nov;41(8):1176–94.

Zaheer A, Singh VK, Qureshi RO, Fishman EK. The revised Atlanta classification for acute pancreatitis: updates in imaging terminology and guidelines. Abdom Imaging. 2013 Feb;38(1):125–36.

CHAPTER 23

ERCP in children

Moises Guelrud[1] & Andres Gelrud[2]

[1] *Division of Gastroenterology, Tufts Medical Center, Tufts University School of Medicine, Boston, USA*
[2] *Interventional Endoscopy of the Center for Endoscopic Research and Therapeutics (CERT), University of Chicago, Chicago, USA*

KEY POINTS

- ERCP is the most demanding endoscopic procedure in children. It is now routinely used for therapeutic purposes.

- ERCP in infants and children is generally performed at a tertiary care facility, or by adult endoscopists who perform a high volume of procedures. A close working collaboration between an adult and a pediatric gastroenterologist is important.

- Personnel with appropriate training in pediatric sedation and monitoring are required for either conscious sedation or general anesthesia.

- Use of a pediatric duodenoscope is mandatory in neonates and in infants younger than 12 months. A standard adult duodenoscope can be used in older children and adolescents.

- In children older than 1 year and adolescents, the rate of successful cannulation of the common bile duct at ERCP is comparable to reports in adults.

- Pancreatitis may be a more common complication of ERCP among children with underlying pancreatitis as compared with those undergoing ERCP for biliary indications.

- ERCP should be considered for all patients with cholangitis or pancreatitis for which an anatomical cause is suspected that might be treated endoscopically.

Introduction

Endoscopic retrograde cholangiopancreatography (ERCP) is the most demanding endoscopic procedure in children. It is the most sensitive and specific technique in the evaluation and treatment of children with suspected disorders of the pancreas and the biliary tract. It is now routinely used for therapeutic purposes [1–5] since magnetic resonance cholangiopancreatography (MRCP) is nowadays the

---

ERCP: The Fundamentals, Second Edition. Edited by Peter B. Cotton and Joseph Leung.
© 2015 John Wiley & Sons, Ltd. Published 2015 by John Wiley & Sons, Ltd.
Companion Website: www.wiley.com/go/cotton/ercp

first-line diagnostic tool for biliopancreatic diseases. The disadvantage is that it is an invasive procedure that frequently needs general anesthesia. The use of this technique in children has been limited. This may be due to the relatively low incidence of diseases, low incidence of clinical suspicion, limited availability of pediatric duodenoscopes, lack of pediatric gastroenterologists well trained in ERCP due to little exposure to the procedure, impression that ERCP in children is technically difficult to accomplish, difficulty in the effective evaluation of the therapeutic result, and because the indications and safety of ERCP in children have not been well defined [6].

Patient preparation

Sedation for ERCP in children

The preparation and sedation of a child undergoing ERCP are similar to those used for upper gastrointestinal endoscopy. Since young children and some adolescents are unable to fully cooperate with procedures under conscious sedation, a state of deep sedation from which the patient is not easily aroused is often required. The endoscopist must choose between conscious sedation and general anesthesia after considering the pertinent risks and taking into account personal skill and experience, expected complexity of the procedure, and, lastly, cost.

Most children can be adequately sedated with a combination of Propofol 1 mg/kg/h and Remifentanil 0.25 μg/kg/min. To obtain adequate sedation, children frequently require much higher doses of midazolam on a milligram per kilogram basis than adults. Postprocedure monitoring is the same as for other endoscopic procedures requiring sedation.

In children younger than 7 years of age, general anesthesia with endotracheal intubation is generally recommended. Younger children have a soft-wall trachea, which, in theory, might be compressed by the endoscope. Prone positioning during ERCP also compromises lung excursion and may cause hypoventilation in a sedated child.

Antibiotic prophylaxis

There are no data to guide antibiotic prophylaxis for ERCP in children. In our experience, routine antibiotic prophylaxis is unnecessary in neonates with cholestasis. Prophylactic antibiotics should be used to prevent endocarditis in susceptible patients in the same manner as for upper gastrointestinal endoscopy. Special situations that require a valvular prosthesis, vascular graft material, indwelling catheters, or transplanted organ in an immunosuppressed patient need individual consideration. Antibiotics are used in the setting of high-grade biliary or pancreatic duct obstruction, biliary or pancreatic duct disruption, and encapsulated pancreatic collections (pseudocyst or walled-off necrosis).

Other medication

Additional medications, which may be useful during ERCP, include glucagon (0.5 mg as an IV bolus) and Buscopan (hyoscine-*N*-butyl bromide) to reduce duodenal motility, and secretin (0.2 µg/kg) to facilitate identification and cannulation of the minor papilla.

Instruments

In neonates and infants younger than 12 months, ERCP is performed with a special Olympus pediatric duodenoscope PJF [7] (Olympus America, Inc., Lehigh Valley, PA), which has an insertion tube diameter of 7.5 mm, a channel of 2.0 mm, and an elevator. A standard adult duodenoscope with an instrument tip outer diameter of 10.5 mm and working channel of 3.2 mm can be used for most children and adolescents. A therapeutic duodenoscope with an instrument tip outer diameter of 12.5 mm and working channel of 4.2 mm can be used in patients between 12 and 17 years. Therapeutic maneuvers, such as placement of endoprostheses and passage of some dilators and retrieval baskets, require instruments with a larger channel.

Technique

ERCP is performed in a radiology suite. Pediatric endoscopy assistants and specially trained nurses can help reduce preprocedure anxiety, monitor the clinical status of the patient, and assist in holding and reassuring, administering medication, handling catheters, and injecting contrast material. The heart rate and oxygen saturation must be continuously monitored. Resuscitation medications and appropriate equipment should be available. Frequently, ERCP is performed on an ambulatory basis. A recovery area equipped with monitors and specialized pediatric nurses familiar with the needs of children is necessary.

The principles of cannulation are those used in adult patients, with the additional limitations of space within the duodenum that depend on age. In young infants, such as those undergoing investigation for neonatal cholestasis, it is important to minimize the procedure time to avoid abdominal overdistension and respiratory compromise. The use of carbon dioxide (CO_2) for insufflation is recommended.

Indications

In general, children with suspected biliary and pancreatic disease should undergo magnetic resonance imaging (MRI) with gadolinium and MRCP with secretin before considering ERCP (which is more often used for therapy).

Biliary indications

The only indication for ERCP in neonates and young infants is cholestasis. Biliary indications for ERCP in children older than 1 year and in adolescents are as follows:
- Known or highly suspected choledocholithiasis
- Known or highly suspected benign or malignant biliary obstruction
- Evaluation of biliary ductal leaks after cholecystectomy or liver transplantation
- Evaluation of abnormal scans (ultrasound, computerized tomography (CT), or MRCP)
- Therapeutic ERCP for other etiologies of obstructive jaundice like parasitic infection (ascaris or fasciola hepatica)

Pancreatic indications

Pancreatic indications for ERCP in children are as follows:
- Recurrent acute pancreatitis from pancreas divisum
- Idiopathic recurrent pancreatitis (selected cases)
- Chronic calcifying pancreatitis with pain for stone extraction
- Chronic pancreatitis with ductal stricture and pain for stent placement
- Evaluation of abnormal scans (ultrasound, CT, or MRCP)
- Treatment of symptomatic pancreatic and peripancreatic fluid collections (pseudocyst or walled-off necrosis)
- Treatment of pancreatic ductal leaks from blunt abdominal trauma

Success rates for ERCP in children

Successful cannulation of the common bile duct in neonates and young infants is lower than that in adults. It varies from 27 to 98% according to the endoscopist experience [7–10]. In our unpublished experience with 184 neonates and young infants with neonatal cholestasis, the procedure was successful technically in 93% of cases. Failure was due to duodenal malrotation in two cases and inability to cannulate in six.

In older children, the success rate for cannulation of the desired duct is 97–98% comparable to that achieved in adults [1–5, 11–18]. Our ERCP success in 220 children older than 1 year was 98%.

Complications

The incidence of complications in pediatric patients is not well established. In neonates and young infants with neonatal cholestasis, there were no major complications in the series reported in the literature [1–5]. In our unpublished experience with 184 neonates and young infants, minor complications without clinical significance occurred in 24 patients (13%). Two neonates had transient narcotic-induced respiratory depression and four young infants had non-narcotic respiratory depression, which resolved with oxygen administration. In 17 patients, minor acute duodenal erosions were observed without clinical consequences. One neonate had abdominal distension for 10 h after completion of ERCP, which resolved without treatment. There were no major complications.

Complications in children older than 1 year vary according to the system studied, biliary or pancreatic. The overall incidence is approximately 5% [1–5]. In our unpublished experience with 220 ERCPs in children older than 1 year, ERCP was performed for diagnostic purposes in 108 cases with two (1.8%) complications. In 112 therapeutic ERCPs, complications occurred in 12 (10.7%).

In a retrospective case-controlled study of 116 children and 116 adults matched for procedure complexity [1], the success and complications of diagnostic and therapeutic ERCP in children and adult patients were compared. Equivalent high rates of technical success and low rates of adverse events were found. The prevalence of post-ERCP pancreatitis was 3.4%. This result is similar to that observed in a review of 343 ERCPs performed in pediatric patients, where post-ERCP pancreatitis, defined by using established criteria, occurred in less than 3% [3].

In a retrospective study of 329 ERCPs, total complications occurred in 32 patients (9.7%) and included cholangitis in 1 patient and pancreatitis in 31. Of 92 diagnostic ERCPs, complications occurred in 5.4%. Of 235 therapeutic ERCPs, complications occurred in 11.1%. Pancreatitis occurred in 5.6% of ERCPs for biliary indications and in 10.6% for pancreatic indications. In patients with manometrically documented sphincter of Oddi dysfunction (SOD), the post-ERCP pancreatitis rates, according to therapies, were 30% (3 of 10 patients) with biliary sphincterotomy alone, 25% (2 of 8) with biliary sphincterotomy followed by a pancreatic duct (PD) stent, 21.4% (3 of 14) with pancreatic sphincterotomy followed by a PD stent, and 20% (5 of 25) with needle–knife dual pancreaticobiliary sphincterotomy over a PD stent. There was no statistically significant difference between biliary sphincterotomy alone and dual sphincterotomy with a prophylactic PD stent [2].

In adults, a single dose of rectal indomethacin immediately after ERCP has been shown to reduce the incidence of pancreatitis [19]. Studies are needed to evaluate the use of prophylactic rectal indomethacin in children. Eventually, it could replace pancreatic stent placement in patients undergoing high-risk ERCP.

Biliary findings

Biliary atresia versus neonatal hepatitis

The differential diagnosis of neonatal cholestasis is critical in the first 2 months of life. In approximately 30% of patients, a specific metabolic or infectious disease can be recognized (Table 23.1).

Discriminating analysis using duodenal drainage, high-quality diagnostic ultrasound, scintigraphy imaging, and liver biopsy permitted accurate diagnosis

Table 23.1 Biliary findings in ERCP in neonates and children.

Congenital anomalies
Biliary atresia versus neonatal hepatitis
Alagille syndrome and paucity syndrome
Congenital hepatic fibrosis
Caroli's disease and Caroli's syndrome
Biliary strictures due to cystic fibrosis
Choledochal cyst
Benign biliary strictures
Acquired diseases
Bile plug syndrome
Primary sclerosing cholangitis
Biliary obstruction due to parasitic infestation
Choledocholithiasis
Benign biliary strictures
Malignant biliary strictures
Common bile duct complications after liver transplantation

of either biliary atresia or neonatal hepatitis in 80–90% of patients [20, 21]. Thus, 10–20% of neonates required laparotomy to establish the diagnosis. In these patients, visualization of a patent biliary tree by ERCP may help.

Clearly, the success of ERCP in this context depends upon the experience of the endoscopist, who must have confidence that nonvisualization of the common bile duct is not related to technical problems and to positioning of the catheter. ERCP is the most direct method of establishing a diagnosis in the hands of skilled endoscopists, and may be appropriate as the first-line test when expertise and equipment are available. The Cholestasis Guideline Committee of the North American Society for Pediatric Gastroenterology, Hepatology, and Nutrition (NASPGHAN) [6] concludes that ERCP is not frequently used because of the cost of instrumentation and the need for technical expertise. The usefulness of ERCP appears to depend on the center and operator. The Committee recommends that a liver biopsy be obtained before subjecting an infant to ERCP. Under selected circumstances, ERCP can clarify the cause of neonatal cholestasis and obviate the need for laparotomy.

ERCP findings

Three types of ERCP findings have been described in patients with biliary atresia [21] (Figure 23.1): Type 1, no visualization of the biliary tree (Figure 23.2); Type 2, visualization of the distal common duct and gallbladder (Figure 23.3); Type 3 is divided into two subtypes: Type 3a, visualization of the gallbladder and the complete common duct with biliary lakes at the portahepatis (Figure 23.4), and Type 3b, in which both hepatic ducts are seen with biliary lakes.

Several authors [8–10, 22] have shown that in half of the patients in whom extensive investigations failed to distinguish intra- from extrahepatic cholestasis, the

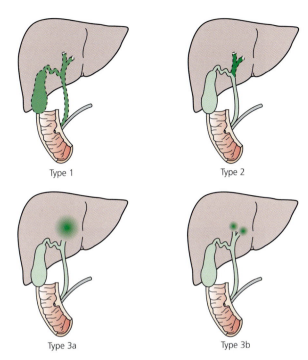

Type 1

Type 2

Type 3a

Type 3b

Figure 23.1 Variants of biliary atresia.

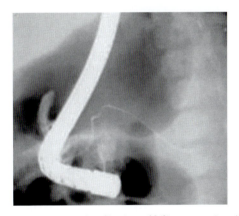

Figure 23.2 Biliary atresia Type 1. No visualization of biliary tree. Opacification of normal pancreatic duct.

biliary tree was opacified, thus avoiding surgery. The diagnosis by ERCP was incorrect in only five (1.6%) patients. When the biliary tree was partially visualized (Type 2 and Type 3), the diagnosis of biliary atresia was made and confirmed by surgery. When the biliary tree was not opacified and only the pancreatic duct was visualized (Type 1), the diagnosis of biliary atresia was suspected and exploratory laparotomy was indicated. The diagnosis by ERCP was incorrect in only five (1.6%) patients.

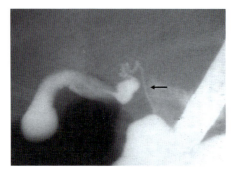

Figure 23.3 Biliary atresia Type 2.Visualization of a narrow and irregular distal common bile duct (*arrow*). Normal cystic duct and gallbladder.

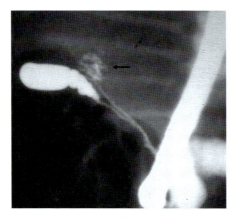

Figure 23.4 Biliary atresia Type 3a in a 25-day-old neonate. Visualization of narrow and irregular distal common bile duct and common hepatic duct with biliary lakes (*arrow*) at the portahepatis.

Miscellaneous genetic cholestatic diseases

In Alagille syndrome, the extrahepatic ducts are normal. ERCP shows marked and diffuse narrowing of the intrahepatic duct and reduced arborization [22, 23]. Congenital hepatic fibrosis is characterized by disordered terminal interlobular bile ducts, which form multiple macroscopic and microscopic cysts (Figure 23.5) that can be demonstrated by ERCP [22]. In Caroli's disease, there are multiple segmental cylindrical or saccular dilatations of small biliary radicles with a normal common bile duct that can be demonstrated by ERCP [22]. Diagnosis of these conditions can be done by MRCP, avoiding needless surgery.

Bile plug syndrome

Bile plug syndrome represents a correctable cause of obstruction of the extrahepatic bile ducts by bile sludge in patients with a normal biliary tract. The diagnosis is suspected by ultrasonography and confirmed by ERCP, which offers

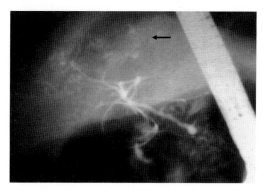

Figure 23.5 Congenital hepatic fibrosis in a 38-day-old infant. Normal extrahepatic ducts. Irregular intrahepatic ducts with multiple small cysts (*arrow*).

therapeutic possibility. Improvements of patients after ERCP suggest that simple irrigation with contrast material may be helpful [22].

Choledochal cyst

Choledochal cyst is a congenital malformation of the biliary tract characterized by saccular dilatation of the biliary tree. Choledochal cyst is primarily a disease of children and young adults, and 60% of reported cases are diagnosed before age 10 [24]. The diagnosis of this congenital malformation of the biliary tract is made by abdominal ultrasound, CT, or MRCP. ERCP confirms the diagnosis and helps surgical planning.

Pathogenesis of choledochal cyst

Many theories have been proposed to explain the development of choledochal cysts. The more generally accepted theory proposes that cysts are acquired. The majority of patients with choledochal cysts have an anomalous pancreaticobiliary union [25–27] located outside the duodenal wall (Figure 23.6) and are not under the influence of the sphincter of Oddi mechanism. According to this theory, there is reflux of pancreatic juice upward into the biliary system that can produce damage to the common duct lining, resulting in saccular dilatation of the duct [28].

The maximum normal length of the common channel in neonates and infants younger than 1 year is 3 mm. It increases with age to a maximum of 5 mm in children and adolescents between 13 and 15 years of age [29].

Classification of anomalous ductal union

There are three types of anomalous ductal union [30]. If it appears that the pancreatic duct is joining the common bile duct, it is denoted as the P–B type. If the common bile duct appears to join the main pancreatic duct, it is denoted as the B–P type, and if there is only a long common channel, it is denoted as the long Y type (Figure 23.7).

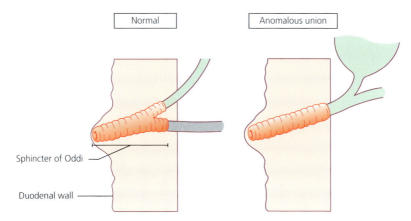

Figure 23.6 The normal pancreaticobiliary union is located within the duodenal wall. The anomalous pancreaticobiliary union is located outside the duodenal wall and is not under the influence of the sphincter of Oddi mechanism.

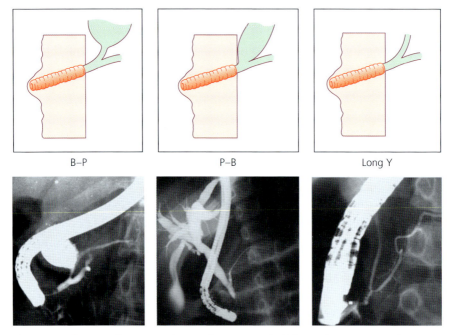

Figure 23.7 There are three types of anomalous pancreaticobiliary union. Type B–P: the common bile duct appears to join the main pancreatic duct. Type P–B: the pancreatic duct joins the common bile duct. Long Y type: there is only a long common channel.

Classification of choledochal cysts

The anatomical classification by Todani *et al.* [31] of bile duct cysts is most often used (Figure 23.8):

Type I   Type I cyst is the most common and accounts for 80–90% of all choledochal cysts [24]. Type I is subdivided into Type A, a typical cyst dilatation of

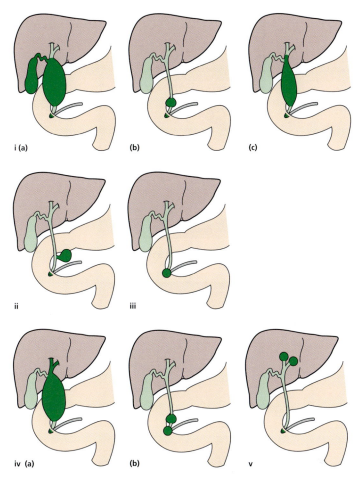

Figure 23.8 Anatomical classification by Todani *et al.* [38] of choledochal cysts. Source: Todani et al 1977 [38]. Reproduced with permission of Elsevier.

the choledochus; Type B, segmental choledochal dilatation; and Type C, diffuse or fusiform dilatation (Figures 23.9 and 23.10).

Type II Type II is a diverticulum anywhere in the extrahepatic duct.

Type III Type III, a choledochocele, involves only the intraduodenal duct.

Type IV Type IV represents multiple intrahepatic and extrahepatic cysts (Figure 23.11).

Type V Type V (Caroli's disease) includes single or multiple intrahepatic cysts.

Choledochocele

Although classified as one of the forms of choledochal cysts, choledochocele is probably not related. It is a rare cause of obstructive jaundice. The diagnosis is established with certainty by ERCP, and it may be effectively treated with endoscopic sphincterotomy [32].

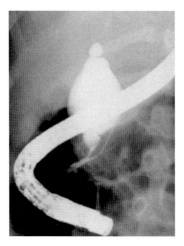

Figure 23.9 Choledochal cyst Type I-C in a 3-year-old female. Note an anomalous Type B–P union.

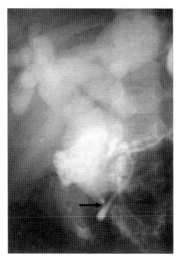

Figure 23.10 Choledochal cyst Type I-C with cystolithiasis (*arrow*).

The presence of a distal bile duct stricture at its point of connection with the pancreatic duct is frequently observed (Figure 23.11). Primary cystolithiasis occurs in 8% of patients and is usually multiple (Figure 23.10), involving intrahepatic and extrahepatic ducts [26].

Patients with long common channel with no cystic dilation in the biliary tree have an increased risk of gallbladder cancer and may develop gallbladder cancer at a younger age [33]. This finding is an indication of prophylactic cholecystectomy.

Treatment of choledochal cysts

The anomalous anatomical configuration of the pancreaticobiliary ductal system observed in most patients with choledochal cysts has certain technical implications with regard to management. In most patients, endoscopic sphincterotomy is

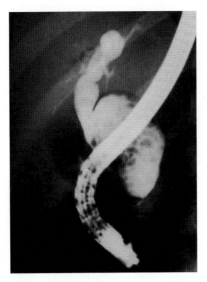

Figure 23.11 Choledochal cyst Type IV-A in a 12-year-old female. Note an anomalous Type B–P union.

probably not indicated, and endoscopic access to the biliary system for removal of stones or sludge is therefore not possible. In selected cases, with fusiform bile duct dilatation and widely dilated common channel, endoscopic sphincterotomy has been attempted, with encouraging results [34]. In patients with Caroli's disease, liver transplantation may be required [35].

Fusiform choledochal dilatation and carcinoma

Fusiform choledochal dilatation, as opposed to cystic dilatation, has been observed to be more commonly associated with low-grade, short strictures located at or distal to the pancreaticobiliary junction. Moreover, carcinoma seldom, if ever, develops in fusiform dilatation [36].

Primary sclerosing cholangitis

In children, primary sclerosing cholangitis is associated with histiocytosis X, immune deficiency states, and, less frequently, patients with reticular cell sarcoma and sickle cell anemia. The association with inflammatory bowel disease is relatively uncommon (14%), suggesting that genetic and immunological features are the most important factors [37].

Most benign biliary strictures in children are due to sclerosing cholangitis. ERCP provides an accurate and sensitive method of diagnosing sclerosing cholangitis. MRCP has been shown to be a useful noninvasive diagnostic technique [38]. The cholangiogram will show pruning of the peripheral biliary tree and areas of stenosis and ectasia. Patients with major ductal strictures are candidates for endoscopic treatment with sphincterotomy and balloon dilatation to relieve the obstruction in order to delay the progression to cirrhosis [2]. However, a

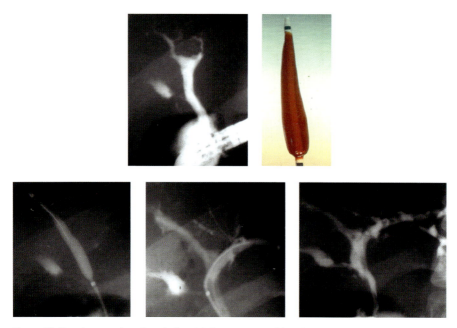

Figure 23.12 Primary sclerosing cholangitis in a 16-year-old male. Severe narrowing of both right and left hepatic ducts without opacification of intrahepatic ducts. A guidewire is introduced into both hepatic ducts. A tapered hydrophilic balloon is fully inflated. Cholangiogram obtained immediately after dilatation shows visualization of irregular areas of stenosis and ectasia of intrahepatic ducts.

dominant stricture that is amenable to therapeutic endoscopic dilation is rare in children. The authors developed a tapered hydrophilic balloon to dilate hepatic duct strictures and to avoid small intrahepatic duct rupture (Figure 23.12) [39].

Parasitic infestation

Ascaris infestation can produce acute biliary obstruction with cholangitis. The worm can be seen with ERCP and can be removed with a tripod basket [22].

Choledocholithiasis

Choledocholithiasis occurs rarely in both infants and children. Conditions associated with the presence of stones include biliary tract malformations such as choledochal cyst, chronic liver disease, hemolysis, infection, prematurity, total parenteral nutrition, and the use of certain medications (e.g., furosemide, ceftriaxone). The diagnostic approach is more difficult, and identification of the cause of obstruction by ultrasonography is often impossible. MRCP is the best noninvasive technique in demonstrating common bile duct stones and is clearly superior to ultrasonography [40]. Gallstones in children are usually black pigment stones consisting of calcium carbonate, which is rarely found in adults [41].

ERCP for stones

The role and value of ERCP and endoscopic sphincterotomy in children with choledocholithiasis are not well established. Sphincterotomy with common bile duct stone removal has been successfully performed in young infants [42], children, and adolescents [2, 43–45]. Endoscopic papillary balloon dilatation with stone extraction is an alternative technique for stone removal. In children, published experience with this technique is limited [45].

Most infants with asymptomatic gallstones and no factors that would make them susceptible to stone formation can be managed conservatively [46]. However, larger stones are less likely to resolve, whereas smaller stones, sludge, and mucus should be able to pass in response to oral feeding without symptoms or complications. In children, sphincterotomy should be reserved for symptomatic patients or those with underlying lithogenic disorders.

A combined endoscopic sphincterotomy with common duct stone extraction followed by laparoscopic cholecystectomy has been successfully reported in children [47]. Although the combined procedure seems to be safe, additional experience is awaited so that the true advantages, limitations, and complications of this approach can be placed into clinical perspective.

Biliary strictures and leaks

Primary stricture

Primary stricture of the common hepatic duct has been reported [48]. Hydrostatic balloon dilatation may be used in the treatment of dominant common duct strictures.

Malignant strictures

Malignant strictures of the common bile duct are uncommon in children and have been successfully bypassed by placement of stents [2–5, 49, 50]. The main indication is to treat the cholestasis prior to starting chemotherapy or undergoing surgery.

Liver transplantation

ERCP is the procedure of choice to treat anastomotic stricture post orthotropic liver transplantation or living related transplantation depending on the type of surgical reconstruction (duct-to-duct anastomosis). An alternative therapy is percutaneous transhepatic cholangiography. ERCP is the procedure of choice in patients with coagulopathy when the biliary tree must be imaged and treated. Biliary strictures can be dilated and stented. The indications for duct-to-duct biliary reconstruction in living donor liver transplantation for small children are still controversial. In a recent study, duct-to-duct anastomosis was compared with Roux-en-Y biliary reconstruction [51]. Living donor liver transplantation was performed in 56 children weighing less than 10 kg. Biliary reconstruction was performed using duct-to-duct procedure in 20 patients and Roux-en-Y in 36 patients. During a minimum of

2 years of follow-up, the incidence of biliary stricture was 5.0% in the duct-to-duct group and 11.1% in the Roux-en-Y group. This study showed that duct-to-duct reconstruction in living donor liver transplantation for small children (weighing less than 10 kg) is a feasible option for biliary reconstruction.

Bile leaks

Bile leaks may be found after blunt abdominal trauma or after cholecystectomy. It can be treated by endoscopic sphincterotomy or with stent placement [52].

Pancreatic findings

Recurrent pancreatitis

ERCP has been found to be useful in the identification of treatable causes in approximately 75% of children with recurrent pancreatitis (Table 23.2) [1–3, 53–56]. Whatever the etiology of pancreatitis, the possibility of an anatomical abnormality amenable to endoscopic therapy or surgery should always be considered.

The timing of performance of an ERCP in children is controversial. In children with idiopathic pancreatitis in whom recovery has occurred with standard medical treatment, there is no consensus as to when an ERCP to look for an obstructive cause is indicated. The potential benefit of proceeding with ERCP after the first episode as opposed to waiting for a second attack of pancreatitis is, of course, in preventing that second episode with its associated morbidity and mortality. No randomized controlled clinical trials have been performed that

Table 23.2 Pancreatic findings in ERCP in children.

Recurrent pancreatitis
Congenital disorders
Biliary anomalies
Choledochal cyst
Anomalous pancreaticobiliary union
Pancreatic anomalies
Pancreas divisum
Annular pancreas
Short pancreas
Cystic dilatation of the pancreatic duct (pancreatocele)
Duodenal anomalies
Duodenal or gastric duplication cysts
Duodenal diverticulum
Acquired disorders
Parasitic infestation: *Ascaris*
Sphincter of Oddi dysfunction
Pancreatic trauma
Acquired immunodeficiency syndrome
Chronic pancreatitis
Pseudocysts

directly address this issue. Although not reported in the literature, it is the experience of the authors that children with normal MRCP after the first episode of pancreatitis should not undergo ERCP.

Choledochal cyst and anomalous pancreaticobiliary union

Choledochal cysts have been associated with recurrent pancreatitis in 6–18% of cases [1, 54, 55]. An anomalous pancreaticobiliary union has been observed in most children with choledochal cysts and recurrent pancreatitis (Figure 23.13) [31, 57]. In this subgroup of patients, SOD has been demonstrated, suggesting that this motor abnormality might be related to the development of recurrent pancreatitis [58]. Moreover, because the sphincter of Oddi muscular segment is located within the duodenal wall, endoscopic sphincterotomy prior to surgery has been performed with excellent results, supporting this theory [58]. Occasionally, pancreatic stones or protein plugs may be endoscopically removed (Figure 23.14) [22]. Choledochocele has been reported in patients with recurrent pancreatitis [22, 59]. Treatment by endoscopic sphincterotomy provides excellent results [55, 60].

Pancreas divisum

Pancreas divisum is a congenital variant caused by failure of fusion of the dorsal and ventral endodermal buds. Each duct drains via its own separate orifice, the major papilla of Vater for the ventral duct of Wirsung, and the minor accessory papilla for the dorsal duct of Santorini.

Prevalence of pancreas divisum

Pancreas divisum is the most common congenital variant of the pancreas. In adults, it has been found in 5–14% of autopsy series and 0.3–8% of ERCP studies [61, 62].

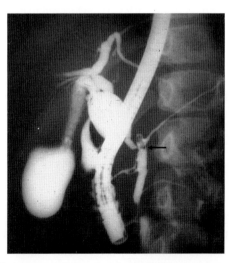

Figure 23.13 Choledochal cyst Type I-A and pancreas divisum in a 5-year-old male with recurrent pancreatitis. A long common channel is observed with pancreatic stones (*arrow*).

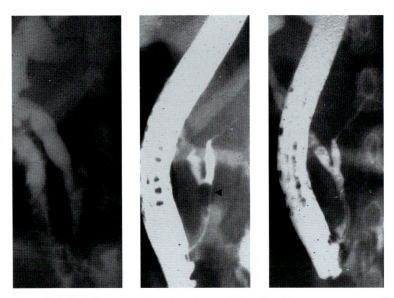

Figure 23.14 Choledochal cyst Type IV-A in a 6-year-old female with recurrent pancreatitis. An anomalous pancreaticobiliary union, long Y type. Stone in the pancreatic duct (*arrow*). After endoscopic sphincterotomy the pancreatic stone is removed with an occlusion balloon (*arrowhead*).

The prevalence of pancreas divisum in children is not known. In our experience with 272 consecutive cases of successful ERCP performed in children, pancreas divisum was found in 9 (3.3%) children [63]. Two patient groups were identified on the basis of the age at which ERCP was performed. Group 1 included 147 neonates or young infants in whom ERCP was performed to evaluate neonatal cholestasis. Two (1.4%) neonates had pancreas divisum, one with neonatal hepatitis and the other with biliary atresia. Group 2 included 125 children older than 1 year in whom ERCP was performed to evaluate pancreatic and biliary disorders. Seven (5.6%) children had pancreas divisum.

Significance of pancreas divisum
The clinical significance of pancreas divisum is controversial. An association between pancreas divisum and pancreatitis has been suggested [61, 62, 64, 65]. However, others have considered it to be a coincidental finding [66, 67]. It appears that the combination of pancreas divisum with minor papilla stenosis would lead to a real functional obstruction. In children with recurrent pancreatitis, pancreas divisum has been found in 9.5% of patients [1, 54, 55, 68, 69].

ERCP diagnosis of pancreas divisum
Cannulation of the major papilla shows a short duct of Wirsung (ventral pancreas) that quickly tapers and undergoes arborization (Figure 23.15). To confirm the diagnosis and proceed with therapy, it is most important to cannulate the minor papilla to demonstrate the dorsal pancreas.

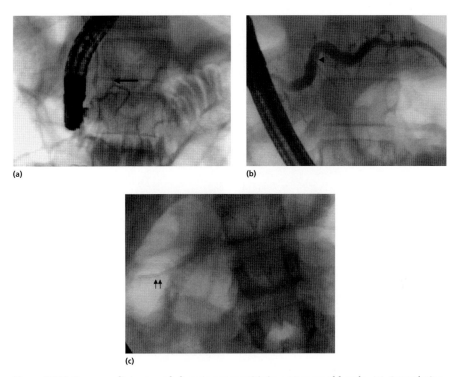

(a)   (b)

(c)

Figure 23.15 Pancreas divisum and chronic pancreatitis in a 12-year-old male. (a) Cannulation of the major papilla shows a normal common duct and a small ventral pancreatic duct (*arrow*). (b) Cannulation of the minor papilla shows a dilated dorsal pancreatic duct (*arrowhead*) with dilated primary and secondary branches. (c) After minor papilla sphincterotomy, a 5 Fr pancreatic stent (*two arrows*) without proximal flaps was left in place for 5 days.

Treatment of pancreas divisum

Surgical minor papilla sphincteroplasty used to be the treatment of choice, with 70% improvement [70]. Endoscopic treatment has been utilized to decompress the dorsal duct by a variety of methods, including endoscopic minor papilla sphincterotomy with insertion of an endoprosthesis.

Endoscopic sphincterotomy of the minor papilla is indicated in patients with documented pancreatitis. It has been attempted in conjunction with temporary stent placement in the dorsal pancreatic duct (Figures 23.16 and 23.17), and has led to improvement in approximately 75% of children [1–3, 55]. Overall, these results indicate that in certain children with recurrent pain or pancreatitis and pancreas divisum, endoscopic therapy can offer complete resolution or improvement of symptoms.

Other pancreatic congenital anomalies

Annular pancreas has been associated with recurrent pancreatitis in children [55, 71]. However, the relationship with pancreatitis is unclear. In 14 cases of annular pancreas reported in the English literature, there were 5 with coexistent

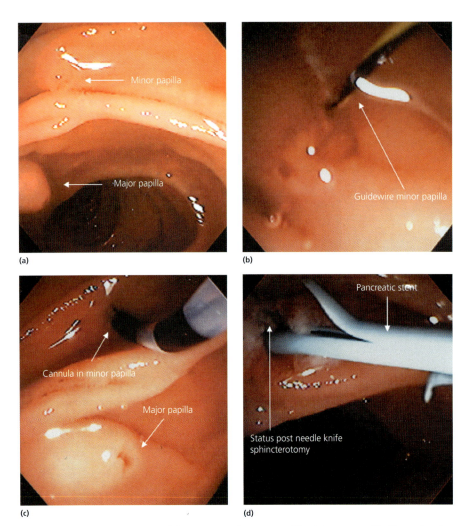

Figure 23.16 Endoscopic view of the major and minor papilla. (a) A tapered balloon (3 Fr) is used to cannulate the minor papilla. (b) A guidewire is introduced into the dorsal pancreas. (c) A 5 Fr pancreatic stent is introduced into the dorsal pancreas. (d) A sphincterotomy of the minor papilla is performed with a needle–knife sphincterotome over the pancreatic stent.

pancreas divisum, suggesting that pancreas divisum occurs more often in the presence of annular pancreas than in the general population [71]. This association may explain pancreatitis in some patients. Annular pancreas can be diagnosed later in life when a patient is admitted with duodenal obstruction.

Other pancreatic congenital anomalies found to cause pancreatitis include short pancreas [54, 72] and cystic dilatation or pancreatocele of the distal pancreatic duct.

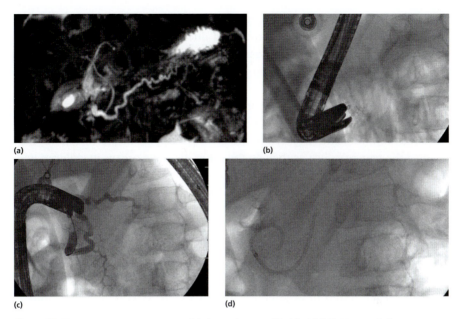

Figure 23.17 Recurrent acute pancreatitis in an 8-year-old girl. (a) MRCP revealed a dilated dorsal duct that drains into the minor papilla consistent with pancreas divisum. (b) Pancreatogram via the major papilla revealed a small ventral duct. (c) Pancreatogram via the minor papilla revealed a dilated dorsal duct without.

Duodenal duplication cyst

Duodenal duplication cyst is a congenital anomaly that has been associated with recurrent pancreatitis due to intermittent obstruction of the pancreatic duct [73]. ERCP has been shown to be useful in the diagnosis as well as for definitive treatment. If the cyst is bulging into the intestinal lumen, a wide cystoduodenostomy can be endoscopically performed, with excellent results [74].

Sphincter of Oddi dysfunction

Sphincter of Oddi manometry is the diagnostic procedure of choice for this functional motor disorder. It was found in children with recurrent pancreatitis [2, 11, 55]. These patients are generally treated by standard biliary sphincterotomy and, in general, they do not respond well [14] presumably because the pancreatic sphincter is not transected. Recurrent attacks of pancreatitis may be attributed to an affected pancreatic sphincter [75]. Dual endoscopic sphincterotomy of the pancreatic and common duct sphincters may be necessary to improve outcome [2, 55]. However, the safety and efficacy of sphincter of Oddi manometry and sphincterotomy in the pediatric population await further study.

Pancreatic trauma

Recent evidence has suggested that it is safe to perform ERCP soon after traumatic pancreatitis and it may be helpful in identifying the need for endoscopic therapy with stent placement or surgery at the same time [76, 77]. Early ERCP may identify the presence and location of duct leakage. Patients with normal pancreatogram are treated conservatively. Surgical resection or reconstruction is reserved for cases in which stenting is impossible or fails.

Acquired immunodeficiency syndrome

Little has been written regarding pancreatic involvement in children with acquired immunodeficiency syndrome (AIDS). Opportunistic infections may involve the pancreas, just as they do the other digestive organs in children with AIDS. Most common are cytomegalovirus and *Cryptosporidium*, followed by *Pneumocystis carinii*, *Toxoplasma gondii*, and *Mycobacterium avium*. ERCP has been shown to be useful in the evaluation and treatment of children with AIDS [78]. Pancreatic duct dilatation in two children with pancreatic duct stricture produced significant clinical improvement of pain.

Chronic pancreatitis

ERCP has been found to be useful in the treatment of chronic pancreatitis in 14–69% of children with recurrent pancreatitis [1–5, 55]. In children with chronic pancreatitis, debilitating pain and recurrent attacks may be caused by strictures of the main duct, pancreatic stones, or pseudocysts that impair the normal outflow of pancreatic secretions. ERCP demonstrates evidence of these abnormalities that can be treated endoscopically [1–5, 18, 55, 79].

Children with chronic pancreatitis frequently have an underlying genetic mutation (PRSS1, CFTR, SPINK1, CTRC, and others) as etiological factor, and endotherapy may be of help but a group of nonresponders with debilitating pain may benefit from total pancreatectomy with islet autotransplantation [69].

Endoscopic treatment of chronic pancreatitis in children

The aim of endoscopic therapy is based on the concept of pancreatic duct decompression. Pancreatic sphincterotomy has been performed to improve pancreatic drainage and to allow intraductal therapeutic maneuvers, severe stenosis has been dilated and bypassed with stents, and obstructing ductal stones have been removed in some cases after fragmentation by electrohydraulic lithotripsy or extracorporeal shock-wave lithotripsy (Figure 23.17). These endoscopic techniques constitute an excellent alternative to relieve frequent recurrent or chronic abdominal pancreatic pain and to avoid early surgical interventions.

Endoscopic pancreatic therapy in childhood is well tolerated, safe, and likely to be technically successful in experienced hands. Overall, there is an 80% short-term symptomatic improvement after pancreatic endoscopic therapy in children with chronic pancreatitis [1–5, 55, 79]. A longer follow-up period will be necessary to determine whether endoscopic success produces long-standing clinical improvement.

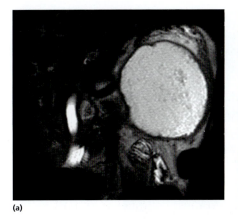
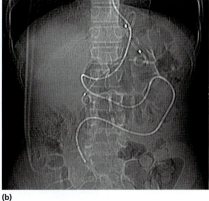

(a)   (b)

Figure 23.18 A 12-year-old girl was kicked by a horse in the abdomen with subsequent development of pancreatitis. Two weeks later the patient was referred for the treatment of symptomatic pseudocyst with likely main pancreatic ductal disruption. (a) MRCP revealed an 8 × 9 × 10 cm peripancreatic pseudocyst compressing the stomach. (b) Treatment with a transgastric 10 Fr × 4 cm double pig tail stent, 5 Fr × 7 cm main pancreatic duct stent and a nasojejunal feeding tube was successfully performed. Six weeks later documentation of complete resolution was obtained by CT and the stent pulled out.

Pancreatic pseudocysts

Pancreatic pseudocysts are common complications of acute and chronic pancreatitis. Most of the pseudocysts resolve spontaneously. Treatment is indicated only in symptomatic patients with abdominal pain, biliary obstruction, or early satiety, and nausea and vomiting suggesting and outlet obstruction (gastric or duodenal). Endoscopy is the treatment of choice with or without endoscopic ultrasound depending on the presence or absence of a good bulge. These techniques have become the first line of therapy when available. An alternative is surgical or percutaneous drainage. Endoscopic methods include endoscopic cystogastrostomy (Figure 23.18), cystoduodenostomy, and transpapillary drainage (Figure 23.19). In adults, successful pseudocyst resolution has been reported in approximately 80% of cases (Figure 23.20) [80]. As with other therapeutic interventions, pediatric experience is limited [81].

Outstanding issues and future trends

ERCP is an established procedure in children. Even though there are an increased number of pediatric gastroenterologists performing ERCP, the number of cases is not enough for them to gain proficiency. Currently, ERCP has become a therapeutic procedure and is rarely used for diagnostic purposes. The adult therapeutic endoscopist is currently working together with the pediatric team

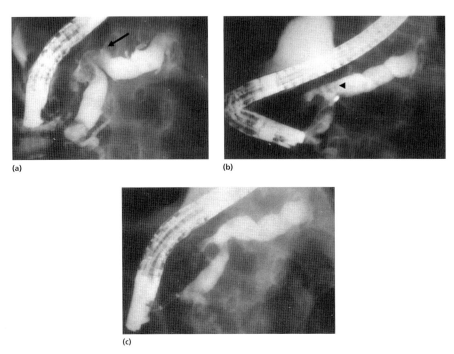

(a) (b)

(c)

Figure 23.19 Chronic pancreatitis in a 14-year-old female with hereditary pancreatitis. (a) Big pancreatic stones at the junction of the head and body of the pancreatic duct (*arrow*). (b) Two days after pancreatic sphincterotomy, followed by extracorporeal shock-wave lithotripsy, multiple small residual stones (*arrowhead*) are retrieved with a Dormia basket. (c) After a month, a follow-up ERCP showed a dilated pancreatic duct without stones.

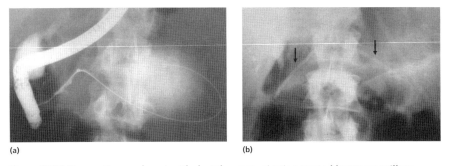

(a) (b)

Figure 23.20 Pancreatic pseudocyst with ductal communication treated by transpapillary pancreatic duct endoprosthesis in a 13-year-old female. (a) After endoscopic sphincterotomy of the biliary and pancreatic sphincters, a guidewire is introduced into the cystic cavity. (b) A 7 Fr stent (arrows) is placed beyond the stricture.

and doing most of these cases. Well-trained pediatric therapeutic endoscopists are needed and few are already in the field with a large number of cases.

This has become more apparent since, nowadays, ERCP is less diagnostic and more therapeutic. It is my belief that, in the future, ERCP in children will be performed by highly trained endoscopists working in tertiary care facilities, which maintain a high volume of such activity. Further studies should be directed to assess the usefulness of MRCP in the diagnosis of biliopancreatic diseases in children. In general, children with suspected biliary and pancreatic disease should undergo MRI with MRCP before ERCP is considered, with the latter being reserved for therapy.

References

1 Varadarajulu S, Wilcox CM, Hawes RH, Cotton PB. Technical outcomes and complications of ERCP in children. *Gastrointest Endosc* 2004;60:367–371.

2 Cheng CL, Fogel EL, Sherman S, *et al.* Diagnostic and therapeutic endoscopic retrograde cholangiopancreatography in children: a large series report. *J Pediatr Gastroenterol Nutr* 2005;41:445–453.

3 Iqbal CW, Baron TH, Moir CR, Ishitani MB. Post-ERCP pancreatitis in pediatric patients. *J Pediatr Gastroenterol Nutr* 2009;49:430–434.

4 Jang JY, Yoon CH, Kim KM. Endoscopic retrograde cholangiopancreatography in pancreatic and biliary tract disease in Korean children. *World J Gastroenterol* 2010;16:490–495.

5 Otto AK, Neal MD, Slivka AN, Kane TD. An appraisal of endoscopic retrograde cholangiopancreatography (ERCP) for pancreaticobiliary disease in children: our institutional experience in 231 cases. *Surg Endosc* 2011;25:2536–2540.

6 Fox VL, Werlin SL, Heyman MB. ERCP in children: a position statement from the North American Society for Pediatric Gastroenterology and Nutrition. *J Pediatr Gastroenterol Nutr* 2000;30:335–342.

7 Guelrud M, Jaen D, Torres P, *et al.* Endoscopic cholangiopancreatography in the infant: evaluation of a new prototype pediatric duodenoscope. *Gastrointest Endosc* 1987;33:4–8.

8 Derkx HH, Huibregtse K, Taminiau JA. The role of endoscopic retrograde cholangiopancreatography in cholestatic infants. *Endoscopy* 1994;26:724–728.

9 Shteyer E, Wengrower D, Benuri-Silbiger I, *et al.* Endoscopic retrograde cholangiopancreatography in neonatal cholestasis. *J Pediatr Gastroenterol Nutr* 2012;55:142–145.

10 Wilkinson ML, Mieli-Vergani G, Ball C, *et al.* Endoscopic retrograde cholangiopancreatography in infantile cholestasis. *Arch Dis Child* 1991;66:121–123.

11 Brown CW, Werlin SL, Geenen JE, Schmalz M. The diagnostic and therapeutic role of endoscopic retrograde cholangiopancreatography in children. *J Pediatr Gastroenterol Nutr* 1993;17:19–23.

12 Buckley A, Connon JJ. The role of ERCP in children and adolescents. *Gastrointest Endosc* 1990;36:369–372.

13 Cotton PB, Laage NJ. Endoscopic retrograde cholangiopancreatography in children. *Arch Dis Child* 1982;57:131–136.

14 Hsu RK, Draganov P, Leung JW, *et al.* Therapeutic ERCP in the management of pancreatitis in children. *Gastrointest Endosc* 2000;51:396–400.

15 Lemmel T, Hawes R, Sherman S, *et al.* Endoscopic evaluation and therapy of recurrent pancreatitis and pancreaticobiliary pain in the pediatric population. *Gastrointest Endosc* 1994;40:A54.

16 Putnam PE, Kocoshis SA, Orenstein SR, Schade RR. Pediatric endoscopic retrograde cholangiopancreatography. *Am J Gastroenterol* 1991;86:824–830.

17 Tagge EP, Tarnasky PR, Chandler J, *et al.* Multidisciplinary approach to the treatment of pediatric pancreaticobiliary disorders. *J Pediatr Surg* 1997;32:158–164.

18 Poddar U, Thapa BR, Bhasin DK, *et al.* Endoscopic retrograde cholangiopancreatography in the management of pancreaticobiliary disorders in children. *J Gastroenterol Hepatol* 2001;16: 927–931.

19 Elmunzer BJ, Scheiman JM, Lehman GA, *et al.* A randomized trial of rectal indomethacin to prevent post-ERCP pancreatitis. *N Engl J Med* 2012;366:1414–1422.

20 (a)Balistreri WF. Neonatal cholestasis. *J Pediatr* 1985;106:171–184. (b)Virginia M, Deborah F, Whitington PF, *et al.* Guideline for the evaluation of cholestatic jaundice in infants: recommendations of the North American Society for pediatric gastroenterology, hepatology and nutrition. *J Pediatr Gastroenterol Nutr* 2004;39:115–128.

21 (a)Sevilla A, Howman-Gile R, Saleh H, *et al.* Hepatobiliaryscintigraphy with SPECT in infancy. *Clin Nucl Med* 2007;32:16–23. (b)Guelrud M, Jaen D, Mendoza S. *et al.* ERCP in the diagnosis of extrahepatic biliary atresia. *Gastrointest Endosc* 1991;37:522–526.

22 Guelrud M, Carr-Locke D, Fox VL. *ERCP in Pediatric Practice: Diagnosis and Treatment.* Oxford: Isis Medical Media Ltd., 1997.

23 Morelli A, Pelli MA, VedovelliA, *et al.* Endoscopic retrograde cholangiopancreatography study in Alagille's syndrome: first report. *Am J Gastroenterol* 1983;78:241–244.

24 Yamaguchi M. Congenital choledochal cyst: analysis of 1433 patients in the Japanese literature. *Am J Surg* 1980;140:653–657.

25 Arima E, Akita H. Congenital biliary tract dilatation and anomalous junction of the pancreaticobiliary system. *J Pediatr Surg* 1979;14:9–15.

26 Oguchi Y, Okada A, Nakamura T, *et al.* Histopathologic studies of congenital dilatation of the bile duct as related to an anomalous junction of the pancreaticobiliary ductal system: clinical and experimental studies. *Surgery* 1988;103:168–173.

27 Ikada A, Nakamura T, Higaki J, *et al.* Congenital dilatation of the bile duct in 100 instances and its relationship with anomalous junction. *Surg Gynecol Obstet* 1990;171:291–298.

28 Babbitt DP. Congenital choledochal cysts: new etiological concept based on anomalous relationship of common bile duct and pancreatic bulb. *Ann Radiol* 1969;12:231–240.

29 Guelrud M, Morera C, Rodriguez M, *et al.* Normal and anomalous pancreaticobiliary union in children and adolescents. *Gastrointest Endosc* 1999;50:189–193.

30 Misra SP, Dwivedi M. Pancreaticobiliary ductal union. *Gut* 1990;31:1144–1149.

31 Todani T, Watanabe Y, Narusue M. Congenital bile duct cyst. *Am J Surg* 1977;134:263–269.

32 Venu RP, Geenen JE, Hogan WJ, *et al.* Role of endoscopic retrograde cholangiopancreatography in the diagnosis and treatment of choledochocele. *Gastroenterology* 1984;87: 1144–1149.

33 Hu B, Gong B, Zhou DY. Association of anomalous pancreaticobiliary ductal junction with gallbladder carcinoma in Chinese patients: an ERCP study. *Gastrointest Endosc* 2003;57: 541–545.

34 Ng WD, Liu K, Wong MK, *et al.* Endoscopic sphincterotomy in young patients with choledochal dilatation and a long common channel: a preliminary report. *Br J Surg* 1992;79:550–552.

35 Yonem O, Bayraktar Y. Clinical characteristics of Caroli's disease. *World J Gastroenterol* 2007;13:1930–1933.

36 Todani T, Watanabe Y, Fujii T, *et al.* Cylindrical dilatation of the choledochus: a special type of congenital bile duct dilatation. *Surgery* 1985;98:964–968.

37 Debray D, Pariente D, Urroas E, *et al.* Sclerosing cholangitis in children. *J Pediatr* 1994;124:49–56.

38 Ferrara C, Valeri G, Salvolini L, Giovagnoni A. Magnetic resonance cholangiopancreatography in primary sclerosing cholangitis in children. *Pediatr Radiol* 2002;32:413–417.

39 Guelrud M, Mendoza S, Guelrud A. A tapered balloon with hydrophilic coating to dilate difficult hilar biliary strictures. *Gastrointest Endosc* 1995;41:246–249.

40 Arcement CM, Meza MP, Arumania S, Towbin RB. MRCP in the evaluation of pancreaticobiliary disease in children. *Pediatr Radiol* 2001;31:92–97.

41 Stringer MD, Taylor DR, Soloway RD. Gallstone composition: are children different? *J Pediatr* 2003;142:435–440.

42 Guelrud M, Daoud G, Mendoza S, *et al.* Endoscopic sphincterotomy in a 6-month-old infant with choledocholithiasis and double gallbladder. *Am J Gastroenterol* 1994;89:1587–1589.

43 Guelrud M, Mendoza S, Jaen D, *et al.* ERCP and endoscopic sphincterotomy in infants and children with jaundice due to common bile duct stones. *Gastrointest Endosc* 1992;38:450–453.

44 Man DW, Spitz L. Choledocholithiasis in infancy. *J PediatrSurg* 1985;20:65–68.

45 Tarnasky PR, Tagge EP, Hebra A, *et al.* Minimally invasive therapy for choledocholithiasis in children. *Gastrointest Endosc* 1998;47:189–192.

46 Wesdorp I, Bosman D, de Graaff A, *et al.* Clinical presentations and predisposing factors of cholelithiasis and sludge in children. *Pediatr Gastroenterol Nutr* 2000;31:411–417.

47 Guelrud M, Zambrano V, Jaen D, *et al.* Endoscopic sphincterotomy and laparoscopic cholecystectomy in a jaundiced infant. *Gastrointest Endosc* 1994;40:99–102.

48 Chapoy PR, Kendall RS, Fonkalsrud E, Ament ME. Congenital stricture of the common hepatic duct: an unusual case without jaundice. *Gastroenterology* 1981;80:380–383.

49 Bickerstaff KI, Britton BJ, Gough MH. Endoscopic palliation of malignant biliary obstruction in a child. *Br J Surg* 1989;76:1092–1093.

50 Guelrud M, Mendoza S, Zager A, Noguera C. Biliary stenting in an infant with malignant obstructive jaundice. *Gastrointest Endosc* 1989;35:259–261.

51 Yamamoto H, Hayashida S, Asonuma K, *et al.* Single center experience and long-term outcomes of duct-to-duct biliary reconstruction in infantile living donor liver transplantation. *Liver Transpl* 2014;20:347–354.

52 Ulitsky A, Werlin S, Dua KS. Role of ERCP in the management of non-iatrogenic traumatic bile duct injuries in the pediatric population. *Gastrointest Endosc* 2011;73:823–827.

53 Blustein PK, Gaskin K, Filler R, *et al.* Endoscopic retrograde cholangiopancreatography in pancreatitis in children and adolescents. *Pediatrics* 1981;68:387–393.

54 Forbes A, Leung JW, Cotton PB. Relapsing acute and chronic pancreatitis. *Arch Dis Child* 1984;59:927–934.

55 Guelrud M, Mujica C, Jaen D, *et al.* The role of ERCP in the diagnosis and treatment of idiopathic recurrent pancreatitis in children and adolescents. *Gastrointest Endosc* 1994;40:428–436.

56 Agarwal J, Nageshwar Reddy D, Talukdar R, *et al.* ERCP in the management of pancreatic diseases in children. *Gastrointest Endosc* 2014;79:271–278.

57 Mori K, Nagakawa T, Ohta T, *et al.* Pancreatitis and anomalous union of the pancreaticobiliary ductal system in childhood. *J Pediatr Surg* 1993;28:67–71.

58 Guelrud M, Morera C, Rodriguez M, *et al.* Sphincter of Oddi dysfunction in children with recurrent pancreatitis and anomalous pancreaticobiliary union: an etiologic concept. *Gastrointest Endosc* 1999;50:194–199.

59 Weisser M, Bennek J, Hormann D. Choledochocele—a rare cause of necrotizing pancreatitis in childhood. *Eur J Pediatr Surg* 2000;10:258–264.

60 Siegel JH, Harding GT, Chateau F. Endoscopic incision of choledochal cysts (choledochocele). *Endoscopy* 1981;13:200–202.

61 Cotton PB. Congenital anomaly of pancreas divisum as a cause of obstructive pain and pancreatitis. *Gut* 1980;21:105–114.

62 Bernard JP, Sahel J, Giovanni M, Sarles H. Pancreas divisum is a probable cause of acute pancreatitis: a report of 137 cases. *Pancreas* 1990;5:248–254.

63 Guelrud M. The incidence of pancreas divisum in children [letter].*Gastrointest Endosc* 1996;43:83–84.

64 Cotton PB. Pancreas divisum. Curiosity or culprit? *Gastroenterology* 1985;89:1431–1435.

65 Richter JM, Shapiro RH, Mulley AG, Warshaw AL. Association of pancreas divisum and pancreatitis, and its treatment by sphincterotomy of the accessory ampulla. *Gastroenterology* 1981;81:1104–1110.

66 Delhaye M, Engelholm L, Cremer M. Pancreas divisum: congenital anatomic variant or anomaly? Contribution of endoscopic retrograde dorsal pancreatography. *Gastroenterology* 1985;89:951–958.

67 Gelrud A, Sheth S, Banerjee S, *et al*. Analysis of cystic fibrosis gener product (CFTR) function in patients with pancreas divisum and recurrent acute pancreatitis. *Am J Gastroenterol* 2004;99:1557–1562.

68 Enestvedt BK, TofaniCh, Lee DY, *et al*. Endoscopic retrograde cholangiopancreatography in the pediatric population is safe and efficacious. *J Pediatr Gastroenterol Nutr* 2013;57: 649–654.

69 Bellin MD, Freeman ML, Gelrud A, Total pancreatectomy and islet autotransplantation in chronic pancreatitis: recommendations from Pancreas Fest. *Pancreatology* 2014;14:27–35.

70 Warshaw AL, Simeone JF, Schapiro RH, Flavin-Warshaw B. Evaluation and treatment of the dominant dorsal duct syndrome (pancreas divisum redefined). *Am J Surg* 1990;159:59–64.

71 Lehman GA, O'Connor KW. Coexistence of annular pancreas and pancreas divisum – ERCP diagnosis. *Gastrointest Endosc* 1985;31:25–28.

72 Yanni GS, Gibbs LH, Nguyen S, Young LW. P0814 pancreatitis in a congenital short pancreas of a child. A case report. *J Pediatr Gastroenterol Nutr* 2004;39:366.

73 Lavine JE, Harrison M, Heyman MB. Gastrointestinal duplications causing relapsing pancreatitis in children. *Gastroenterology* 1989;97:1556–1558.

74 Johanson JF, Geenen JE, Hogan WJ, Huibregtse K. Endoscopic therapy of a duodenal duplication cyst. *Gastrointest Endosc* 1992;38:60–64.

75 Guelrud M, Siegel JH. Hypertensive pancreatic duct sphincter as a cause of pancreatitis. Successful treatment with hydrostatic balloon dilatation. *Dig Dis Sci* 1984;29:225–231.

76 Rescorla FJ, Plumley DA, Sherman S, *et al*. The efficacy of early ERCP in pediatric pancreatic trauma. *J Pediatr Surg* 1995;30:336–340.

77 Canty TG, Weinman D. Treatment of pancreatic duct disruption in children by an endoscopically placed stent. *J Pediatr Surg* 2001 Feb;36(2):345–348.

78 Yabut B, Werlin SL, Havens P, *et al*. Endoscopic retrograde cholangiopancreatography in children with HIV infection. *J Pediatr Gastroenterol Nutr* 1996;23:624–627.

79 Kozarek RA, Christie D, Barclay G. Endoscopic therapy of pancreatitis in the pediatric population. *Gastrointest Endosc* 1993;39:665–669.

80 Cremer M, Deviere J, Engelholm L. Endoscopic management of cysts and pseudocysts in chronic pancreatitis: long-term follow-up after 7 years of experience. *Gastrointest Endosc* 1989;35:1–9.

81 Makin E, Harrison PM, Patel S, Davenport M. Pancreatic pseudocysts in children: treatment by endoscopic cyst gastrostomy. *J Pediatr Gastroenterol Nutr* 2012;55:556–558.

SECTION 4

Quality and Safety

CHAPTER 24

Adverse events: definitions, avoidance, and management

Peter B. Cotton[1] & Mohammad Yaghoobi[2]

[1] *Digestive Disease Center, Medical University of South Carolina, Charleston, USA*
[2] *Advanced Endoscopy Program, Division of Gastroenterology and Hepatology, Medical University of South Carolina, Charleston, USA*

KEY POINTS

- Endoscopists' experience, preprocedure risk assessment, early detection, and appropriate management of the adverse events of ERCP are the keys to minimize the risks.

- Acute pancreatitis is the most common serious post-ERCP adverse event. Multiple patient- and procedure-related risk factors are identified. Prophylactic pancreatic stent placement and rectal nonsteroidal anti-inflammatory drugs (NSAIDs) decrease the rate of post-ERCP pancreatitis. The decision on using either or both methods should be individualized based on risk factors and expertise.

- Perforation can occur as a result of guidewire penetration, sphincterotomy, luminal trauma, or stent migration. Conservative management is appropriate in most cases but most luminal perforations need surgical and/or endoscopic intervention.

- Infection should be suspected when fever occurs following ERCP. Cholangitis when the procedure fails to provide drainage is the most worrisome infection but nosocomial infection, cholecystitis, or pancreatic sepsis can occur. Adequate drainage and antibiotic prophylaxis in high-risk patients decrease the risk.

- Bleeding is considered an adverse event when it is evident after termination of ERCP. Coagulopathy is the most common risk factor. Correcting coagulopathy, endoscopic and endovascular examination and/or treatment, and surgery are the mainstay of management.

- Cardiopulmonary, sedation-related, and stent-related complications are other adverse events. Rarely, death can occur as a consequence of post-ERCP complications.

- The risk of medico-legal action after an adverse event is greatly reduced if the endoscopist and team communicate well and sympathetically with the patient and family before and after the procedure.

ERCP: The Fundamentals, Second Edition. Edited by Peter B. Cotton and Joseph Leung.
© 2015 John Wiley & Sons, Ltd. Published 2015 by John Wiley & Sons, Ltd.
Companion Website: www.wiley.com\go\cotton\ercp

There are several reasons why patients (and family members) may be unhappy after their endoscopic retrograde cholangiopancreatography (ERCP) procedures. They may be technically unsuccessful, completed but clinically unhelpful, or be complicated by an adverse event. Customers may be unhappy even when the procedures are entirely successful, if the process is inefficient or the staff unsympathetic.

Our main goal in this chapter is to describe adverse events, their avoidance and management.

Adverse events

There are many ways in which ERCP procedures may not go smoothly, with a spectrum of severity from fairly trivial "incidents" (such as transient bleeding, which stops or is stopped during the procedure) to life-threatening complications (such as a perforation). Most adverse events are recognized during or shortly after procedures, but they can happen beforehand (e.g., as a result of some aspect of preparation), and some are apparent only later (e.g., delayed bleeding after sphincterotomy).

The level of severity at which an unwanted incident becomes an adverse event statistic is an arbitrary decision, but important, since definitions are essential if meaningful data are to be collected and compared. A consensus workshop in 1991 proposed a simple definition that the event was significant enough to require admission to hospital for treatment (or prolongation of existing admission). It also suggested some levels of severity, mainly determined by the length of admission. Those guidelines have been used widely, and were updated in 2010 by a multidisciplinary workshop sponsored by American Society for Gastrointestinal Endoscopy (ASGE) (covering all types of endoscopic procedures). It proposed a new definition.

Definition: an adverse event is one that
- Prevents completion of the planned procedure (because of an event, not simply for technical reasons), or
- Within 14 days, has clinical results that need treatment involving
  - Unplanned or prolonged hospital admission, or
  - Another procedure (requiring sedation/anesthesia), or
  - Consultation with other specialist

Incidents therefore are unplanned events that do not reach this threshold. Some should be documented (e.g., episodes of hypoxia or transient bleeding) for quality improvement purposes.

The workshop refined the grading of event severity, as shown in Table 24.1.

Table 24.1 Severity grading for adverse events.

Consequence	Grade				
	Incident	Mild	Moderate	Severe	Fatal
procedure completed, no sequelae	X				
procedure aborted (or not started)		X			
post-procedure medical consultation		X			
unplanned anesthesia/ventilation support			X		
unplanned hospital admission ≤3 nights		X			
unplanned admission 4–10 nights			X		
unplanned admission >10 nights				X	
ICU admission				X	
transfusion			X		
repeat endoscopy for AE			X		
interventional radiology for AE			X		
surgery for AE				X	
permanent disability (specify)				X	
death					X

Overall rates and factors affecting them

The chance of suffering an adverse event depends on many clinical and technical factors, which will be discussed. In general terms, pancreatitis occurs in about 1 in 20 procedures, and bleeding, perforation, infection, and cardiopulmonary problems each in about 1 in 100 cases. Procedure-related death is a very rare event.

An important issue affecting the accuracy of reported data is the method of collection. Retrospective studies are known to underestimate complication rates, since many delayed events are missed. This may apply particularly to the centers catering to large volumes (who publish) since the encounters are often brief and most patients return home, often some distance away, for further care. The most reliable data come from prospective studies, which include a routine follow-up visit or call, but this is labor-intensive and rarely done outside of research studies.

Details of the predictors of risks for specific events, methods to minimize them, and recommendations for management are given later. General risks include the skill of the individual endoscopist (and team), the clinical status of the patient, and the precise nature of the procedure.

Expertise

There are now many series showing that more experienced endoscopists (and centers) have more success and lower rates of complications than those who are less active, even when dealing with more complex cases. This fact has important implications for training, credentialing, and informed consent. Failures carry risks of the subsequent needed interventions as well.

General patient-related issues

Much attention has been paid to analyzing the characteristics of patients that may affect the risk of performing ERCP [1, 2]. These must be recognized before planned procedures, and some can be mitigated, as outlined in Chapter 5(Joe R).

Many studies now testify to the safety of performing diagnostic and therapeutic procedures in infants, children, and the elderly. However, a Norwegian prospective multicenter cohort study on 2808 patients (half older than 70) identified age as an independent predictor of severe post-ERCP adverse events [3].

Adverse events are more likely to occur in patients who are already severely ill, for example, with acute cholangitis [4], and in those with substantial comorbidities. The most important comorbidities are cardiopulmonary fragility (posing risks for sedation and anesthesia), immunosuppression, and coagulopathies (including therapeutic anticoagulation) [1, 2]. The American Society of Anesthesiologists (ASA) score is used as a broad guide to the risk for sedation and anesthesia.

ERCP appears to be safe when needed in pregnancy. With suitable precautions, patients with implanted pacemakers or defibrillators can be treated safely.

Procedure indication and specific techniques

Complexity and risk in general travel together, as enshrined in the scale described in Chapter 1. Thus, ampullectomy and pseudocyst drainage are likely more risky than simple bile duct stone extraction. It has become clear that performing ERCP procedures in patients with obscure abdominal pain ("suspected sphincter dysfunction") is especially dangerous. This was emphasized strongly by the National Institutes of Health (NIH) State-of-the-Science Conference on ERCP in 2002 [5]. Sadly, it is true that "ERCP is most dangerous for those who need it least" [6].

The precise therapeutic intervention, for example, sphincterotomy, influences the likely risk. These will be discussed within each event category.

Pancreatitis

Pancreatitis is the most common complication of ERCP and sphincterotomy.

Definitions

Serum amylase and lipase levels can be shown to rise in almost every patient if measured within a few hours of ERCP, even sometimes when the pancreatic duct has not been opacified. While this indicates some irritation of the pancreas, it does not constitute clinically relevant pancreatitis. The 1991 consensus workshop suggested this working definition of post-ERCP pancreatitis [7]: "Pancreatitis after ERCP is a clinical illness with typical pain, associated with at least a threefold increase in serum amylase (or lipase) at 24 h, with symptoms impressive enough to require admission to hospital for treatment (or extension of an existing or planned admission)." Severity was graded as mild if hospitalization is needed for less than 3 nights, moderate if 4–9 nights, and severe if more than 10 nights, or if patients require intensive care or surgical treatment. These categories have been widely used in subsequent endoscopic series.

Incidence and severity

The reported incidence of pancreatitis ranges widely, from less than 1% up to as high as 40%. This huge variation can be attributed to different definitions, different methods for data collection, and especially to differing case mixes. Ranges of 2–9% are representative of more recent prospective series, mostly using consensus definitions [8]. A population-based study of 97 810 ERCPs in Canada reported a pancreatitis rate of 2.2%, with greater risk in younger patients and in women [9]. Most cases are mild (<3 days in hospital), about 20% moderate (3–10 days), 5% severe, and 1% fatal. A relatively similar rate of 3.1% has been reported in another large multicenter prospective study on 2808 ERCPs [3].

Risk factors

Any ERCP procedure can cause pancreatitis, but certain factors are well known to increase the risk.

Patient factors. It is now abundantly clear that pancreatitis is most likely to occur in younger patients with a healthy pancreas, such as women with obscure abdominal pain and "suspected sphincter of Oddi dysfunction." The consensus panel at the 2002 NIH State-of-the-Science Conference on ERCP made the following statement: "It is precisely the typical SOD patient profile (young, healthy female) that is at the highest risk for ERCP-induced severe pancreatitis and even death." A meta-analysis including 10 997 patients showed a rate of 10.3% in those with sphincter of Oddi dysfunction (SOD) as compared to only 3.9% in those without the condition [10]. There is also an increased risk in patients with prior attacks of acute pancreatitis (both spontaneous and ERCP-induced). Conversely, the risk is less in patients with chronic pancreatitis. A normal-sized bile duct was earlier believed to increase the risk of post-ERCP pancreatitis, but this is a surrogate for sphincter dysfunction, and does not apply to patients with stones.

Techniques. Pancreatitis is more likely to occur with aggressive manipulation of the pancreatic orifice [8], and with repeated injections of contrast, sometimes evidenced by acinarization or the appearance of a urogram. The importance of increased pressure in the duct is supported by the old observation that postprocedure pancreatitis is less likely in patients who have a patent duct of Santorini.

For a long time, it was believed that sphincter manometry was a potent cause of pancreatitis. However, it is now clear that manometry is simply a surrogate for SOD, which is the real culprit [11].

Several studies now indicate that standard biliary sphincterotomy does not markedly increase the overall risk of pancreatitis.

In the hands of experts (who publish), access precut sphincterotomy appears to be both useful and safe, at least when used for good (biliary) indications [12]. However, many series document a significantly increased risk of pancreatitis when precutting is performed. In a large prospective multicenter analysis, the complication rate was 24.3% after precutting, with 3.6% severe pancreatitis [13].

Pancreatic sphincterotomy is being performed increasingly in referral centers for many different indications and is identified as a risk factor (OR: 3.1) [13]. Later univariate analysis in a prospective Italian multicenter study showed an incidence of 3.9% for those undergoing pancreatic sphincterotomy as compared to only 0.6% in controls ($p = 0.03$) [14]. The suggestion that pure cutting current could reduce the risk of pancreatitis has not been proven in most of the published studies.

Balloon dilation of the biliary sphincter is used to assist the removal of very large stones. It has also been advocated as an alternative to sphincterotomy for routine stone extraction, in the hope of reducing the (small) short- and long-term risks. Early case series gave encouraging results, but the technique can cause pancreatitis. Many randomized studies have been performed to compare the risk with that of standard sphincterotomy. Some involved older patients, often with dilated ducts and large stones, and showed that the short-term risks of sphincterotomy and of balloon dilation were similar. However, the concept of sphincter preservation is most attractive in younger patients with smaller stones and relatively normal ducts. A major multicenter US study in these types of patients (in the context of laparoscopic cholecystectomy) showed a marked increase in the risk of pancreatitis, with two deaths [15]. This has led to a consensus, at least in the United States, that the balloon technique should be considered now only in special circumstances, such as coagulopathy and maybe Billroth II patients. This restrictive recommendation could change with further progress in preventing pancreatitis, for example, by combining balloon dilation with pharmacological or stenting prophylaxis. The balloon technique is widely used in Asian countries with the rate of adverse events comparable with sphincterotomy in a prospective randomized trial [16]. A Cochrane systematic review on 15 randomized controlled trials (1768 participants) comparing two technics concluded that balloon dilation was statistically associated with less successful stone removal (relative risk 0.90), higher rates of mechanical lithotripsy (relative risk 1.34), and higher risk of pancreatitis (relative risk 1.96) but statistically significant lower rates of bleeding and less short-term and long-term infection. There was no statistically significant difference with regard to mortality, perforation, or total short-term complications [17].

Table 24.2 Risk factors for pancreatitis after ERCP.

Increased risk?	Patient-related	Procedure-related
Yes	Young age	Pancreatography
	Female	Pancreatic sphincterotomy
	Suspected SOD	Balloon dilation of intact sphincter
	Recurrent pancreatitis	Difficult cannulation
	No chronic pancreatitis	Precut (access) sphincterotomy
	Prior post-ERCP pancreatitis	
Maybe	No stone	Pancreatic acinarization
	Normal bilirubin	Pancreatic brush cytology
	Low-volume endoscopist	Pain during ERCP
No	Small/normal bile duct	Therapeutic versus diagnostic
	Periampullary diverticulum	Biliary sphincterotomy
	Pancreas divisum	Sphincter manometry
	Contrast allergy	Intramural contrast injection
	Prior failed ERCP	

Temporary stenting of the biliary sphincter has been used as a therapeutic trial in patients with suspected sphincter dysfunction. This technique is a potent cause of pancreatitis and should be avoided.

Combining patient and technique factors. Many of these risk factors are additive [8]. For instance, precutting in suspected sphincter dysfunction resulted in a complication rate of 35.3% in one series, with no fewer than 23.5% graded as severe [13]. In another study from the same group, a woman with a normal serum bilirubin, bile duct stone, and easy cannulation had a 5% risk of pancreatitis. This increased to 16% if cannulation proved difficult, and to 42% if no stone was found (i.e., suspected SOD) [11]. These are the unfortunate patients who are still developing severe pancreatitis after ERCP, and who feature in lawsuits [17]. A summary of risk factors for post-ERCP pancreatitis is shown in Table 24.2 [19].

Prevention of post-ERCP pancreatitis

The only way to prevent pancreatitis is not to perform ERCP, an option that should always be considered and discussed carefully in cases where the risks are predicted to be high, and the benefits uncertain. **When ERCP is indicated, there are some sensible precautions to be taken.**

Techniques. Attention to the mechanical factors discussed ealier can reduce the risk. Gentle intelligent probing for the desired duct with minimal injections of contrast will help. The endoscopist who personally injects the contrast has better control of this important variable. Probing with a guidewire rather than contrast may be prudent, but reduced risk has not been proven. Wire-guided cannulation was superior to contrast-assisted technique in a meta-analysis of 12 randomized trials with regard to the cannulation rates (84% vs. 77%, respectively) and lower rate of post-ERCP pancreatitis (3.5% vs. 6.7%, respectively) [20]. However, a more recent prospective nonrandomized study comparing two techniques revealed a rate of 5.2% using guidewire and 4.4% using contrast and failed to show a significant difference. The overall rates of post-ERCP pancreatitis were similar with both techniques in high-risk patients versus low-risk patients [21].

Extensive studies have not shown any consistent benefit for one or other contrast agent for ERCP.

It is also important to know when to abort a procedure. Failure to complete an ERCP may feel bad, but severe pancreatitis feels much worse, to both endoscopist and patient. Persisting, and using more dangerous approaches like precutting, can be justified only when there is a strong indication for the procedure, that is, good evidence for biliary (or pancreatic) pathology, and a likelihood of needing endoscopic therapy.

When manometry is performed, an aspirating catheter system should be used.

The type of current used for sphincterotomy does not appear to be a big factor influencing the pancreatitis rate, but it is clearly wise to avoid excessive coagulation near the pancreatic orifice.

Pharmacological prophylaxis. The list of pharmacological agents that have been proposed and tested for prophylaxis of post-ERCP pancreatitis is long and varied [8, 22, 23]. It includes antibiotics, heparin, corticosteroids, nifedipine, octreotide and somatostatin derivatives, trinitrin, lidocaine spray, gabexate, secretin, topical epinephrine, and cytokine inhibitors. Among all these, there is strong evidence only for rectal diclofenac or indomethacin. A large US multicenter double-blind randomized controlled trial on rectal indomethacin in 602 high-risk patients showed a significant risk reduction of 46% in those who received it [24]. A meta-analysis of four randomized controlled trials later showed that periprocedural administration of rectal indomethacin significantly reduce the rate of post-ERCP pancreatitis including moderate to severe pancreatitis to half in both high-risk and low-risk patients [25]. The latest recommendation from the European Society of Gastrointestinal Endoscopy is the routine use of rectally administered diclofenac or indomethacin immediately before or after ERCP to prevent post-ERCP pancreatitis [26]. Interestingly, a network meta-analysis showed that rectal NSAIDs were superior to pancreatic duct stenting and was not inferior to the combination of rectal indomethacin and prophylactic pancreatic stent placement for the prevention of post-ERCP pancreatitis [27]. A more recent network meta-analysis concluded that topical epinephrine and rectal NSAIDs were the most efficacious agents in preventing post-ERCP pancreatitis [28].

A pilot study on 62 average-risk patients showed that aggressive hydration was associated with a lower rate of post-ERCP pancreatitis (0% vs. 17%, $p = 0.016$) [29]. This interesting observation needs confirmation before it can be recommended in routine practice.

Pancreatic stenting. There is strong evidence that temporary stenting of the pancreatic duct can reduce the risk of pancreatitis after ERCP in high-risk patients, for example, those with suspected or proven sphincter dysfunction, at least in expert centers based on a meta-analysis of 14 randomized controlled trials [OR: 0.39 (0.29–0.53), $p<0.001$] [30]. Stents of 3–5 Fr guage are used, either short (3–5 cm) or deep into the duct (8–10 cm). Lack of internal flaps allows the stents to migrate out into the intestine within a few weeks (checked by abdominal X-ray). One important caveat is that additional skills are required to pass small guidewires deep into the pancreatic duct, so that the safety and value of the method are unproven in less experienced hands. Because of this and since more recent studies, as discussed earlier, have shown higher efficacy and cost-effectiveness as well as lower adverse events associated with rectal indomethacin as compared to pancreatic prophylactic stent placement or the combination of both methods, the use of prophylactic pancreatic stent placement may decrease [29, 31].

Recognition and management

Many patients experience some epigastric distress and bloating within 1–2 h after ERCP. Usually, this is due to excessive air insufflation, which settles quickly (and can be prevented by using CO_2 instead of air). Pancreatitis usually becomes evident after a delay of 4–12 h, and is characterized by typical pancreatic-type pain, often associated with nausea and vomiting. Patients have tachycardia, epigastric tenderness, and absent or diminished bowel sounds. Serum levels of amylase and lipase are elevated, but leukocytosis is more predictive of severity than the enzyme levels.

Perforation is the most important alternative diagnosis, which should always be considered if there is marked distress very soon after the procedure and abdominal tenderness (especially if the serum levels of amylase/lipase are not impressive). Abdominal radiographs may be diagnostic in some cases, but computed tomography (CT) is more sensitive.

The spectrum of severity and treatment of patients with pancreatitis after ERCP is the same as for pancreatitis occurring spontaneously. Adequate analgesia and aggressive fluid replacement are key. CT scanning is indicated within 24 h if there is suspicion of perforation, and after a few days if clinical progress is slow or if fever develops (Figure 24.1). Antibiotics are usually not given unless pancreatic infection is proven by percutaneous aspiration. The rare patient who develops a pseudocyst or pancreatic necrosis may require percutaneous or endoscopic drainage, or surgical debridement, and may require transfer to a tertiary center.

Conclusion

Pancreatitis is now the commonest complication of ERCP, and can be devastating. Skillful technique, pharmacological prophylaxis, and the use of small pancreatic stents will keep the risk of pancreatitis below 5% in most circumstances, but cannot yet eliminate it.

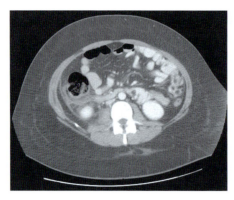

Figure 24.1 CT scan of severe pancreatitis, taken 1 week after ERCP.

Perforation

Four different types of perforation can occur during ERCP:
- Perforation of ducts or tumors by guidewires and other instruments—perhaps better called "penetrations"
- Retroduodenal perforation related to sphincterotomy
- Perforation of the lumen of the esophagus, stomach, duodenum, or small intestine
- Perforation due to stent migration

Duct and tumor "penetrations"

Guidewires and accessories passed over them (such as sphincterotomes, catheters, and dilators) can pass through the wall of the biliary or pancreatic ductal system (or indeed the raw area of a fresh sphincterotomy) [32]. This occurs perhaps most often when attempting to cannulate a patient with a tumor involving the region of the papilla. These incidents are rarely reported, and so their frequency is unknown. They are more likely to occur with vigorous probing in difficult cases, especially when there is distortion by tumor or sharp ductal deviation for other reasons. Rigid guidewires may be more dangerous. Often it is safer to proceed with a "flipped"-tip wire, which tends to find the lumen more easily.

Ducts have also been disrupted occasionally by overaggressive balloon dilatation of biliary (and pancreatic) strictures. The radiographic appearances may appear somewhat alarming when contrast is injected.

The risk of this event can be reduced by careful insertion of instruments while being aware of the potential problem. Recognition is usually straightforward, and the problem can be defused satisfactorily by finding the correct lumen, and by completing the procedure (e.g., by stenting). It is very unusual indeed for a patient to have any adverse consequences.

Sphincterotomy-related perforation

Perforation occurs after about 1% of biliary sphincterotomies and is always retroduodenal. It is defined by the presence of air (and/or contrast) in the retroperitoneum. However, routine CT scans in asymptomatic patients after uncomplicated sphincterotomy have shown small quantities of periuodenal or retroperitoneal air in up to 30% of patients [33], so there are more asymptomatic "microperforations" than is commonly appreciated. Therefore, it is challenging to interpret the finding of a small amount of free air on CT scans in patients with symptomatic post-ERCP pancreatitis.

Risk factors and prevention. It is assumed that perforation is more likely with larger and repeat biliary sphincterotomies, and that cutting beyond "1–2 o'clock" is more risky. It is not reported more frequently in patients with peripapillary diverticula.

As discussed earlier, precut sphincterotomy appears to be relatively safe and useful in expert hands, with restricted indications, but it is clearly more dangerous in routine practice, and when used, for instance, in patients with suspected sphincter dysfunction [13, 34]. A meta-analysis of six trials comparing early precut versus persistent attempts at standard cannulation showed that the overall rate of adverse events was 5% after early precut, not significantly different from 6% in the control group [35]. Precut-related perforations feature prominently in medico-legal cases involving ERCP.

Perforation also appears to be more likely in patients with suspected SOD [13]. This may simply be due to the smaller (often normal) size of the ducts, or because patients with bile duct stones are somehow protected (due to the distorting/fibrotic effect of recurrent stone impaction or passage). It has been reported occasionally after forceful extraction of large stones and even after balloon dilatation of the sphincter to remove stones without sphincterotomy. Perforation after pancreatic sphincterotomy (at the main or minor papilla) is extremely rare. Moreover, adding cholangioscopy to ERCP does not seem to significantly increase the risk of perforation [36].

Clearly, the best way to reduce the risk of causing perforation at sphincterotomy is to minimize the use of higher-risk techniques, such as cutting too far, cutting "off-line," extending prior sphincterotomies, and precutting.

Recognition. Perforation may become obvious during the procedure itself, when unusual territory is encountered or when the radiographs show contrast in nonanatomical shapes around the duodenum. This is best recognized by inflating and then aspirating air to show that the odd radiographic shape does not change (which does change if the contrast is in the duodenum). Occasionally, if sufficient air has been insufflated after the perforation, fluoroscopy may show air around the right kidney and along the lower edge of the liver (Figure 24.2).

Most cases of perforation are not recognized until after the procedure, when the patient complains of epigastric pain. The differential diagnosis is pancreatitis, which is far more common. Perforation should always be considered when the pain starts almost immediately after the procedure (pancreatitis may not develop for 4–12 h), when symptoms are more severe than anticipated and when accompanied by guarding and tachycardia. Rarely, patients may develop subcutaneous emphysema, pneumo-mediastinum, or pneumo-thoraces after a few hours. The white blood count usually rises quickly. Finding a normal or only slightly

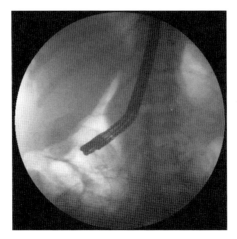

Figure 24.2 Abdominal radiograph at ERCP showing retroperitoneal air.

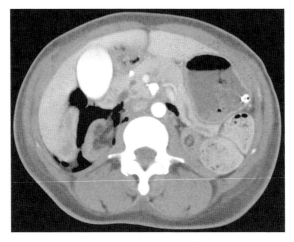

Figure 24.3 CT scan showing retroperitoneal air after perforation.

elevated serum level of amylase or lipase in patients with impressive abdominal pain should raise suspicion of perforation.

A plain abdominal X-ray may show retroduodenal air, but CT scanning is more definitive (Figure 24.3) and should be performed within 24 h in any patient with severe abdominal symptoms after sphincterotomy.

Management. Perforation is a life-threatening event; prompt recognition and efficient management are very important [28]. Patients should have nothing by mouth and be administered with adequate intravenous fluids (and nutrition as necessary), and are usually given antibiotics. Some experts recommend placement of a gastric or duodenal drainage tube. A few endoscopists have suggested placing a biliary stent or nasobiliary drain to reduce contamination of the retroperitoneum, but this is not proven or standard practice, and the additional manipulation may make matters worse. Some experts have treated sphincterotomy perforations effectively with clips [38].

Surgery. Most surgeons equate perforation with immediate operation. However, surgeons exploring such cases are often unable to find the site of perforation, and end up simply leaving retroperitoneal drains. Many series show that most (reported) retroduodenal perforations have been managed conservatively. An important caveat is that conservative therapy seems to be effective only when perforation is recognized early. Despite the dominance of nonoperative treatment for perforation, it is wise to obtain a surgical opinion at the earliest possible stage. Patients should be managed jointly on a daily basis. Conservative management is usually effective if started early, but intervention (percutaneous or surgical) may be required in the ensuing days or weeks if fluid collections/abscesses develop in the right renal or pericolic areas. Operating at a later stage is often difficult because of infection; it may be necessary to perform diversionary procedures as well as multiple drains. In one report on 9314 ERCPs, only 14% of patients with sphincterotomy-related perforation needed surgery, and no deaths were reported [32].

Luminal perforation

Endoscopic perforation can occur anywhere that endoscopes travel. The lateral-viewing nature of the duodenoscope may perhaps increase the risk of perforation in elderly patients with pharyngeal diverticula. In the absence of pathology, it is difficult to conceive how endoscopic perforation could occur in the esophagus or stomach, but such events have been reported [32]. It has also happened rarely in the duodenum, when attempting to negotiate a stricture or marked distortion by tumor. The first therapeutic video-duodenoscopes had a long distal tip, which caused perforations during forceful stone extraction maneuvers.

Perforation of the afferent loop is a definite risk during endoscopy of patients after Billroth II gastrectomy (and more complex bypass procedures after bariatric interventions). Perforation usually occurs as a result of stretching of loops rather than penetration of the endoscopic tip. It can be avoided largely by careful endoscopic technique.

Recognition and management. Diagnosis of luminal perforation is usually obvious, either during the procedure or because of obvious patient distress and clinical signs in the chest or abdomen afterward. Radiographs show air in the peritoneum or mediastinum. Prompt surgical consultation is mandatory and operation is usually effective. A few episodes have been treated conservatively with or without endoscopic clipping.

Stent migration perforation

There have been rare reports of penetration and even perforation of the duodenum, small bowel, and colon by stents that have migrated from the bile duct. Almost all of these have been "straight" 10 Fr gauge stents. Those that have migrated down from the bile duct and penetrated the opposite duodenal wall can sometimes be managed simply by endoscopic extraction. Others have required surgical intervention.

Infection

ERCP differs from most other endoscopies in that it risks contaminating territory that is usually sterile. In addition, when bile is infected (e.g., in patients with stones or blocked stents), biliary manipulation may disseminate the infection locally or systemically. By consensus, infection is defined as "an otherwise unexplained fever of greater than 38 °C lasting 24–48 h after ERCP." The reported incidence of clinical infections after ERCP is low, ranging from 0.7 to 1.6% in various modern series [13]. However, asymptomatic bacteremia rates of up to 27% have been reported. Enteric bacteria are responsible for most post-ERCP infections.

Nosocomial infection. Infections with Pseudomonas, Klebsiella, and Serratia are still being described after ERCP, due to faulty endoscope reprocessing. The organisms are often resistant to antibiotics, and the results can be devastating.

Cholangitis. Bacteremia and septicemia occur when the bile is infected and drainage is compromised. Up to 90% of post-ERCP cholangitis cases happen after failure to provide adequate drainage in patients with biliary stones or strictures. Sepsis is a particular risk after ERCP management of hilar tumors and sclerosing cholangitis, where it may prove impossible to provide complete drainage of all obstructed segments. This is a good reason for obtaining detailed anatomical imaging (by CT and/or magnetic resonance cholangiopancreatography (MRCP)) beforehand to assist therapeutic planning.

Cholecystitis. Cholecystitis has occurred after ERCP; presumably, this is more likely when there is cystic duct compromise by stone or tumor (or occasionally after stenting). It is managed by standard percutaneous or surgical techniques.

Pancreatic sepsis. This has occurred as part of severe pancreatitis after ERCP, and in patients with pseudocysts, due to incomplete drainage.

Prevention of infection

The risk of introducing or stirring up infection when the bile is infected can be minimized by adhering to disinfection protocols, by reducing the biliary pressure (by aspirating bile before injecting much contrast), and by ensuring adequate drainage by removing all obstructing stones or placing appropriate stents.

Prophylactic antibiotics. Most experts recommend giving antibiotics before procedures when failure of complete drainage is predictable (e.g., complex hilar tumors, sclerosing cholangitis, and pseudocysts), and to give them intravenously immediately after any procedure in which drainage fails. A meta-analysis of seven trials failed to show a significant reduction in the rate of post-ERCP cholangitis after antibiotic prophylaxis in unselected patients or those with suspected biliary obstruction [39]. Some have advocated mixing antibiotics with the contrast media, but this practice has never been validated. ASGE recommends antibiotic prophylaxis before an ERCP in patients with known or suspected biliary obstruction when there is a possibility of incomplete drainage, those with communicating pancreatic cysts or pseudocysts, and before transpapillary or transmural drainage of pseudocysts, but not in patients with biliary obstruction when it is likely that an ERCP will accomplish complete biliary drainage. Antibiotics should be continued after a failed drainage or in post-transplantation biliary strictures [40].

Delayed infection

The commonest cause of delayed biliary sepsis is a blocked stent. Patients can become seriously ill quickly with septic cholangitis. For this reason, patients and their caregivers must be fully informed about this risk and instructed to make contact as soon as symptoms develop. For the same reason, it is common practice to change plastic stents routinely (at 3–4 months), especially in patients with benign biliary strictures. The need to do so in patients with malignant disease (as opposed to waiting for obstructive symptoms) has not been validated in controlled studies, but is still common practice.

Bleeding

Cutting procedures such as sphincterotomy, ampullectomy, and pseudocyst drainage can inevitably cause immediate or delayed bleeding. Some oozing is common, but clinically significant bleeding is now rare. Bleeding has also occurred after balloon dilation after sphincterotomy for removal of large stones.

Definition and incidence. Bleeding is defined in clinical terms. Even impressive immediate bleeding is not counted if it stops spontaneously or can be stopped by endoscopic manipulation during the procedure. Thus, bleeding becomes an adverse event statistic only if the planned procedure (e.g., stone extraction) cannot be completed as a result, or if it is evident afterward (hematemesis or melena or symptomatic drop in hemoglobin) and is sufficient to require in-hospital care and/or another procedure (e.g., repeat endoscopy or angiography). By these definitions, bleeding occurs after only about 1% of sphincterotomies (and more often after ampullectomy). It was much more common in the early days [7, 41].

Risk factors for bleeding, and avoidance

Bleeding is certainly more likely to occur in patients with coagulopathy and/or portal hypertension, renal failure, and apparently also when sphincterotomy is repeated. There is no evidence that the risk is greater in patients taking aspirin and other agents affecting platelet function, although it is still common practice to ask patients to discontinue their use. Delayed clinical bleeding may or may not be more common when there has been some immediate oozing [42].

Prevention. Coagulopathies should be corrected wherever possible. Anticoagulants should be discontinued according to latest ASGE guidelines. The need for temporary heparin coverage, and the duration, has been defined based on the perceived risk of bleeding and potential for thromboembolic events if anticoagulants are stopped [43]. Sphincterotomy (but not ERCP) is considered a high-risk procedure. Sphincterotomy should always be performed in a controlled manner, with blended current, avoiding the "zipper" cut. The type of current used may be relevant. One study showed that the ERBE generator reduced bleeding visibly at the time of endoscopy, but not the risk of clinically defined bleeding. Another study utilizing initial cutting current (to reduce the risk of pancreatitis) did show a slightly increased risk of bleeding. Balloon dilatation of the sphincter can be used instead of sphincterotomy for extracting some stones in patients with irreversible coagulopathy or severe portal hypertension.

Management. Bleeding during or immediately after sphincterotomy (Figure 24.4) usually stops spontaneously, and (unless there is a pumping vessel) it is usually not necessary to take any dramatic action. Bleeding that persists can almost always be controlled endoscopically, using epinephrine injection, balloon tamponade, or clips. It may be useful (with unimpressive bleeding) first to spray the site with about 10 ml of a dilute (1:100 000) solution of epinephrine. This often stops oozing temporarily, at least enough to see exactly where the bleeding is coming from. If the bleeding is impressive, or if oozing persists, balloon tamponade is a useful next step. A retrieval balloon is overinflated in the bile duct, and then pulled down forcefully to compress the bleeding site between the balloon and the endoscope tip for 5 min. If that fails, we inject epinephrine

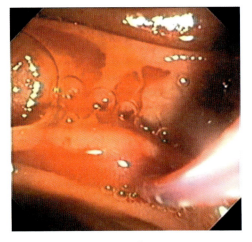

Figure 24.4 Bleeding immediately after starting sphincterotomy.

(diluted 1:10 000) using a standard sclerotherapy needle. Up to 5 ml can be injected in aliquots of 1 ml, taking care not to compromise the pancreatic orifice. For this reason, it is wise to inject just outside the top edges of the sphincterotomy, rather than within it. If there has been much manipulation, it may also be sensible to place a small protective pancreatic stent (if possible). Very rarely, bleeding is profuse, and endoscopic vision is quickly lost. Expert angiographic management can be effective. Surgical oversewing would seem logical when all else fails, but rebleeding may occur.

While significant bleeding is usually manifested by hematemesis and/or melena, occasional patients can present with biliary pain and cholangitis if bleeding fills the bile duct.

Delayed bleeding can occur up to 2 weeks after sphincterotomy, and should be treated like any other episode of bleeding. Restarting warfarin or heparin within 3 days post sphincterotomy has been shown to increase this risk [43, 44]. It is important to confirm the source of bleeding, since patients occasionally bleed from other lesions.

Basket impaction

Baskets may become impacted during attempts to remove large stones from the bile duct. Usually, this situation can be rectified quickly by disengaging the stone or by crushing it with a "rescue" lithotripsy sleeve (Chapter 16). To prevent this problem, it is wise to use a mechanical lithotripsy system initially when approaching stones >1 cm in diameter. Baskets should be used sparingly and with great caution in the pancreatic duct. They are effective for the removal of soft stones (protein plugs) and mucus, but calcified pancreatic stones are very resistant to mechanical lithotripsy. There is a risk that the basket will break inside the duct and remain impacted.

Cardiopulmonary complications and sedation issues

Cardiopulmonary events can occur during or after any endoscopic procedure [45], and myocardial ischemia has been studied specifically during ERCP. Transient hypoxia and cardiac dysrhythmias occur occasionally during ERCP procedures, but are usually recognized and managed appropriately without clinical consequences. Very rarely, they may result in severe decompensation during or after procedures, and are a significant cause of the rare fatalities attributable to ERCP.

Risk factors for cardiopulmonary complications include known or unsuspected premorbid conditions, and problems related to sedation and analgesia. Oversedation can be a serious problem, especially in the elderly and frail, and particularly if monitoring is inadequate (in a darkened room).

Cardiopulmonary complications can be largely avoided by careful preprocedure evaluation, appropriate collaboration with anesthesiologists (and cardiologists) when dealing with high-risk patients (ASA grades III and higher), formal training of endoscopists and nurses in sedation and resuscitation, and careful monitoring. Propofol-based sedation or adding capnography reduces episodes of hypoxia and apnea when using opioids and benzodiazepine [46, 47].

Aspiration pneumonia has been described after all types of endoscopic procedures; the incidence is unknown, but it is probably more common than recognized, since the onset may be delayed.

Late complications of stents

Biliary and pancreatic stents can cause problems through local trauma, blockage, and migration. Much depends on their size, nature, and position.

Blockage of plastic biliary stents is inevitable after a few months, and can cause serious cholangitis. A host of ingenious attempts to prevent this phenomenon over two decades have so far been unavailing (Chapter 3). It is common practice to reduce the infection risk by recommending the routine exchange of plastic biliary stents at about 3 months. It is perhaps legitimate to await events in patients with malignant disease if they (and their caregivers) are well informed about the first symptoms (usually shaking chills) and the need for urgent action. Expandable metal stents usually last much longer, but the consequences of blockage are equally serious.

Plastic stent migration. Straight stents that migrate outward may cause damage to the duodenum or distal intestine. Stents that migrate inward can be difficult to retrieve, especially in the pancreatic duct [48]. Most migrated stents can be teased out of the papilla with a retrieval balloon, or grasped with foreign body forceps, snare, or basket. Rarely, surgery is needed to rectify these situations.

Duct damage due to plastic stents. The presence of a stent in the bile duct for many months may cause some wall irregularity and thickening. This can be seen radiologically (and can cause diagnostic difficulty at endoscopic ultrasound (EUS)), but has no clinical relevance. However, stent-induced duct damage is a serious problem in the pancreas [49], especially when the duct is initially normal. Irritation by the tip of the stent (especially at a duct bend) or by internal flaps often causes wall irregularity and clinically significant narrowing. Relatively stiff pancreatic stents of 7 and even 10 Fr can be used legitimately in some patients with established chronic pancreatitis for the management of stones or strictures. However, when stenting seems to be indicated in relatively normal ducts, it seems wise to use smaller (3 or 5 Fr) and softer stents for only a few weeks [49]. The length of a pancreatic stent should be chosen so that the inner tip is in a straight part of the duct.

Metal stents migration, blockage removal. Fewer adverse events have been reported with metallic stents than with plastic ones. One reason might be that they are used mainly for palliative purposes. Moreover, they have not yet been studied as widely as plastic stents. However, most of the adverse events that were reported for plastic stents could be seen with metallic stents including migration (more with covered ones), occlusion, and duodenal ulceration [50, 51].

Late complications of sphincterotomy

There has been much interest in the possible long-term adverse consequences of biliary sphincterotomy [52]. When performed for "papillary stenosis," there is a significant risk of further biliary-type symptoms, whether due to restenosis or an incorrect diagnosis (Chapter 17).

Sphincterotomy leads almost inevitably to bacterial contamination of the bile, which may be a potent promoter of pigment stone formation. One study showed a significant increase in the incidence of cholangiocarcinoma after surgical sphincteroplasty, but a cohort study in Scandinavia found no such association after endoscopic sphincterotomy [53]. Many patients have been followed for periods of 10 years or more after sphincterotomy for stones. The chance of further biliary problems in these studies ranges from 5 to 24%, with an average of about 10%. The Amsterdam study had the highest figure (24%) and all but one of the patients had recurrent stones [54]. In other series, some patients had episodes of cholangitis without stones, and even cholangitis without stenosis of the sphincterotomy.

Most of these long-term complications of sphincterotomy are easily managed endoscopically, remembering that repeat incisions do carry a slightly greater risk. A few patients continue to re-form stones every 6–12 months despite apparently adequate drainage, and may need to be scheduled for repeated endoscopic "biliary laundry."

The main risk of pancreatic sphincterotomy appears to be restenosis, which occurs in at least 20% of reported cases (Chapters 6–8). It is usually treated endoscopically, but strictures that occur beneath the papilla can be challenging even for surgical repair. Hopefully, better techniques (and new stents) may reduce this risk in the future.

Stenosis of the pancreatic orifice causing recurrent pancreatitis has been reported as a late complication of biliary sphincterotomy.

Rare complications

Many other untoward events have followed ERCP. These include the following:
- **Gallstone ileus** after removing large stones.
- **Musculoskeletal injuries** (e.g., dislocation of the temporomandibular joint or shoulder, dental trauma).

- **Opacification of blood vessels**. The portal venous system and lymphatics have been seen while injecting contrast through tapered-tip catheters. The contrast moves rapidly on fluoroscopy. If air is injected as well, the appearances on CT scan are alarming, but no sequelae have been reported.
- **Portal vein air or bile embolism** with fatality reported due to cardiac or brain air embolism [55]. This is potentially a concern with direct cholangioscopy.
- **Antral sinus infection** after prolonged nasobiliary drainage.
- **Renal dysfunction** with the use of nephrotoxic medications (such as gentamycin).
- **Impaction or fracturing of nasobiliary and nasopancreatic drains**.
- **Allergic reactions to iodine-containing contrast agents.** Allergic reactions have happened, even with the very small doses that enter the bloodstream during ERCP. Endoscopy units should have policies in place to deal with patients who claim to be allergic.
- **Increased cholestasis** in patients with sclerosing cholangitis.
- **Splenic injury** has been reported several times during ERCP.
- **Distant abscesses** have occurred in the spleen and kidney, and no doubt elsewhere.
- **Hemolysis** due to G6PD deficiency and hemolytic–uremic syndrome has been reported.
- **Dissemination of pancreatic cancer** was reported after sphincterotomy.
- **Pseudoaneurysm** of a branch of the pancreatico–duodenal artery developed after needle–knife sphincterotomy.

Deaths after ERCP

The literature reporting deaths after ERCP is difficult to analyze as the series contain different spectra of patients and procedures, and some do not distinguish between 30-day mortality and events attributable to the procedure itself. One paper illustrates the difficulty in attributing mortality between concurrent illness, active complications, and complications due to other procedures required after ERCP failure. Data collected for the consensus conference in 1991 reported 103 deaths after 7729 sphincterotomies (1.3%). The largest meta-analysis to date included 21 prospective studies with 16 885 patients and reported ERCP-related mortality of 0.33% (CI: 0.24–0.42) [56].

The causes of death in all of the reported series cover the spectrum of the commonest complications, with approximately equal numbers resulting from pancreatitis, bleeding, perforation, infection, and cardiopulmonary events. Delay in diagnosis of perforation is mentioned as a contributing cause in several publications [57]. Of nine fatalities resulting in claims to insurance in Denmark, seven were attributable to pancreatitis (two of which had undergone precutting) [58].

Care after ERCP

Admission? Keeping patients in hospital overnight means that staff can ensure adequate fluid intake (mainly intravenously), and can quickly detect and pay appropriate attention to any symptoms that may herald important complications. However, overnight observation adds costs, and can add other burdens for patients and their families. Several studies have evaluated factors predicting the need for admission [59]. Admission is unnecessary in the majority of standard-level procedures (simple biliary stones and stents), but seems wise when the risk is predicted to be higher than average (e.g., sphincter dysfunction management), when the procedure has been difficult in some way, or when the patient is frail or has no responsible accompanying person. Staying overnight in a local hotel is an appropriate compromise option for patients who live more than an hour or two away.

    Early refeeding? Patients are often keen to catch up on the meals that they have missed as a result of the procedure, but it has been our practice to recommend taking fluids only until the next morning, when the main risk of pancreatitis has passed. However, a trial suggested that early refeeding is not detrimental [60].

Managing adverse events

Each event requires specific skillful recognition and management, but there are several important general guidelines.

Prompt recognition and action

The keys to effective management are early recognition and prompt focused action. Delay is dangerous both medically and legally. Patients in pain and distress after procedures should always be examined carefully and never be simply "reassured." Get appropriate laboratory studies and radiographs, consult the extensive literature, and do not hesitate to seek advice from other experts in the relevant fields. It is wise to consult an (informed) surgeon early on for anything that might remotely require surgical intervention. Sometimes it may be appropriate to offer transfer of care of the patient to a specialty colleague or to a larger medical center, but, if this happens, try to keep in touch, and to show continuing interest and concern. Apparent abandonment alienates patients and their relatives, and may lead to initiation of legal action.

Professionalism and communication

Endoscopists often feel devastated when serious complications occur. Some distress is understandable and worthy, and it is important to be sympathetic, but it is equally important to be composed and matter of fact. Excessive apologies may give an unfortunate impression. Poor communication is the basis for much unhappiness, and many lawsuits. Remember that the truly informed patient and any accompanying persons have been told already that complications can happen. This is an integrally important part of the consent process. So it is appropriate and correct to address suspected complications in that spirit. "It looks as if we have a perforation here. We discussed that as a remote possibility beforehand, and I am sorry that it has occurred. Here is what I think we should do." It is also wise to contact and inform other interested relatives, referring physicians, supervisors, and your risk management advisers.

Documentation

Document what has happened carefully and honestly in real time. Don't even think of adding notes retrospectively. The results of many lawsuits hang on the quality of the documentation, or lack of it.

Learning from lawsuits

Fortunately, most complications do not result in legal action. Despite the fact that ERCP is the most dangerous of the routine endoscopic procedures, there are more claims after colonoscopy and upper endoscopy [61]. There are several reasons why patients (or their survivors) may initiate a claim [18].

Communication

Inadequate education in the consent process (Chapter 4) is often a major issue. Too often we hear that "we would never have consented to the procedure if we had known that this might happen." Good communication after an adverse event is equally important. Show that you care. Litigants are sometimes simply (and justifiably) angry if they get the impression that you do not.

Standard-of-care practice

Once a lawsuit has been filed, the key issue is whether the endoscopist (and others involved) practiced within the "standard of care." This is defined as what reasonable colleagues would do in similar circumstances (and is expressed in court by what expert witnesses opine).

Indications. Was the ERCP procedure really indicated? The task clearly is to balance the possible benefits against the potential risks [62]. Although professional societies publish guidelines for the use of ERCP, the devil is in the details: for example, how much elevation of liver tests or increased duct size constitutes "objective evidence of pathology." In practice, the validity of the decision to proceed will be judged by the severity of the symptoms, by the thoroughness of prior treatment and investigations, and by the process of communication. Were the symptoms (or other signs of pathology) really that pressing?

Had less invasive approaches (nowadays including MRCP) been exhausted, or at least considered and discussed?

For less experienced endoscopists, consideration of alternatives (especially for higher-risk procedures) should include possible referral to an expert center.

Technique. Was there an obvious deviation from customary practice, like placing a 10 Fr stent in a normal pancreatic duct? Did the level of suspicion of pathology really justify a precut? Was there radiological evidence for overmanipulation of the pancreas, overinjection (e.g., acinarization), or injection into a branch duct? The notes of the procedure nurse may contain important evidence, like excessive sedation or contrast, or documentation of patient distress. Pretty endoscopic photographs may also be incriminating, for example, if they show sphincterotomy in an unusual direction.

Postprocedure care. Was the patient appropriately monitored, discharged in good condition, and properly advised? Was action taken promptly when unexpected symptoms developed? Was the endoscopist available to advise? Among the most common errors are delay in action (particularly in considering and managing perforation) and inadequate fluid resuscitation in patients with pancreatitis.

Risks for endoscopists and staff

The endoscopy unit is not a dangerous place, but there are a few risks for the ERCP endoscopist and staff. The possibility of transmission of infection exists, but should be entirely preventable with standard precautions (gowns, gloves, and eye protection) and assiduous disinfection protocols. Certain immunizations are also appropriate. Rarely, staff may become sensitive to materials used in the ERCP process, such as glutaraldehyde or latex gloves. The risks of radiation are minimized by appropriate education, shielding, and exposure monitoring. Some older endoscopists have neck problems caused by looking down fiberscopes, a situation aggravated by ERCP rooms where the video and X-ray monitors are not side by side. Busy ERCP practitioners sometimes also complain of "elevator thumb."

Conclusion

After more than 40 years, the risks of ERCP and its therapeutic procedures are now well documented. Pancreatitis is the commonest, but bleeding, perforation, infection, and sedation-related events still occur. There are a host of rare complications. An experienced team, understanding and managing the main risk factors, can keep these events to a minimum but cannot eliminate them [37]. Making sure that patients understand what they are accepting is of crucial importance. Careful and caring management of patients when adverse events occur can minimize the medico-legal risk.

References

1 Romagnuolo J, Cotton PB, Eisen G, et al. Identifying and reporting risk factors for adverse events in endoscopy. Part I: cardiopulmonary events. Gastrointest Endosc 2011;73(3):579–85.

2 Romagnuolo J, Cotton PB, Eisen G, et al. Identifying and reporting risk factors for adverse events in endoscopy. Part II: noncardiopulmonary events. Gastrointest Endosc 2011;73(3): 586–97.

3 Glomsaker T, Hoff G, Kvaløy JT, et al.; Norwegian Gastronet ERCP Group. Patterns and predictive factors of complications after endoscopic retrograde cholangiopancreatography. Br J Surg 2013;100(3):373–80.

4 Leung JW, Chung SC, Sung JJ, Banez VP, Li AK. Urgent endoscopic drainage for acute suppurative cholangitis. Lancet 1989;1(8650):1307–9.

5 Cohen S, Bacon BR, Berlin JA, et al. National Institutes of Health State-of-the-Science Conference Statement: ERCP for diagnosis and therapy, January 14–16, 2002. Gastrointest Endosc 2002;56:803–9.

6 Cotton PB. ERCP is most dangerous for people who need it least. Gastrointest Endosc 2001;54(4):535–6.

7 Cotton PB, Lehman G, Vennes J, et al. Endoscopic sphincterotomy complications and their management: an attempt at consensus. Gastrointest Endosc 1991;37:383–93.

8 Freeman ML, Guda NM. Prevention of post-ERCP pancreatitis: a comprehensive review. Gastrointest Endosc 2004;59(7):845–64.

9 Urbach DR, Rabeneck L. Population-based study of the risk of acute pancreatitis following ERCP. Gastrointest Endosc 2003;57(5):AB116.

10 Masci E, Mariani A, Curioni S, Testoni PA. Risk factors for pancreatitis following endoscopic retrograde cholangiopancreatography: a meta-analysis. Endoscopy 2003;35(10):830–4.

11 Freeman ML, DiSario JA, Nelson DB, et al. Risk factors for post-ERCP pancreatitis: a prospective, multicenter study. Gastrointest Endosc 2001;54(4):535–6.

12 Cotton PB. Precut papillotomy: a risky technique for experts only. Gastrointest Endosc 1989;35:578.

13 Freeman ML, Nelson DB, Sherman S, et al. Complications of endoscopic biliary sphincterotomy. N Engl J Med 1996;335:909–18.

14 Testoni PA, Mariani A, Giussani A, et al.; SEIFRED Group. Risk factors for post-ERCP pancreatitis in high- and low-volume centers and among expert and non-expert operators: a prospective multicenter study. Am J Gastroenterol 2010;105(8):1753–61.

15 DiSario JA, Freeman ML, Bjorkman DJ, et al. Endoscopic balloon dilation compared with sphincterotomy for extraction of bile duct stones. Gastroenterology 2004;127:1291–9.

16 Fujita N, Maguchi H, Komatsu Y, et al.; JESED Study Group. Endoscopic sphincterotomy and endoscopic papillary balloon dilatation for bile duct stones: a prospective randomized controlled multicenter trial. Gastrointest Endosc 2003;57(2):151–5.

17 Weinberg BM, Shindy W, Lo S. Endoscopic balloon sphincter dilation (sphincteroplasty) versus sphincterotomy for common bile duct stones. Cochrane Database Syst Rev 2006;4:CD004890.

18 Cotton PB. Analysis of 59 ERCP lawsuits; mainly about indications. Gastrointest Endosc 2006;63(3):378–82.

19 Cotton PB, Garrow DA, Gallagher J, Romagnuolo J. Risk factors for complications after ERCP: a multivariate analysis of 11,497 procedures over 12 years. Gastrointest Endosc 2009;70(1):80–8.

20 Tse F, Yuan Y, Moayyedi P, Leontiadis GI. Guide wire-assisted cannulation for the prevention of post-ERCP pancreatitis: a systematic review and meta-analysis. Endoscopy 2013;45(8):605–18.

21 Mariani A, Giussani A, Di Leo M, et al. Guidewire biliary cannulation does not reduce post-ERCP pancreatitis compared with the contrast injection technique in low-risk and high-risk patients. Gastrointest Endosc 2012;75(2):339–46.

22 Freeman ML. Prevention of post-ERCP pancreatitis: pharmacologic solution or patient selection and pancreatic stents. Gastroenterology 2003;124(7):1977–80.

23 Andriulli A, Leandro G, Niro G, et al. Pharmacologic treatment can prevent pancreatic injury after ERCP: a meta-analysis. Gastrointest Endosc 2000;51:1–7.

24 Elmunzer BJ, Scheiman JM, Lehman GA, et al.; U.S. Cooperative for Outcomes Research in Endoscopy (USCORE). A randomized trial of rectal indomethacin to prevent post-ERCP pancreatitis. N Engl J Med 2012;366(15):1414–22.

25 Yaghoobi M, Rolland S, Waschke KA, et al. Meta-analysis: rectal indomethacin for the pre-vention of post-ERCP pancreatitis. Aliment Pharmacol Ther 2013;38(9):995–1001.

26 Dumonceau JM, Andriulli A, Deviere J, et al.; European Society of Gastrointestinal Endoscopy. European Society of Gastrointestinal Endoscopy (ESGE) Guideline: prophylaxis of post-ERCP pancreatitis. Endoscopy 2010;42(6):503–15.

27 Akbar A, Abu Dayyeh BK, Baron TH, et al. Rectal nonsteroidal anti-inflammatory drugs are superior to pancreatic duct stents in preventing pancreatitis after endoscopic retrograde cholangiopancreatography: a network meta-analysis. Clin Gastroenterol Hepatol 2013;11(7):778–83.

28 Akshintala VS, Hutfless SM, Colantuoni E, et al. Systematic review with network meta-analysis: pharmacological prophylaxis against post-ERCP pancreatitis. Aliment Pharmacol Ther 2013;38(11–12):1325–37.

29 Buxbaum J, Yan A, Yeh K, et al. Aggressive hydration with lactated ringer's solution reduces pancreatitis after endoscopic retrograde cholangiopancreatography. Clin Gastroenterol Hepatol 2014;12(2):303–7.

30 Mazaki T, Mado K, Masuda H, Shiono M. Prophylactic pancreatic stent placement and post-ERCP pancreatitis: an updated meta-analysis. J Gastroenterol 2014;217(5):788–801.

31 Elmunzer BJ, Higgins PD, Saini SD, et al.; United States Cooperative for Outcomes Research in Endoscopy. Does rectal indomethacin eliminate the need for prophylactic pancreatic stent placement in patients undergoing high-risk ERCP? Post hoc efficacy and cost-benefit analyses using prospective clinical trial data. Am J Gastroenterol 2013;108(3):410–5.

32 Enns R, Eloubeidi MA, Mergener K, et al. ERCP-related perforations: risk factors and management. Endoscopy 2002;34(4):293–8.

33 Genzlinger JL, McPhee MS, Fisher JK, et al. Significance of retroperitoneal air after endo-scopic retrograde cholangiopancreatography with sphincterotomy. Am J Gastroenterol 1999;94(5):1267–70.

34 Cotton PB. Needleknife precut sphincterotomy: the devil is in the indications. Endoscopy 1997;29:888.

35 Cennamo V, Fuccio L, Zagari NM et al. Can early precut implementation reduce ERCP-realted complication risk? Meta-analysis of randomized controlled trials. Endoscopy 2010; 42(5):381–8

36 Hammerle CW, Haider S, Chung M, et al. Endoscopic retrograde cholangiopancreatography complications in the era of cholangioscopy: is there an increased risk? Dig Liver Dis 2012;44(9):754–8.

37 Balmadrid B, Kozarek R. Prevention and management of adverse events of endoscopic ret-rograde cholangiopancreatography. Gastrointest Endosc Clin N Am 2013;23(2):385–403.

38 Lee TH, Han JH, Park SH. Endoscopic treatments of endoscopic retrograde cholangiopancre-atography-related duodenal perforations. Clin Endosc 2013;46(5):522–528.

39 Bai Y, Gao F, Gao J, et al. Prophylactic antibiotics cannot prevent endoscopic retrograde chol-angiopancreatography-induced cholangitis: a meta-analysis. Pancreas 2009;38(2):126–30.

40 Anderson MA, Fisher L, Jain R, et al.; ASGE Standards of Practice Committee. Complications of ERCP. Gastrointest Endosc 2012;75(3):467–73.

41 Vaira D, D'Anna L, Ainley C, et al. Endoscopic sphincterotomy in 1000 consecutive patients. Lancet 1989;2:431–4.

42 Wilcox CM, Canakis J, Monkemuller KE, et al. Patterns of bleeding after endoscopic sphincterotomy, the subsequent risk of bleeding, and the role of epinephrine injection. Am J Gastroenterol 2004;99:244–8.

43 Anderson MA, Ben-Menachem T, Gan SI, et al.; ASGE Standards of Practice Committee. Management of antithrombotic agents for endoscopic procedures. Gastrointest Endosc 2009;70(6):1060–70.

44 Hussain N, Alsulaiman R, Burtin P, et al. The safety of endoscopic sphincterotomy in patients receiving antiplatelet agents: a case-control study. Aliment Pharmacol Ther 2007;25(5):579–84.

45 Lee JF, Leung JWC, Cotton PB. Acute cardiovascular complications of endoscopy: prevalence and clinical characteristics. Dig Dis 1995;13(2):130–5.

46 Riphaus A, Stergiou N, Wehrmann T. Sedation with propofol for routine ERCP in high-risk octogenarians: a randomized, controlled study. Am J Gastroenterol 2005;100(9):1957–63.

47 Qadeer MA, Vargo JJ, Dumot JA, et al. Capnographic monitoring of respiratory activity improves safety of sedation for endoscopic cholangiopancreatography and ultrasonography. Gastroenterology 2009;136(5):1568–76.

48 Johanson JF, Schmalz MJ, Geenen JE. Incidence and risk factors for biliary and pancreatic stent migration. Gastrointest Endosc 1992;38:341–6.

49 Rashdan A, Fogel E, McHenry L, et al. Pancreatic ductal changes following small diameter long length unflanged pancreatic stent placement [Abstract]. Gastrointest Endosc 2003;57:AB213.

50 Kahaleh M, Tokar J, Conaway MR, et al. Efficacy and complications of covered Wallstents in malignant distal biliary obstruction. Gastrointest Endosc 2005;61(4):528–33.

51 Ee H, Laurence BH. Haemorrhage due to erosion of a metal biliary stent through the duodenal wall. Endoscopy 1992;24(5):431–2.

52 Park SH, Watkins JL, Fogel EL, et al. Long-term outcome of endoscopic dual pancreatobiliary sphincterotomy in patients with manometry-documented sphincter of Oddi dysfunction and normal pancreatogram. Gastrointest Endosc 2003;57(4):483–91.

53 Karlson BM, Ekbom A, Arvidsson D, et al. Population-based study of cancer risk and relative survival following sphincterotomy for stones in the common bile ducts. Br J Surg 1997; 84:1235–8.

54 Bergman JJGHM, van der Mey S, Rauws EAJ, et al. Long-term follow-up after endoscopic sphincterotomy for bile duct stones in patients younger than 60 years of age. Gastrointest Endosc 1996;44(6):643–9.

55 Finsterer J, Stöllberger C, Bastovansky A. Cardiac and cerebral air embolism from endoscopic retrograde cholangio-pancreatography. Eur J Gastroenterol Hepatol 2010;22(10):1157–62.

56 Andriulli A, Loperfido S, Napolitano G, et al. Incidence rates of post-ERCP complications: a systematic survey of prospective studies. Am J Gastroenterol 2007;102(8):1781–8.

57 Howard TJ, Tan T, Lehman GA, et al. Classification and management of perforations complicating endoscopic sphincterotomy. Surgery 1999;126(4):658–65.

58 Trap R, Adamsen S, Hart-Hansen O, Henriksen M. Severe and fatal complications after diagnostic and therapeutic ERCP: a prospective series of claims to insurance covering public hospitals. Endoscopy 1999;31(2):125–30.

59 Linder JD, Tarnasky P. There are benefits of overnight observation after outpatient ERCP. Gastrointest Endosc 2004;59(5):AB208.

60 Barthet M, Desjeux A, Gasmi M, et al. Early refeeding after endoscopic biliary or pancreatic sphincterotomy: a randomized prospective study. Endoscopy 2002;34(7):546–50.

61 Gerstenberger PD, Plumeri PA. Malpractice claims in gastrointestinal endoscopy: analysis of an insurance industry data base. Gastrointest Endosc 1993;39(2):132–8.

62 Cotton PB. Is your sphincterotomy really safe—and necessary? Gastrointest Endosc 1996;44(6):752–5.

CHAPTER 25

ERCP: Quality issues and benchmarking

Peter B. Cotton

Digestive Disease Center, Medical University of South Carolina, Charleston, USA

KEY POINTS

- ERCP practitioners vary in expertise, which affects the likelihood of success and of adverse events.
- Potential patients deserve to have information about the quality of services on offer.
- Practitioners should be encouraged to provide the information by using established quality metrics in report cards and participating in benchmarking exercises.
- The results of ERCP procedures depend also on the quality of the facility and assisting team, which can also be measured and recorded.

Endoscopic retrograde cholangiopancreatography (ERCP) has become enormously popular throughout the world because of its tremendous clinical value. The problem is that the benefits are maximized only when procedures are performed at an optimal level of quality, which is not always the case. Technical failures and serious complications can occur in the best of hands, but are more likely when procedures are performed by endoscopists with inadequate expertise, both technical and clinical. Practitioners, patients, and payers should all be interested in enhancing the quality of endoscopy, and documenting it.

The professional organizations associated with endoscopy and their leaders have increasingly embraced the quality improvement paradigm that is advancing through medicine. Professional societies interested in gastroenterology and endoscopy throughout the world have produced helpful reports and guidelines. The problem is that most of the thoughtful conclusions and well-meaning documents from these organizations have had little impact so far in the real world. Quality is often discussed, but measurement is spotty, and certainly not mandated. Few hospital privileging bodies follow published guidelines for credentialing.

ERCP: The Fundamentals, Second Edition. Edited by Peter B. Cotton and Joseph Leung.
© 2015 John Wiley & Sons, Ltd. Published 2015 by John Wiley & Sons, Ltd.
Companion Website: www.wiley.com\go\cotton\ercp

We all need to agree on the metrics of endoscopic performance, to develop the infrastructure to collect and analyze the data, and use the resulting knowledge to stimulate improvements in practice. Patients will benefit.

What is quality endoscopy?

Society (i.e., the informed patient) expects that our procedures will be done for the right reasons, and that they will be performed expeditiously, skillfully, successfully, safely, and comfortably. These expectations can be expanded to make a list of desirable characteristics for all types of endoscopic procedures:
- Correct indications—adherence to published guidelines
- Appropriate environment, support team, and behavior
- Well-prepared and informed patients
- Strategies to minimize risk, including patient preparation and monitoring
- Appropriate use of medications, including sedation/analgesia
- Correct selection of equipment
- Comfortable intubation
- Complete survey of the relevant areas
- Recognition of all abnormalities (and photo documentation)
- Appropriate tissue sampling as needed
- Application of indicated therapy
- Avoiding, recognizing, and managing complications
- Reasonable duration
- Smooth recovery, explanation, and discharge
- Detailed and clear recommendations and follow-up plans
- Integrated pathology results and communications
- Complete documentation

Many organizations and groups have explored these quality issues and their metrics [1–6]. The report from the National Institutes of Health (NIH) "state of the science" conference on ERCP made many comments on quality issues [7].

ERCP is a team event, as emphasized in other chapters, but we will address separately the quality aspects of endoscopists and the units in which they work.

How to recognize and measure excellence in endoscopists?

There are some factors of the ERCP endoscopist that make a good outcome more likely. Formal endoscopic training and extensive experience do not guarantee quality practice, but they certainly make it more likely. Thus, documentation of these and related elements should be a part of any assessment of endoscopic performance. Appropriate metrics could include the following:

- Specialty training and certification (place and dates)
- Training and maintenance of competence in life support and sedation
- Evidence for relevant continuing education
- ERCP lifetime numbers, total last year
- Spectrum of practice in last year (complexity grades)

The proof of quality comes from documentation of performance. There is no substitute for collecting relevant data (23). Trainees in most countries are now expected to maintain logbooks of their procedural activity during training, and the American Society for Gastrointestinal Endoscopy (ASGE) and other authorities have recommended that endoscopists should collect data prospectively on their endoscopic practice and performance [3]. This translates into "endoscopy report cards," which I have advocated for many years [8].

Report cards and benchmarking performance

Report cards cannot include all of the data elements that have been listed in various well-meaning publications. Items should be selected based on ease of data collection, and by assumed relative importance. Some items are easily recorded and already appear in most procedure reports (e.g., indication, anatomical extent, duration, diagnosis, immediate unplanned events). Other items are more subjective (e.g., lesion interpretation) or more difficult to record (e.g., delayed complications, endoscopist-specific patient satisfaction). Some items would appear to be more important markers of quality than others. For ERCP, selective cannulation rates and rates of adverse events are obvious key parameters [9].

Benchmarking means comparing the performance of an individual endoscopist with that of his or her peers and "competitors." This requires an organization as well as motivation.

The ERCP quality network project

With the support of Olympus America, we set up a pilot project to test the practicality and acceptability of collecting and comparing data on the practice and quality of ERCP procedures by individual endoscopists [10]. Baseline information included the experience and practice environment of the endoscopists. Data on each procedure were loaded onto a secure web site, prospectively, either directly or via a single-paper data sheet. The data points included the indications, complexity grade, American Society of Anesthesiologists (ASA) grade, sedation/anesthesia, admission policy, scope and fluoroscopy times, and success rates for individual technical procedures such as deep biliary cannulation, sphincterotomy,

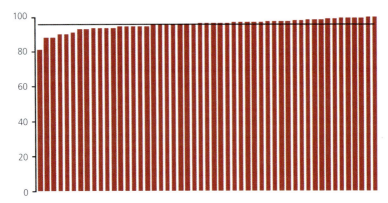

Figure 25.1 Median reported biliary cannulation rates for individual endoscopists in the ERCP quality network.

and stenting. Immediate and delayed complications were noted. There were no patient identifiers. The data were analyzed automatically, and results posted immediately on the web site. Contributors could view a summary of their own performance (report card) and compare it with that of all other contributors to the system (benchmarking), not identified by name. More than 150 ERCPists from several countries entered data on over 20 000 cases. An example of an output, mean biliary cannulation rates per endoscopist, is shown in Figure 25.1. It is perhaps surprising (but encouraging) that some endoscopists were prepared to submit data showing rather low success rates.

This pilot study demonstrated that certain physicians are prepared, even enthusiastic, to share their data, and to compare their performance with peers. A similar exercise for colonoscopy (GI Quality Improvement Consortium (GIQUIC)) was set up by the ASGE and the American College of Gastroenterology (ACG) [11]. Incorporation of ERCP in that project is under consideration.

What performance level is good enough? Who decides?

The ERCP quality project confirmed the obvious fact that endoscopists vary in their levels of performance, even among those comfortable enough to share their data. Not all patients can be managed by the superexperts. The issue then is who decides what constitutes acceptable performance, and what that should be. Professional organizations initially guessed (far too low) the "numbers" needed to achieve competence, but have recently concentrated on what might be *acceptable* performance, that is, the skill level that would justify independent practice (completion of formal training). The latest ASGE report on ERCP quality

[12] paints a broad canvas: "Successful cannulation rates at or above 95% are consistently achieved by experienced endoscopists, and rates at or above 80% are a goal of training programs. ... Thus, although >90% is an overall appropriate target for successful cannulation, rates of >85% should be achievable for most endoscopists." It goes on to say that "[t]echnical success for common (biliary) procedures should be achievable in >85% of cases."

Who is going to do your ERCP?

Are we all comfortable with the fact that many ERCP procedures are done by marginal endoscopists, especially bearing in mind that the less experienced also have more complications? I have written on this topic elsewhere [13]. Would you let your recent trainee lose on your family? Would you yourself submit to an 80–85% ERCPist, or allow your mother to do so? This level of performance would be acceptable, maybe life-saving, in an urgent and remote situation, but certainly not for an elective procedure when experts are available nearby. I would suggest that 95% is an appropriate target, at least for the basic-level biliary procedures. How can patients make an informed judgment since they have no way of telling the difference between an 85 and a 95% performer? Those of us in health care have ways of knowing who is "good" and who is not, but most of our customers do not. They rely on advice from their primary care givers (and friends), and the honesty and communication skills (sometimes inadequate) of their proposed endoscopists. I believe that we need to do better, and there are only two ways forward. One is for professional societies (and the payers) to set the bar higher, and to press for a certificate or diploma to be granted only after a formal examination. This would be resource-intensive, and not without controversy, but exams are the recognized method for assuring a reasonable level of knowledge and performance in many other fields. The diploma would be based on data from report cards, an examination of core knowledge, observation of a few cases, and, possibly, some work on simulators. This exercise would require agreement on how to "score" the more subjective elements of a procedure. The second method—and a step toward the first—is to encourage or mandate report cards, as described earlier, and to educate the public to ask for them.

How to move forward now?

The quality network project showed that data can be collected, shared, and compared by a small number of enthusiastic volunteers, with some commercial support. What might motivate the main body of practitioners? Ultimately, informed consumers will drive this agenda. Practitioners with poor outcomes, or those who choose not to provide data, will be disadvantaged. Keeping a report card will provide a competitive advantage. It should provide some medico-legal protection, and will eventually be a crucial tool in the evolving use of "pay for performance" in the United States. The increasing use of electronic endoscopy reporting systems will make this process easier, even automatic.

There still needs to be a sophisticated central agency to collect, analyze, and distribute the data. This will require ongoing financial support. What would practitioners be willing to pay? Cost is not the only deterrent. Skeptics will always doubt the accuracy of the data, and will say (correctly) that report cards as currently proposed focus only on technical skills, while knowledge and judgment are also important determinants of the outcome of procedures. These are challenges to be solved, not avoided.

How to recognize and measure excellence in endoscopy units?

Patients hope and usually assume that their procedures will be "done well," and are often more concerned about their safety, comfort, and dignity, and the efficiency of the process. Indeed, patients are obviously much better able to assess these elements than the technical aspects performed while they are sedated. Endoscopists (however talented) cannot work without good facilities, equipment, and a team of well-trained and motivated staff, as described in an earlier chapter. While endoscopists have responsibility for all of these elements, and can influence the way the rest of the team functions, there are important quality elements of the endoscopy unit and staff that can be considered separately.

It is not difficult to list features of endoscopy units that may affect the quality of the ERCP procedures being performed in them.

1 Years unit existed
2 Nature; hospital, freestanding endoscopy clinic, or office
3 Accreditation agency (and most recent rating)
4 Name of medical director
5 Name of nurse manager
6 ERCP volumes last calendar year, by complexity grade
7 Number of procedure rooms and patient bays
8 Total number of nursing staff (and training levels)
9 Written policies and systems for
   • Sedation and monitoring
   • Cleaning and disinfection
   • Risk reduction
   • Patient recall for surveillance
   • Tracking pathology results
   • Quality improvement

10 Safety data
- Pancreatitis rates
- Infection rates
- Unplanned intubations
- Unplanned admissions

11 Communications and feedback
- Patient satisfaction data
- Staff satisfaction data

An "Endoscopy Unit Report Card" could be developed by picking a selection of these criteria. As part of the Endoscopy Modernization process in Britain, a "Global Rating Scale" for endoscopy units was developed by Dr Roland Valori [14]. The system is supported by a comprehensive knowledge base and useful improvement tools. Sequential measurements in almost all the British endoscopy units over 8 years have shown gratifying and progressive improvement in the results. In the United States, the ASGE initiated an "Endoscopy Unit Recognition Program" [1]. This is voluntary and generic, but items specific to ERCP are being added. This program is popular and many hundreds of units are now officially recognized. Emphasis is placed on quality improvement projects and processes.

Conclusion

No one involved in endoscopy doubts the importance of ensuring the highest possible quality of our processes and procedures. Many patients assume that any doctor offering a procedure is competent to do it, and that all facilities are equally safe (although some may look less appealing). The very simplicity of endoscopy as a "walk-in, walk-out" procedure can lull patients and practitioners alike into a sense of false security. Bad things can and do happen. Our profession must work harder to encourage the collection and dissemination of performance data. The fact that some endoscopists will be reluctant to document and advertise their performance should not stop us from doing the right thing. We should wear our data plainly and proudly as badges of quality. It is the right thing to do, and will pay huge dividends eventually.

References

1 www.bsg.org.uk. Accessed August 8, 2014.
2 www.asge.org. Accessed August 8, 2014.
3 www.acg.org. Accessed August 8, 2014.
4 www.thejag.org.uk. Accessed August 8, 2014.
5 www.conjoint.org.au. Accessed August 8, 2014.
6 Faigel DO, Cotton PB; World Organization of Digestive Endoscopy. The London OMED position statement for credentialing and quality assurance in digestive endoscopy. Endoscopy 2009;41:1069–74.

7 Cohen S, Bacon BR, Berlin JA, et al. NIH State of the Science Conference Statement; ERCP for diagnosis and therapy. Gastrointest Endosc 2002;56:803–9.

8 Cotton PB. How many times have you done this procedure, doctor? Am J Gastroenterol 2002;97:522–3.

9 Johanson JF, Cooper G, Eisen GM, et al. Quality assessment of ERCP. Gastrointest Endosc 2002;56(2):165–9.

10 Cotton PB, Romagnuolo J, Faigel DO, et al. The ERCP quality network: a pilot study of benchmarking practice and performance. Am J Medical Quality 2013;28(3):256–60.

11 www.giquic.gi.org. Accessed August 8, 2014.

12 Baron TH, Petersen BT, Mergener K, et al. Quality indicators for endoscopic retrograde cholangiopancreatography. Am J Gastroenterol 2006;101:892–7.

13 Cotton PB. Are low-volume ERCPists a problem in the United States? A plea to examine and improve ERCP practice-NOW. Gastrointest Endosc 2011;74(1):161–6.

14 www.globalratingscale.com. Accessed August 8, 2014.

Index

Page numbers in *italics* refer to illustrations; those in **bold** refer to tables

ERCP: The Fundamentals, Second Edition. Edited by Peter B. Cotton and Joseph Leung.
© 2015 John Wiley & Sons, Ltd. Published 2015 by John Wiley & Sons, Ltd.
Companion Website: www.wiley.com\go\cotton\ercp

405